ADOLESCENTS AT RISK

Also from Nancy Boyd-Franklin

Black Families in Therapy, Second Edition:
Understanding the African American Experience
Nancy Boyd-Franklin

Therapy in the Real World:
Effective Treatments for Challenging Problems
Nancy Boyd-Franklin, Elizabeth N. Cleek,
Matt Wofsy, and Brian Mundy

ADOLESCENTS AT RISK

Home-Based Family Therapy and School-Based Intervention

Nancy Boyd-Franklin
Brenna Hafer Bry

THE GUILFORD PRESS
New York   London

In loving memory of Dave Bry (1970–2017)

Copyright © 2019 The Guilford Press
A Division of Guilford Publications, Inc.
370 Seventh Avenue, Suite 1200, New York, NY 10001
www.guilford.com

Printed in the United States of America

This book is printed on acid-free paper.

Last digit is print number: 9   8   7   6   5   4   3   2   1

Library of Congress Cataloging-in-Publication Data is available
from the publisher.

978-1-4625-3653-5 (paperback)
978-1-4625-3654-2 (hardcover)

About the Authors

Nancy Boyd-Franklin, PhD, is an African American clinical psychologist and family therapist and is a Distinguished Professor in the Graduate School of Applied and Professional Psychology at Rutgers, The State University of New Jersey. Her outstanding contributions have been recognized with awards from many professional organizations, including the American Family Therapy Academy, the Association of Black Psychologists, the American Psychological Association (Divisions 45 and 43), the Association of Black Social Workers, and the American Psychiatric Association, and she has received an honorary doctorate from the Phillips Graduate Institute. Dr. Boyd-Franklin is the author or coauthor of numerous articles and books, including *Black Families in Therapy, Second Edition: Understanding the African American Experience*, and *Therapy in the Real World: Effective Treatments for Challenging Problems*.

Brenna Hafer Bry, PhD, is Professor Emerita in the Graduate School of Applied and Professional Psychology at Rutgers, The State University of New Jersey, where she served as Department Chair and Director of Clinical Training. Her research has focused on risk factors that predict adolescent conduct problems. She discovered that the probability of youths' future problems increases as their number of risk factors increases, and that their probability of future problems can be reduced by reducing their number of risk factors. She subsequently developed and evaluated the Achievement Mentoring Program, a school-based intervention that reduces numbers of risk factors, which she is currently disseminating. Dr. Bry is a recipient of the Prevention Science Award from the Prevention Research Society.

Preface

In 2000, we published our book *Reaching Out in Family Therapy: Home-Based, School, and Community Interventions* (Boyd-Franklin & Bry, 2000), which introduced our concept of reaching out to youth and families in their homes, schools, and communities. Initially, we proposed a second edition of our earlier book, but during the writing process we realized that the challenges in working with at-risk adolescents with many different presenting problems have increased significantly during the last 19 years. It became clear that the book we were writing far surpassed what could be expected in a second edition. We therefore decided to write a new book that incorporated and expanded upon our earlier ideas.

This new book represents an evolution in our thinking, our work, and the field. Other models of treatment, including a number of evidence-based approaches, have been developed in home-based family therapy. In addition, Brenna Bry's Achievement Mentoring Program has been adopted in a number of school systems throughout the United States and in Ireland. There has also been a growing research base. We wanted to incorporate these changes into this new volume.

It is important to note, however, that many of the ideas delineated in our earlier book are still guiding this work. In addition to writing 11 new chapters, we have expanded and updated four chapters from the earlier book (Chapters 3, 5, 6, and 9) to include current ideas, concepts, authors, and references. For example, Chapter 3, "Cultural, Racial, and Socioeconomic Issues," includes additional material on the challenges facing at-risk adolescents and their families, most notably a discussion of the impact on African American youth and families of the increasing numbers of Black men and women killed by the police. Home-based family therapists, other clinicians, teachers, counselors, achievement mentors, and school administrators will appreciate the careful discussion of the ways in which families may be helped to address their fears and protect their children.

Chapter 5, "Multigenerational Patterns in Families of At-Risk Adolescents," allows those who work with at-risk youth and their families to look beyond the current presenting problems and to explore the intergenerational processes that may be operating in these situations. It expands upon our original discussion of multigenerational crises that many of these families face, including teenage pregnancy, drug and alcohol abuse, and juvenile delinquency. In addition to these issues, this new book addresses physical and sexual abuse, domestic violence, and gang involvement.

Chapter 6, "An Overview of the Multisystems Model and Home-Based Family Therapy," builds upon the cornerstone of the original book—effective treatment often involves providing interventions at many system levels in the lives of these adolescents and their families. This aspect of our Multisystems Model is described in detail. This chapter also expands the description of home-based family therapy provided in the original book to include current issues and case examples. Finally, Chapter 9, "Supervision and Training of Home-Based Family Therapists," further develops our concept of frontline supervision and describes an active model of supervision that engages clinicians directly as they learn to enter the homes and communities of clients who may be culturally, racially, and socioeconomically different from them.

The first chapter of our current book describes our guiding concepts and gives an overview of the ways in which the material from our earlier work has been integrated with the new material, which includes such relevant topics as the risk and protective factors impacting at-risk adolescents and their families, the challenges in working with kinship care families, and a full chapter devoted to a Multisystems Model case example. In addition, a chapter has been devoted to a description of multisystemic therapy (MST; Henggeler, Schoenwald, Borduin, Rowland, & Cunningham, 2009), a home-based family intervention for at-risk youth with antisocial behaviors, which, like our approach, provides treatment at many different system levels but was developed independently from our interventions. Parts III and IV are also totally new to this book. Chapter 10 explores the issues of school engagement, disengagement, and dropouts, and introduces a learning theory framework. Chapters 11–14 describe the Achievement Mentoring Program, including a full-chapter case example (Chapter 13). The final chapter of the book, Chapter 15, discusses the research on MST and Achievement Mentoring that is most relevant to practitioners and educators.

Acknowledgments

We would like to give our special thanks to Jim Nageotte, Senior Editor at The Guilford Press, who has guided us and been an amazing support to us throughout the entire publication process. His wisdom and intuitive editorial sense are always appreciated. Senior Production Editor Anna Nelson and Senior Assistant Editor Jane Keislar have also been a great help to us in the final part of this journey. The copy editor, Betty Pessagno, did a terrific job on the final editing. Throughout this entire process, our wonderful personal editor, Hazel Staloff, has provided exceptional editing, and her input has been invaluable in the preparation of this book; she has incredible patience and has encouraged us from start to finish. We would like to also give special thanks to Armani Wynn and Sydney Brinson, who did research for the book and whose excellent computer skills were greatly appreciated.

Nancy Boyd-Franklin: I would like to give thanks to God for the opportunity to write this book and to work with my coauthor, Brenna Bry. My special thanks to my husband and soulmate, Dr. A. J. Franklin, who has given me so much love and support throughout our 40 years together. This book has been particularly challenging, and his encouragement made it possible. I also want to thank all of the children of my heart: Deidre, Tunde, Remi, and Jay, my daughter-in-law Debbie, and my wonderful grandchildren, Kyra, Kayla, Kaylan, Jelani, Ajahni, and Adia, who bring so much joy to my life. I am grateful to my mother, Regina Boyd, who prayed for me and proofread every one of my earlier books; I honor her memory and feel certain that she was looking down from heaven during the writing of this book. I would also like to give a very personal thank you to my "sister friends": Rosemary Allwood, Jo

Ann Tatum, Paulette Hines, Brenna Bry, Hazel Staloff, Shalonda Kelly, and Janis Sanchez Hucles, for all of their love and support. Last but not least, I would like to thank all of the clients and families that I have worked with over the years, and all of the clinicians and student therapists whom I have supervised, for the inspiration they have provided and for their contributions to the case examples in this book.

Brenna Hafer Bry: First, I gratefully acknowledge my friend, colleague, codirector of our integrated home-based family therapy and school-based achievement mentoring initiative, and coauthor, Nancy Boyd-Franklin. Nancy is a gifted clinical trainer, consummate scholar, and valued friend who continually "reaches out." Regarding achievement mentoring, I appreciatively acknowledge my children, David and Deborah, and my mentee, Shakira, for teaching me more through their responses to my parenting and mentoring than any book or training program could have done. Their spontaneous, energetic efforts to become effective people confirmed my faith that every youth can develop beyond any adult's goals for them, if youth are acknowledged, praised, and provided engaging choices.

Next, I am beholden to three visionary members of the Monmouth County, New Jersey, Board of Drug Abuse Services who hypothesized in 1972 that adolescent conduct problems could be prevented by school-based intervention for adolescents at risk. Dr. Gerry Weinberger, Dr. Sandra Wolman, and Robert Ansell, Esq., persuaded elected officials to fund the development and rigorous evaluation of such a program in both urban and suburban schools. I was hired to conduct the experiment, and the Achievement Mentoring Program resulted.

Accordingly, I respectfully appreciate the several thousand students who, since 1973, have participated in the Achievement Mentoring Program, as well as their parents. Witnessing adolescents develop confidence, competence, and trust in themselves and others continues to inspire me today and makes this work indescribably fulfilling. Furthermore, I honor the hundreds of adults who enthusiastically have served as achievement mentors. Every one of them has made the Program better by offering creative insights during training workshops, sharing weekly successes and dilemmas, and devotedly implementing the Program during extremely challenging workdays.

The Achievement Mentoring Program never could have garnered the respect and reliable outcomes it enjoys without foundational empirical studies. Thus, I am forever indebted to the Rutgers and Irish researchers who conducted etiological studies of at-risk adolescents and their families, as well as program evaluations of intervention effects. At the risk of forgetting someone, I will acknowledge them by name:

Neil Bien, David Russell, Robert Pandina, Georgann Witte, Seth Warren, Magda Pedraza, Juliet Sternberg, Greer Melidonis, Elizabeth Turk-Karan, Juliet Beier, Charlena Sears, Monica (Leccese) Walsh, (Dennis) Mac Greene, Shaun Whittaker, Karen Krinsley, Bernetta Brown, Alice Alexander, Mary Parker, Damaris Miranda, Rosemary Parece, David Brantley, Nicole Attaway, Phuong-Anh Urga, Lisa (Pugh) House, Ayorkor Gaba, Laura (Vangsness) Holt, Angela (Chiong) Ziskis, Lolalyn Clarke, (Andrea) Lynne Taylor, Valerie Johnson, Sean McDonnell, Alex Kelly, Patricia Simon, Mina Yadegar, and Mason Shepherd.

Based on their support for and weekly knowledge of mentees' and mentors' activities, research assistants substantially improved Program procedures too: Helen Stanley, Frances George, Patricia (Trish) McKeon, Cathy Conboy, Karen Bisgay, RandiLynne Lieberman, Ruben Lelah, Elizabeth (Miller) Cleek, Denise Bethea, Vanessa Ramirez, Ratesha Berthier, (Umaima) Mimi Ahmed, Majella Butler, Ellen Twist, Devanshi Mehta, Mina Yadegar, Gabriela (DeCandia) Brown, Angelo Alago, Jared Ramos, Caitlin O'Donnell, Lindsay Shouldis, and Leah Shaw. Finally, the contributions of Achievement Mentoring and Targeted Family Intervention trainers and supervisors are so engrained in Program concepts and methods that I cannot separate theirs from my own. They are Nancy Boyd-Franklin, Meir Winokur, Claire Fishman, Nancy Bloom, Rita Johnson, Sherry Barr, Laura Fenster Rothschild, Scott Albert, Christine Harris, Michael Logan, and Paul Johnston. Helping at-risk adolescents requires a team effort, and our team excels!

Contents

CHAPTER 1

Introduction and Overview of the Book

This book draws upon our collective experience of more than 40 years each of clinical work, supervision, and the development of programs that reach out to at-risk adolescents and their families in their homes, schools, and communities. Throughout our careers, we have witnessed many professionals such as therapists, counselors, clinical program directors, and school personnel (i.e., teachers, counselors, mentors, principals, and other administrators), who have been well trained to work with adolescents and families, become demoralized as they discover that their clients, students, and families often do not choose to participate in available programs. Many of these at-risk adolescents and their families are not self-referred and may not trust or believe in therapy or in school-based interventions. This response to participation in these programs is unfortunate because the trajectory for too many at-risk youth starts with school failure and all too often ends with involvement in the juvenile justice system. As a result, many of these adolescents are not well served by the very systems that are in place to help them. This book is dedicated to mental health and school-based professionals who are committed to reversing this process by reaching out to these adolescents and ensuring that they can overcome challenges, achieve their potential, and realize their life goals.

The number of at-risk youth in this country, particularly among ethnic minority groups and those from poor families, has continued to rise. These adolescents are at risk for school disengagement, academic failure, dropping out of school, behavior and conduct problems, school and community violence, involvement with delinquent peers, juvenile delinquency, gang involvement, drug and alcohol abuse, incarceration,

1

family conflict, child abuse and neglect, removal from their families, teenage pregnancy, and other serious issues.

With these risks in mind, we have developed effective strategies for reaching out to engage these adolescents through their families and their schools. This new book builds on the ideas we first introduced in *Reaching Out in Family Therapy: Home-based, School and Community Interventions* (Boyd-Franklin & Bry, 2000). In order to address the needs of at-risk adolescents in different settings, this book presents the evolution of our reaching-out model in two different approaches: home-based family therapy and the implementation of the school-based Achievement Mentoring Program for at-risk students. The reaching-out approach is essential for programs serving a population that is often facing complex, multiple, and overwhelming life challenges, such as poverty, racism, discrimination, unsafe communities, violence, homelessness, and struggling schools. With these complex issues in mind, we have incorporated the Multisystems Model as a core principle in our work to empower these adolescents and their families, and to assist service providers in coordinating care and avoiding redundancy in interventions.

THE MULTISYSTEMS MODEL

The Multisystems Model is a problem-solving approach that helps adolescents and families with multiple problems to focus and prioritize their issues, and that allows clinicians to maximize the effectiveness of their interventions (Boyd-Franklin, 1989, 2003; Boyd-Franklin & Bry, 2000; Boyd-Franklin, Cleek, Wofsy, & Mundy, 2013). This model was introduced by Boyd-Franklin (1989) in her book, *Black Families in Therapy: A Multisystems Approach*, which was the first to combine a Multisystems Model with a multicultural approach to the treatment of African American families. It represents a combination of structural family therapy (Minuchin, 1974; Nichols, 2011), strategic (Haley, 1976), and behavioral/family systems (Robin & Foster, 2002) approaches.

Our Multisystems Model incorporates multiple systemic levels, including the individual, family, extended family, "nonblood kin" and other close friends, peers of the adolescents, church and community resources, and other outside systems (see Chapter 6). This outside systems level deserves particular emphasis here because therapists and school personnel often discover that many of the adolescents and families with whom they work are dealing with multiple complex problems and have a preexisting involvement with an array of agencies, systems, and institutions, including schools, medical or health care providers, mental health agencies, child welfare or protective services, welfare programs, housing authorities, courts, and the juvenile justice system. To further complicate matters, individual family members may have separate relationships with such agencies, institutions, and systems, many of which may be negative and most of which will have a considerable impact on the therapeutic relationship, the outcome of therapy, and the adolescent's performance in school. The Multisystems Model covers these various systems and also includes a final level that addresses societal forces that impact these youth and their families on a systemic level: poverty, racism, discrimination, immigration policies, homophobia, ageism, and sexism, among others.

A number of researchers and clinical scholars (Aponte, 1995; Boyd-Franklin, 1989, 2003; Boyd-Franklin & Bry, 2000; Boyd-Franklin et al., 2013; Bronfenbrenner, 1977; Henggeler et al., 2009) have developed different pragmatic approaches to understanding complex ecosystems and have encouraged therapists to intervene at multiple systemic levels. It is extremely helpful in work with poor families, including those who are White, who may simultaneously confront a staggering number of problems. In addition, because the Multisystems Model recognizes the impact of the dual sociopolitical stressors of poverty and racism or prejudice, it is particularly useful in work with African American, Latino, and other ethnic minority families and communities (Boyd-Franklin, 1989, 2003; Boyd-Franklin & Bry, 2000; McGoldrick & Hardy, 2008) (see Chapter 3).

In addition to our Multisystems Model, this book also discusses multisystemic therapy (MST) (Henggeler et al., 2009; Henggeler & Sheidow, 2012), an evidence-based, home-based family therapy that also incorporates multisystemic levels in its treatment approach (see Chapter 7).

REACHING OUT

The Multisystems Model is a useful theoretical framework for schools and clinical programs that recognize that at-risk adolescents and their families may need a different level of reaching out in order to engage them in their services. In schools, these at-risk youth who are disengaged from the school culture and who may be experiencing academic failure and behavior problems may require special efforts to engage them in their school work and reverse the trajectory that may be leading them toward dropping out of school. The Achievement Mentoring Program is a proven form of such special efforts to reach out (see Chapters 11–15). For clinicians who do home- or office-based clinical work, the Multisystems Model allows them to conceptualize the realities of their clients' lives in a more complete and complex way. By incorporating the process of reaching out (i.e., outside the office), this approach can allow the clinician to observe and intervene directly in the various systems that either support or hinder their clients' progress toward achieving therapeutic change (Boyd-Franklin, 1989, 2003; Boyd-Franklin & Bry, 2000; Boyd-Franklin et al., 2013; Henggeler et al., 2009).

In office-based family therapy, we frequently work with only an isolated subsystem of a complex family household and extended family network, not engaging with individuals who often have a great deal of power either to produce or to sabotage change (Boyd-Franklin, 1989, 2003; Boyd-Franklin & Bry, 2000; Haley, 1976; Minuchin, 1974; Nichols, 2011). By reaching out to the family's environment and significant others in home-based work, however, we have the opportunity to engage and form a therapeutic alliance with fathers, boyfriends, and other key extended family members, such as grandparents, who often do not come in for office-based sessions.

Reaching out also has a broader meaning that extends beyond the family and extended family. Too often a clinician or family therapist "joins" only with those present in treatment. This may be a serious error, particularly with poor African American and Latino clients and families. Our approach encourages therapists to actively intervene in the multiple settings that are significant in their clients' lives (Boyd-Franklin, 1989, 2003; Boyd-Franklin & Bry, 2000; Boyd-Franklin et al., 2013). This outreach may take place in a client's home; school; or, if it is convenient or useful to the intervention, at a local facility or institution, such as a church, community center, or another common meeting place.

Strategies for Clinicians in Office-Based Work

Many office-based clinicians may be motivated to make home- and community-outreach efforts, but feel constrained by workplace practices that often restrict treatment to agency premises and by insurance plans that do not cover home- or community-based services. For therapists in these situations, the benefit from even one well-timed home-based family session can increase the impact of ongoing office-based work. For example, a key family member resistant to attending an office session may be amenable to a home-based session, and such participation can facilitate his or her "buy-in" and support of the therapeutic process (Boyd-Franklin, 1989, 2003; Boyd-Franklin & Bry, 2000). Targeted reaching out can also be useful in crises or major therapeutic efforts that require the participation of a large number of family and extended family members.

Clinicians have often told us that paying a brief lunch-hour visit to a child's school avoided hours of wasted time engaged in "telephone tag." Although a large caseload may prevent such visits on a regular basis, one carefully planned meeting may allow a clinician to connect with a principal, teacher, or counselor who has the power to make major decisions in a youth's life (see Chapter 8).

KEY CONCEPTS

The key concepts described in this section represent the guiding themes and values in our work that are incorporated in chapters throughout this book:

• The *multisystems* or *ecological approach to service delivery* (Boyd-Franklin, 1989, 2003; Boyd-Franklin & Bry, 2000; Boyd-Franklin et al., 2013). The Multisystems Model allows us to view clients and families in their full ecological and systemic context, including the many different institutions, agencies, and systems that have an impact on them (see Chapter 6). In addition, see Chapter 7 for a description of multisystemic therapy (MST) (Henggeler et al., 2009).

• *Cultural sensitivity and competence* (Boyd-Franklin, 2003; Falicov, 2005, 2014; McGoldrick, Giordano, & Garcia-Preto, 2005). Each intervention must be tailored to and sensitive to the cultural realities of the family.

• *Emphasis on strengths* (Boyd-Franklin, 2003; Boyd-Franklin & Bry, 2000; Henggeler et al., 2009). The emphasis is on identifying the strengths in the adolescent, parent, caregiver, family, school, and community that can be utilized to produce change.

• *Empowerment of families, particularly parents or caregivers* (Berg, 1994; Boyd-Franklin, 2003; Boyd-Franklin & Bry, 2000; Henggeler et al., 2009). This approach emphasizes empowering families to take charge of their own lives. The clinician should not take over the job of the parents or caregivers.

• *The importance of reaching out to schools and to at-risk adolescents in schools.* The importance of contacting schools as a part of the Multisystems Model (Boyd-Franklin & Bry, 2000) is addressed from the perspective of family therapists and other clinicians (see Chapters 6 and 8). Part III of this book provides an in-depth discussion of the Achievement Mentoring Program, a school-based program that reaches out to adolescents who present with school disengagement and academic failure and who are at risk for dropping out (see Chapters 10 through 14).

• *Proactive and active interventions* (Boyd-Franklin & Bry, 2000; Bry, 1994). Rather than accepting the situation and waiting for change to occur, the role of the clinician or the achievement mentor in this model is active and proactive. The therapist reaches out to family members and initiates contact and changes within systems, such as schools, child protective services, the juvenile justice system, the police, and the courts; the achievement mentor reaches out to the adolescents in the school and to their teachers and parents.

• *Value of support* (Boyd-Franklin & Bry, 2000; Henggeler et al., 2009). Throughout this book, we emphasize the importance of support and support networks in the lives of adolescents, parents, and families.

• *Community involvement* (Boyd-Franklin & Bry, 2000; Swenson, Henggeler, Taylor, & Addison, 2005). As key community members and organizations can be helpful to the process of change, reaching out extends to the communities in which the families live. For example, a church might provide a location for a family support group, a school might provide an after-school tutoring program, and a community center in a low-income housing project might provide general equivalency diploma (GED) courses or job training.

• *Prevention* (Boyd-Franklin & Bry, 2000; Bry, 1994). One of the most useful applications of the Multisystems Model and the process of reaching out involves interventions with adolescents who are at risk for conduct disorder, dropping out of school, drug or alcohol abuse, school or community violence and/or gang involvement or other criminal activity. These negative outcomes can be prevented if targeted interventions begin at an early stage.

OVERVIEW OF THE BOOK

When we embarked on this project, our goal was to create a comprehensive resource that could serve as a guide for both beginning and experienced therapists in many different types of agencies and clinics, as well as for school personnel interested in implementing the Achievement Mentoring Program in their schools. With this objective in mind, we have divided this book into four parts: (I) an in-depth description of at-risk adolescents and their families; (II) discussions of the Multisystems Model and home-based family therapy; (III) an analysis of the risk factors for adolescents in the schools and an exploration of the Achievement Mentoring Program, including the process of mentoring and the competencies of mentors; and (IV) a research chapter documenting the evidence base for home-based family therapy interventions and Achievement Mentoring programs.

Part I: At-Risk Adolescents and Their Families

Chapter 2 discusses risk and protective factors at all multisystems levels including the individual, the family, peers, the school, and the community, and provides a comprehensive discussion of the types of issues presented by at-risk adolescents that may result in school dropout, such as school disengagement, academic failure, truancy, and behavioral and conduct problems in the school. (School-related risk factors are discussed in more detail in Part III, Chapter 10.) Also discussed are presenting problems related to conduct disorder and antisocial behaviors, including violence, involvement with delinquent peers, juvenile delinquency, drug and alcohol abuse, and gang involvement.

In Chapter 3, we discuss the importance of understanding the cultural, racial, and socioeconomic factors present in the lives of at-risk adolescents and their families. This chapter focuses primarily on the cultural strengths of African American and Latino families and on our interventions with poor and working poor families from many cultures, including White families. Case examples are included in order to illustrate culturally competent clinical work and school interventions.

It is important for clinicians and school personnel to understand the complex family situations of these young people. In many families of at-risk adolescents, kinship caregivers (e.g., grandmothers, grandfathers, aunts, uncles, older siblings, and close family friends) assume parental roles when biological parents are unable to care for their children properly due to serious issues, such as the parents' abuse or neglect of the children, drug or alcohol abuse, serious mental illness, or incarceration. In addition, in African American, Latino, and many other ethnic minority families, kinship care—or "taking in children" in times of need—is a cultural strength and an expectation. Chapter 4 offers an in-depth discussion of at-risk youth from kinship care families, many of whom are referred by child welfare agencies or child protective services. This chapter clarifies the distinctions between (1) formal kinship caregivers, who are licensed by the states and receive the same financial compensation as nonfamilial foster parents, monitoring by child protective workers, and services and referrals if necessary; and (2) the far more common situation of informal kinship caregivers, who raise the children and adolescents of extended family members or close friends and receive no financial assistance, with the result that many are living in poverty. A number of case examples illustrate the significant issues commonly presented by at-risk adolescents from kinship care families.

Chapter 5 focuses on multigenerational patterns of families in crisis. Many at-risk adolescents have families that experience one or more multigenerational family patterns of teenage pregnancy, child abuse, domestic violence, juvenile delinquency, gang involvement, drug and alcohol abuse, and other issues. This chapter offers case examples highlighting the nature of these issues and potential complications (such as toxic secrets and repeated crises), and provides guidelines that will be helpful to new and experienced therapists, school counselors, and achievement mentors when working with such families.

Part II: The Multisystems Model and Home-Based Family Therapy

Part II focuses on many different aspects of the Multisystems Model. Chapter 6 introduces the reader to the Multisystems Model, discusses the application of this model in home-based family treatment, and describes the different systems levels in which at-risk adolescents and their families are embedded (i.e., individual, family household, family subsystems, extended family, nonblood family, friends, and the adolescents' peers, schools, churches, communities, and community agencies, as well as external systems, such as child protective services, the police, the courts, and the juvenile justice system) (Boyd-Franklin, 1989, 2003; Boyd-Franklin & Bry, 2000; Boyd-Franklin et al., 2013). The chapter also addresses societal forces such as poverty, racism, discrimination, immigration policies, and sexism. As therapists begin to identify presenting problems, this model allows them to explore the strengths of the client, his or her family, and the broader social network at all systems levels that can be utilized for change, together with the ways in which each level may contribute to the problems. This chapter then discusses the importance of reaching out to families in home-based family therapy. We introduce our model, which includes the initial interview, the process of joining or engaging family members, identifying and prioritizing problems and goals, and problem-solving interventions.

A number of evidence-based home-based family therapy models have been developed. Chapter 7 provides an in-depth description of multisystemic therapy (MST) (Henggeler et al., 2009), which is the evidence-based model most consistent with our approach. It provides home-based family therapy to at-risk youth and their families, and it intervenes at many systemic levels. Although MST and our approach were developed independently, the two models have many features in common. Both are discussed in this book in order to expose home-based family therapists to a number of interventions that will help them to provide effective treatment to these families.

Although we have presented numerous illustrative examples throughout this book, the entirety of Chapter 8 is devoted to a comprehensive

Multisystems Model case example. In this chapter, therapists are guided through the multiple interventions involving home-based family therapy and comprising different multisystems levels in the treatment of an at-risk adolescent from an immigrant Latino family. Therapists will gain a greater degree of cultural competence in work with presently undocumented immigrant families who are fearful of deportation. Like many at-risk adolescents, this client presents with serious school problems, including academic failure; truancy; fighting in the school and community; close associations with delinquent, gang-involved peers; and involvement with the juvenile justice system. Therapists will learn culturally sensitive techniques for joining with and engaging the parents and empowering them to effectively monitor the youth's behavior despite their long hours in the workplace. Interventions with the school, the courts, and the probation system are described. In addition, the therapist empowers the parents to identify social supports such as extended family members, their pastor, and church family members to help them. Among the most important aspects of this case are (1) the negative consequences arising out of the adolescent's involvement with delinquent, gang-involved peers; and (2) the therapist's empowering the family to identify prosocial peers and activities in the school and the community so that the at-risk adolescent's trajectory can be reversed.

Like the Multisystems Model of treatment, our model of supervision is an active one involving outreach. Chapter 9 explores the process of the supervision and training of home-based family therapists within the Multisystems Model. We view training and supervision as "antidotes" to the burnout that frontline family therapists often experience, and as keys to the empowerment of clinicians to do this work effectively (Boyd-Franklin, 1989, 2003; Boyd-Franklin & Bry, 2000; Boyd-Franklin et al., 2013). The chapter discusses the value of group supervision in providing support for therapists, in addition to contributing to team building within a program or an agency. Frontline supervision and the involvement of other clinicians through the supervisory group process empower clinicians to intervene successfully in the crises that are prevalent among many at-risk adolescents and their families. Supervisory challenges in this type of work are discussed in detail.

Part III: Achievement Mentoring—An Evidence-Based, School-Based Intervention

In Part III, Chapters 10 through 14 address different aspects of the school-based Achievement Mentoring Program for at-risk adolescents. Since schools afford the greatest long-term, continuous access to adolescents, Chapter 10 presents a strong argument for addressing the needs of at-risk youth through a school-based program. School disengagement is a serious risk factor for at-risk students, which manifests as increasingly poorer grades, more disciplinary referrals, heightened negative feelings about teachers and peers, and fewer beliefs in self-efficacy (Reschly & Christenson, 2012). This chapter discusses these risk factors and the role of school engagement and a sense of belonging in the school as protective factors that prevent students from dropping out of school.

Chapter 11 offers a detailed description of the Achievement Mentoring Program, an evidence-based program for disengaged, at-risk pre-adolescents and adolescents, the purpose of which is to increase the skills necessary for school engagement and to change habits that interfere with acquiring knowledge and succeeding in school (Bry, 1982, 2001a; Clarke, 2009; Holt, Bry, & Johnson, 2008; Taylor, 2010). This chapter also demonstrates how repeated corrective experiences with nonparental adult mentors over time can reengage students in the process of learning.

In order for achievement mentors to improve school engagement and the academic performance of at-risk students, they must receive training in the competencies necessary to connect with these adolescents, some of which are specific communication skills. Chapter 12 describes these communication skills, which include asking open-ended questions; active listening; interviewing teachers about mentees in their classrooms; praising; reporting teacher feedback; Motivational Interviewing; helping mentees shape a small, feasible next step to take each week; and working with the adolescents to plan details of that step's implementation.

In order to illustrate the process, Chapter 13 presents an Achievement Mentoring case example that details the progress and challenges presented over time from the perspectives of both the adolescent and the mentor. The involvement of the ongoing Achievement Mentoring trainer, teachers, school administrators, and parents is also discussed. In addition, this case example presents the outcomes of this intervention.

Chapter 14 describes the training methods, ongoing coaching, and organizational supports that enable mentors to learn to do the program in their school settings as it was designed. Attaining maximum results requires achievement mentors to implement the Program with a high level of competence and fidelity, which may be difficult to do given the challenges and stresses involved in addressing the behavioral habits and skill deficits of at-risk adolescents in schools with limited resources. This chapter describes the ongoing training, consultation, and professional development that are so crucial in Achievement Mentoring.

Part IV: Research

In the last 40 years, there has been increasing scientific evidence of the benefits to at-risk adolescents of home-based family therapy,

Achievement Mentoring, and the two interventions in combination. Chapter 15 reviews research supporting the effectiveness of these interventions, so that home-based family therapists and achievement mentors can be encouraged in their belief that they are making a difference in adolescents' lives in the face of ongoing challenges. There are relevant studies as well that point to essential program components, exactly how successful families and adolescents change during the interventions, characteristics of typical providers and adolescents served, necessary organizational supports, and views of the interventions from adolescents, parents, teachers, providers, and administrators. This updated review of the research is directed especially at program directors, who must select evidence-based approaches to address their specific schools' or communities' needs, as well as at those who write grant proposals to obtain funding.

CONFIDENTIALITY OF CLIENTS AND STUDENTS

One strength of this book is its extensive use of case material. In order to protect the confidentiality of clients and students, all identifying details have been changed in all of the cases we present. In some instances, we have created composite cases in which details from more than one case have been combined in order to further disguise the identities of the individuals involved.

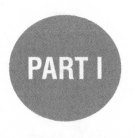

PART I

AT-RISK ADOLESCENTS AND THEIR FAMILIES

CHAPTER 2

At-Risk Adolescents and Their Families

Behaviors, Risk, and Protective Factors

TYPES OF AT-RISK BEHAVIOR

At-risk behaviors and risk factors were defined by Kazdin, Kraemer, Kessler, Kupfer, and Offord (1997) as "those conditions that are associated with a higher likelihood of negative outcomes" (as cited in Stoddard et al., 2013, p. 58). Patterns in adolescents that may be considered at risk include (1) antisocial behavior (Farrington, 2007; Henggeler et al., 2009; Swenson et al., 2005); (2) substance abuse (Monahan, Rhew, Hawkins, & Brown, 2014), including alcohol use (Johnston, O'Malley, Bachman, & Schulenberg, 2011) and drug use (Chassin, Hussong, & Beltran, 2009); (3) conduct disorder (Dixon, Howie, & Starling, 2004; Pliszka, Sherman, Barrow, & Irick, 2000); (4) delinquency (Thornberry & Krohn, 2003); (5) criminal behavior (Farrington, 2007); (6) youth violence (Massetti et al., 2011; Stoddard et al., 2013); and (7) community violence (Goddard, 2014; Gorman-Smith, Henry, & Tolan, 2004; McMahon et al., 2013). Many adolescents present with co-occurring antisocial behaviors. For example, research studies have identified the co-occurrence of peer delinquency and peer substance abuse among at-risk youth (Monahan et al., 2014). Similarly, a number of researchers have discussed the co-occurrence of conduct disorder and substance abuse (Abrantes, Hoffman, & Anton, 2005; Pliszka et al., 2000).

Adolescents whose behavior falls into the above categories may also be at high risk for dropping out of school. Additional factors, such as school disengagement, academic failure (i.e., not being promoted and repeating grades), and in-school behavioral problems, can also increase the risk for school dropout. Dropping out of school may also be associated with other negative conditions, such as (1) delinquent behaviors (Bridgeland, Dilulio, & Morison, 2006), (2) substance abuse (Bachman et al., 2008), (3) alcohol abuse and dependence (Muthén & Muthén, 2000), (4) welfare dependence (Waldfogel, Garfinkel, & Kelly, 2007), (5) incarceration (Lochner & Moretti, 2004), and (6) unemployment (Symonds, Schoon, & Salmela-Aro, 2016). Although there is a great deal of co-occurrence between these problems, this chapter provides a brief discussion of some of the school risk and protective factors. Chapter 10 presents a more comprehensive discussion of school-related issues, such as school engagement and disengagement, academic failure, and behavior problems that may lead adolescents to drop out of school.

The present chapter focuses on four main areas of adolescent antisocial behaviors: delinquency, youth violence, community violence, and substance abuse. Hawkins, Catalano, and Miller (1992) and Hawkins et al. (2000) have noted that numerous research studies have consistently identified similar risk factors related to antisocial behaviors. With this consideration in mind, the second part of the chapter focuses on risk factors at the following levels: individual, family, peer, school, and community. Research has also identified protective factors related to at-risk areas that can make a difference in the outcome for at-risk youth and can contribute to more prosocial behaviors (Hawkins, Catalano, Kosterman, Abbott, & Hill, 1999). The last part of this chapter concentrates on these protective factors and the resilience of many of these adolescents.

ADOLESCENT ANTISOCIAL BEHAVIORS
Delinquency and Youth Violence

Juvenile delinquency includes a range of crimes committed by adolescents that primarily fall into two categories: violence against a person (i.e., fighting, weapon use, shootings, stabbings, murder, etc.) or crimes against the property of others (i.e., shoplifting, vandalism, burglary, theft, car theft, etc.). There is often a progression in offenses. For example, an adolescent may start with fighting with peers and escalate to more serious and more deadly forms of youth violence. Similarly, an adolescent may start with shoplifting and escalate to more serious forms of theft (Thornberry & Krohn, 2003). This section begins with an overview of delinquency and ends with a specific emphasis on youth violence.

Delinquent Behavior

A number of researchers have addressed the complex issues involved in juvenile delinquency (Bartollas & Schmalleger, 2014; Siegel & Welsh,

2014; Thornberry & Krohn, 2003). Howell et al. (2013) and Loeber and Farrington (2012) have studied the trajectory from juvenile to adult crime. Thornberry, Huizinga, and Loeber (2004) identified three different pathways into juvenile delinquent behavior: (1) childhood aggression based in conflicts with authority before the age of 12 that progress to truancy and different forms of aggression; (2) minor covert acts prior to adolescence that progress to property damage and more serious forms of delinquency; and (3) the most overt pathway, aggression initially directed toward persons, leading to fighting and then to more serious forms of violence. Exhibiting problematic behavior in childhood does not necessarily dictate a progression toward delinquency. Some youth stop such behaviors as they enter adolescence, and others may have only a brief period of involvement during their teenage years. Those who progress to more serious forms of violence and other types of delinquency in their later adolescence and early adulthood may also be likely to demonstrate other forms of antisocial behavior, such as engaging in substance abuse and acting out in school, and may also exhibit mental health problems (Thornberry et al., 2004).

Youth Violence

The prevalence of youth violence in the United States has reached alarming levels. In 2006, homicide was the second most common cause of death for 15- to 19-year-olds, the third most common cause among 10- to 14-year-olds, and the fourth most common cause among 5- to 9-year-olds, according to the National Center for Injury Prevention and Control (2010). The Centers for Disease Control and Prevention (CDC; 2009) reported that in the same year, 2006, a total of 5,958 adolescents between the ages of 10 and 24 were murdered, or an average of 16 per day. The statistics are even more alarming for ethnic minority youth. For those aged 10–24, homicide is the leading cause of death for African Americans; the second leading cause of death for Latinos/Hispanics; and the third most common cause for Asian/Pacific Islanders, Native Americans, and Alaska natives (CDC, 2009).

Parker and Tuthill (2006) reported, however, that over 50% of adolescents arrested for violent acts in schools were White. Massive public attention has focused on the alarming and increasing number of school shootings with multiple victims, for example, Columbine High School in 1999, Sandy Hook Elementary School in 2012, and Marjory Stoneman Douglas High School in Parkland, Florida in 2018. The overwhelming percentage (90%) of perpetrators of school shootings have been White males (Parker & Tuthill, 2006). These incidents of mass violence have led to strong cries for gun control legislation. Although most of the research on youth violence has focused on ethnic minorities in urban areas, Guerra and Smith (2006) have indicated these school shootings have underscored that adolescents are at risk for violence across ethnic and racial groups, across socioeconomic levels, and in suburban and rural areas as well as inner-city communities. This argues strongly for mental health services in all schools that can help to identify and treat at-risk youth.

In spite of all of these disturbing statistics on youth violence, the vast majority of violent acts occur in the community, not in schools. Basch (2011) has pointed out that "[h]omicide remains a rare event in school settings" (p. 620). Statistics on other crimes that occur in school are also a serious concern, however. According to the National Center for Education Statistics' *Indicators of School Crime and Safety* (2007), cited by Basch (2011):

> Recent national data indicate that among students aged 12–18, approximately 628,200 violent crimes and 868,100 thefts occurred [in school]. Physical fighting was more commonly reported by Blacks and Hispanics (44.7% and 40.4% respectively) than Whites (31.7%). In-school threats and injuries were nearly twice as prevalent in cities as in suburbs and towns or rural areas (10% vs. 6% and 5% respectively). (p. 619)

Community Violence and Gangs

Community violence, a particularly dangerous form of violence, is often associated with groups of adolescents composed of delinquent peers (Dodge, Dishion, & Lansford, 2006), and in some cases, gangs (Thornberry & Krohn, 2003). In addition, a number of researchers have demonstrated that increasingly dangerous antisocial behaviors, delinquency, violence, and drug use are committed by youth who are involved in gangs and other groups of delinquent peers (Dishion, Ha, & Veronneau, 2012; Dodge et al., 2006; Henggeler et al., 2009; Swenson et al., 2005; Thornberry & Krohn, 2003). As they age, adolescents who have demonstrated a propensity for associating with delinquent peers are more at risk for recruitment by gangs in their communities. A report from the Office of Juvenile Justice and Delinquency Prevention (Snyder & Sickmund, 2006), stated that 8% of adolescents in a national sample indicated gang membership by age 17. Not surprisingly, cities with significantly more gang involvement also show higher rates of youth membership. Ironically, as major cities have increased arrests and pressure on gang members, gangs have expanded their recruitment into smaller cities, suburban, and rural areas. Many of these communities are in complete denial of the presence of gangs in their midst until gang-related shootings begin to occur in larger numbers. For example, MS 13, a violent gang originating in El Salvador, is known for murders and drug trafficking. Many

Americans were surprised to learn of the stronghold this gang has established on Long Island in parts of Suffolk County, New York. MS 13, like many other major gangs, operates in 42 states and Washington, DC, in many different types of communities. Many of these gangs begin recruitment in elementary school and initiate gang members in middle and high school ("What to Know about MS 13," 2017).

A number of longitudinal studies have examined the involvement of at-risk adolescents in gangs. Thornberry, Krohn, Lizotte, Smith, and Tobin (2003) reported that the participants who had joined gangs constituted approximately 30% of their sample and became gang members between the ages of 14 and 18. The vast majority of delinquent and criminal acts, drug sales, illegal gun possession, and arrests are attributable to gang members. According to Massetti et al. (2011):

> Gang members are responsible for a large proportion of *all* violent offenses committed in adolescence [Thornberry, 1998; Thornberry et al., 2004]. Furthermore, youth perpetrate violence at substantially higher levels when they are in a gang than in the years before or after membership [Thornberry, 1998; Thornberry et al., 2003; Thornberry et al., 2004]. These increased rates of violence are also found for youth who affiliate with gangs but are not members themselves [Curry, Decker, & Egley, 2002]. (p. 1419)

Gang membership was not a long-term commitment for most of the participants in the Thornberry et al. (2003) study, as discussed earlier. Half of the boys and two-thirds of the girls reported that their gang involvement was relatively brief and lasted approximately one year. Very few (7%) indicated that they had remained in the gang for as long as 4 years (Thornberry et al., 2003).

Paradoxically, certain interventions designed to help at-risk adolescents may achieve the opposite result (Dodge et al., 2006). For example, education programs, such as special education classes and alternative schools; community-based interventions; juvenile justice programs where adolescents are in detention centers and correctional facilities; and mental health programs, such as therapy groups or residential treatment centers, often isolate at-risk adolescents in groups. When these adolescents have long periods of unstructured time interacting with each other, they are likely to be at greater risk for expanding their involvement in delinquent activities.

Substance Abuse

Wagner and Waldron (2001) provided a very useful model of the continuum of adolescent substance use and abuse. Henggeler, Cunningham,

Rowland, Schoenwald, and Associates (2012) have summarized this continuum as follows:

1. *Abstinence*—no substance use.
2. *Experimental use*—typically minimal use in the context of recreational activities.
3. *Early abuse*—more established use, greater frequency of use, often more than one drug used, negative consequences of use beginning to emerge.
4. *Abuse*—history of frequent use [and] negative consequences have emerged.
5. *Dependence*—continued regular use in spite of negative consequences, considerable activity devoted to seeking and using drugs. (p. 11)

Researchers have noted that the majority of adolescents have used some substances (Henggeler et al., 2012; Liddle & Rowe, 2010; Wagner & Waldron, 2001). With this fact in mind, treatment intervention is usually given to adolescents at the early abuse, abuse, or dependent levels (Henggeler et al., 2012; Wagner & Waldron, 2001).

Wagner and Waldron (2001) and Henggeler et al. (2012) offered additional guidelines in determining whether a referral should be made for treatment: (1) particularly dangerous drugs, such as heroin or crack cocaine, are being used; (2) the person beginning to experiment with alcohol or marijuana is extremely young (i.e., a child or a preadolescent); (3) the adolescent has abused large quantities of a substance given the significant risk involved; and (4) the adolescent is using substances while driving or in school.

As indicated earlier, substance abuse often co-occurs with other at-risk or antisocial behaviors. Thus, it is important for a therapist to do a very careful assessment of the adolescent's actual use; involvement with substance-abusing peers; and reports of family, friends, school officials, or members of the community who are concerned about use or the possibility of abuse (Henggeler et al., 2012; Swenson et al., 2005).

RISK FACTORS

As Swenson et al. (2005) have demonstrated, there is considerable overlap between the risk factors for antisocial behaviors such as delinquency, violence, gangs, and substance abuse. These risk factors may derive from different areas of the adolescent's life, including at the (1) individual level (e.g., personal characteristics, mental health problems, attention-deficit/

hyperactivity disorder [ADHD], impulsivity, poor academic achievement, antisocial behavior at an early age); (2) the family level (e.g., poor parental monitoring; family conflict and disruptions; lack of family connectedness; parental or caregiver mental health, substance abuse, or other antisocial problems); (3) the peer level (e.g., involvement with delinquent peers or gangs or with substance-using peers); (4) the school level (school disengagement, dropout, academic failure, truancy, frequent out-of-school suspensions (see Chapter 10), placement in an alternative class or school with other at-risk students (Dodge et al., 2006); and (5) the community level (e.g., high crime and drug involvement, poverty, availability of guns, community violence, lack of community cohesion) (Henggeler et al., 2009; Swenson et al., 2005). This section reviews the literature and research on each of these risk factors for adolescent at-risk behaviors.

Individual Risk Factors

Risk factors at the individual level have been identified by researchers (Massetti et al., 2011) as including (1) impulsive behavior; (2) hyperactivity; (3) inattention; (4) poor academic achievement (Massetti et al., 2011); (5) learning problems; (6) antisocial behavior; (7) hopelessness; (8) observation of violence; (9) drug and alcohol abuse (Stoddard et al., 2013); and (10) victimization, which includes physical, sexual, and severe emotional abuse and neglect (Massetti et al., 2011). Child abuse and trauma have all been shown to increase the risk for youth violence and delinquency (Massetti et al., 2011, p. 1418). In addition, risk factors (i.e., risk taking, thrill seeking, and drug dealing) have been shown to cluster together for some adolescents (Massetti et al., 2011, p. 1417).

Individual risk factors, such as substance use and abuse and aggression, are influenced by cognitive and behavioral factors. For example, cognitive and behavioral factors can contribute to denial about the extent of substance use and abuse (Henggeler et al., 2012; Swenson et al., 2005; Wagner & Waldron, 2001), and cognitive and behavioral factors and beliefs about aggression can impact youth violence (McMahon et al., 2013). Research by McMahon et al. (2013) has shown that greater exposure to violence and aggressive beliefs are related to more aggressive behavior. They indicate that "[a]ggressive children tend to believe that aggression is a legitimate and acceptable behavior that will lead to increased status and that negative consequences are minimal" (p. 408). These adolescents may therefore be more likely to resort quickly to violent behaviors and less likely to remove themselves from potentially aggressive situations (McMahon et al., 2013).

Impulsivity and conditions such as ADHD can contribute to many antisocial behaviors, including violence and substance abuse (Barkley, 2013; Barkley & Robin, 2014; Henggeler et al., 2009, 2012; Swenson et al., 2005). Impulsivity has been shown to lead to aggressive behavior. McMahon et al. (2013) indicated that "[i]mpulsive youth may be less likely to engage in the necessary precautions to avoid potential conflicts and may not consider consequences of their behavior" (p. 418).

Family Risk Factors

Parenting and family risk factors have been identified as contributing to a number of antisocial behaviors, including substance abuse, poor school performance, truancy, violence, and delinquency (Henggeler et al., 2009; Swenson et al., 2005). Research has consistently shown that poor parental or caregiver monitoring of children and adolescents can lead to negative outcomes for adolescents (Dishion, Nelson, & Kavanagh, 2003; Veronneau, Dishion, Connell, & Kavanagh, 2016). Poor parental monitoring and supervision has been identified by researchers as one of the strongest predictors of violence and delinquency (Massetti et al., 2011, p. 1418). Adolescents who have low parental monitoring are also at risk for early autonomy, as some parents of high-risk adolescents feel overwhelmed and withdraw from them, concluding that any efforts they could undertake to influence these youth would be futile, particularly as their problem behaviors escalate (Connell, Klostermann, & Dishion, 2011; Dishion, Nelson, & Bullock, 2004). Early autonomy can also increase the likelihood that at-risk adolescents will begin to associate with deviant peers (Connell et al., 2011).

In addition to poor parental monitoring, research studies have identified the following family risk factors for youth violence: (1) problematic parent–child relationships, (2) a history of criminal behavior by parents, (3) conflicts within the family, (4) family disruption and instability (Massetti et al., 2011), and (5) aggressive behavior within the family and positive attitudes toward violence by family members (Herrenkohl et al., 2000; Stoddard et al., 2013). Some parents may punish their children when they do not engage in fighting, at least with respect to defending themselves when attacked. Harsh parental discipline, particularly physical abuse, can also be predictive factors for physical aggression in young males (Massetti et al., 2011). Herrenkohl et al. (2000) found that parental criminality and antisocial behavior were predictors of youth violence. In their longitudinal study, Murray and Farrington (2010) found that parental substance abuse and a history of antisocial behavior are strong predictors of juvenile delinquency, youth violence, and adolescent substance abuse. Parental incarceration has also been identified as a strong predictor in meta-analyses (Murray & Farrington, 2005). In their meta-analysis of parental factors that predict violence and delinquency, Hoeve et al. (2009) identified psychological control, rejection, and hostility (Massetti et al., 2011), in addition to confirming the importance of parental monitoring.

Domestic violence and violence between parents have been identified by Herrenkohl et al. (2000) as risk factors for juvenile delinquency and antisocial behavior. Instability and family disruptions, such as homelessness, unemployment, removal of children by child welfare authorities, and parental drug addiction or chronic alcoholism, can lead to delinquency and adolescent substance abuse. Massetti et al. (2011) have offered a possible explanation for the wide-ranging impact on children caused by family disruption: "Family disruption causes a constellation of multiple stressors for youth, including parental conflict, parental loss, reduced financial resources, and deterioration in child rearing practices" (p. 1419). Similarly, Keller, Catalano, Haggerty, and Fleming (2002) found that in families with substance-abusing parents, more disruptions led to greater delinquency among their children.

Peer Risk Factors

Peer relationships, among the most important interpersonal connections in the lives of children and youth, become increasingly influential during adolescence (Massetti et al., 2011; Stoddard et al., 2013). Research has shown that involvement with delinquent or antisocial peers, particularly those with gang affiliation or membership, increases the risk for (1) violence and delinquency in adolescents (Dodge et al., 2006; Henggeler et al., 2009); (2) weapon carrying (Stoddard et al., 2013); (3) criminal activity (Ferguson & Meehan, 2010); and (4) substance abuse (Obando, Trujilio, & Trujilio, 2014; Wagner & Waldron, 2001). In fact, research has demonstrated that association with delinquent peers is a greater predictor of violence in youth than individual and family factors (Dodge et al., 2006). Similarly, involvement with substance-abusing peers is also a greater predictor of substance abuse (Obando et al., 2014; Wagner & Waldron, 2001). Massetti et al. (2011) cited Svensson's (2003) research finding that an adolescent's association with delinquent peers, combined with family risk factors, such as lack of parental affection and monitoring, "can substantially increase the risk for violence and delinquency" (p. 1419). There are also gender differences in delinquent peer affiliations. While delinquent boys usually associate with similar boys, delinquent girls relate to both sexes (Svensson, 2003). When these girls have older boyfriends, their level of risk increases (Massetti et al., 2011).

Peer pressure can play a major role in leading adolescents to engage in increasingly risky behaviors. For example, young adolescents may feel pressured by their peers to become involved in fighting and weapon carrying. As peers escalate their delinquent behaviors and criminal activity, the youth are placed at greater risk (Stoddard et al., 2013). Similarly, young adolescents may be pressured by substance-using peers to try entry-level drugs, such as alcohol and marijuana. Continued involvement with these peers may lead to increased pressure to experiment with more dangerous substances, such as heroin and crack cocaine. As stated earlier, given the danger and serious level of risk associated with these substances, even initial experimentation warrants intervention (Henggeler et al., 2012; Wagner & Waldron, 2001). In addition, the importance of gang membership as a powerful risk factor for delinquency in youth cannot be overstated (Thornberry et al., 2003).

School-Related Risk Factors

School-related risk factors, such as academic failure, attention and learning problems, school disengagement, lack of involvement in or connection to school activities, truancy and absenteeism, and school dropout (Henry, Knight, & Thornberry, 2012), can put students at risk for involvement in youth violence (Basch, 2011), substance abuse, and antisocial behavior (Obando et al., 2014). Similarly, adolescents who engage in aggression, fighting, or bullying in school and in the community are less likely to experience a positive connection to the school, and these behaviors can affect school adjustment (Basch, 2011).

Students involved with youth violence often experience academic difficulties very early in the educational process—that is, the third through fifth grades (Schwartz & Gorman, 2003). At-risk adolescents often can be characterized by disruptive behavior in the classroom. As these students' behavior can interrupt teaching and impede the learning process for others in the class (Basch, 2011), they often receive repeated in-school and out-of-school suspensions. When time spent out of the classroom accumulates, the possibility of educational losses, academic failure, grade retention, and school dropout increases. (See Chapter 10 for further discussion of school-related risk factors.)

Exposure to violence in the community and in school can affect students in different ways (Schwartz & Gorman, 2003). For example, some students are more likely to exhibit internalizing behaviors, such as withdrawal, isolation, depression, sadness, or anxiety (Basch, 2011). For others, the same circumstances can result in externalizing at-risk behaviors, such as youth violence, community violence, disruptive behaviors, conduct disorders (Basch, 2011; Schwartz & Gorman, 2003), and substance abuse (Henry et al., 2012; Liddle & Rowe, 2010; Wagner & Waldron, 2001). Students at either end of the spectrum of internalizing or externalizing behaviors can experience interference with cognitive development that may negatively impact their academic achievement (Basch, 2011).

A negative school climate, described by Bradshaw, Waasdorp, Debnam, and Johnson (2014) as a school rife with bullying, aggression, and drug use—all of which lead students to perceive a lack of safety in the school—can also be a risk factor for many adolescents. A lack of: (1) engagement and connection between students and teachers; (2) a process to engage students in the value of academic achievement; (3) clear and fair rules and consequences; (4) an orderly physical environment, but rather one characterized by chaos and disorder; and (5) parental involvement with the school can all be risk factors for academic failure, as well as serious antisocial behavior in students (Bradshaw et al., 2014).

Community Risk Factors

Rates of youth violence and delinquency vary considerably across environments and may be related to the social, economic, and demographic characteristics of the community (Herrenkohl et al., 2000; Massetti et al., 2011). Massetti et al. (2011) have identified community risk factors as including poverty and economic deprivation; social and community disorganization; high quantities of drugs, alcohol, and guns; and higher crime rates.

The connection between community violence and adolescents' aggressive behavior is well documented (McMahon et al., 2013). Research has shown that African American adolescents who grow up in low-income urban neighborhoods are more at risk for aggression because of their greater exposure to community violence (Brezina, Agnew, Cullen, & Wright, 2004); and these individuals—perceiving themselves to be surrounded by danger—may see no option other than fighting in order to protect themselves (Latzman & Swisher 2005).

GENDER DIFFERENCES

In recent years, the rates of violence conducted by female adolescents have been increasing (Massetti et al., 2011). While some of the rate increases may be attributed to changes in laws and policies, the proportion of females involved in some form of youth violence is substantial and should be addressed (Massetti et al., 2011). However, when Massetti et al. (2011) reviewed the current research on antisocial behaviors and violence prevention, they confirmed that, despite some recent increased interest in addressing violence prevention among girls, the vast majority of research has focused on boys. The rationale for the focus on boys is that boys are involved in the greatest amount of youth violence. A national study on juvenile crime reported that males were responsible for 83% of arrests for violent crimes and 93% of those arrests were for murder (Massetti et al., 2011). However, gender discrepancies are not as extreme when less severe criminal activity is studied. For example, the Centers for Disease Control and Prevention (2009) reported that 39.9% of high school boys and 22.9% of high school girls had been in a fight in the year studied, and weapon carrying was also reported by 27.1% of males and 7% of females. Although these statistics demonstrate that boys are in the majority in terms of youth violence reports, girls are at risk as well, particularly in communities in which there are high rates of violence (Massetti et al., 2011). Another gender discrepancy can be found in the research on risk and protective factors that has focused largely on boys. Even in studies that include both males and females in their samples, the differences by gender have not been examined for the most part (Massetti et al., 2011).

As indicated in this discussion, hyperactivity, inattention, and impulsivity are risk factors for antisocial behavior, youth violence, academic failure, and substance abuse. Girls present with significantly lower rates of these issues (Massetti et al., 2011). Although poor academic achievement has consistently been identified as a risk factor for violence and delinquency in adolescents, some studies have indicated that it is a higher predictor of risk for boys (Junger-Tas, Ribeaud, & Cruyff, 2004), while others have contradicted those results, stating the need for more research in this area (Massetti et al., 2011).

Despite the general paucity of research on youth violence among girls, some studies have examined issues unique to girls. For example, girls who experience puberty at a younger age than average are more likely to become involved in violence, delinquency, and increased substance use later in adolescence (Massetti et al., 2011). Researchers have found one possible explanation for these results: girls who experience early puberty may receive more attention from older boys, who then put the girls at increasing risk for delinquency, violence, risky sexual activity, and substance abuse. In addition, girls are more likely to experience sexual abuse and rape than boys (although boys are victims of sexual abuse and rape as well). According to the studies of sexual abuse conducted with girls in the juvenile justice system (Hennessey, Ford, Mahoney, Ko, & Siegfried, 2004), sexual abuse places them at a greater risk for involvement in youth violence. Religiosity was identified as a protective factor for girls, but not for boys, in at-risk communities in the Longitudinal Study of Adolescent Health (Massetti et al., 2011). Resilience and other factors that protect adolescents against the development of academic failure, school disengagement, and antisocial and other at-risk behaviors are discussed in the next section.

RESILIENCY THEORY

Two children or adolescents can grow up in the same community with dangerous levels of violence, and whereas one may succumb to the risk factors and become involved in youth aggression, the other may avoid negative behaviors and issues of violence, delinquency, substance abuse, teenage pregnancy, academic failure, and school dropout. Resiliency theory offers an explanation for the divergent outcomes in that protective factors (e.g., self-efficacy, parental monitoring, close family relationships, and involvement in a violence prevention program) "can help reduce the burden of cumulative risk for youth violence" (Stoddard et al., 2013, p. 57). Thus, resiliency theory provides an important perspective for researchers, clinicians, teachers, and school administrators to adopt.

Research has shown that a major protective factor for at-risk adolescents is the presence of a nonparental caring adult, such as a mentor, in their lives (Holt et al., 2008). School-based mentoring has been shown to increase adolescents' (1) school engagement; (2) connection to the school environment, particularly to teachers (Holt et al., 2008); and (3) sense of school belonging (Portwood, Ayers, Kinnison, Waris, & Wise, 2005). All three are protective factors for students who are at risk of dropping out of school (see Chapter 10).

Resilience theory is particularly relevant when working with African American, Latino, and other poor, inner-city adolescents. A large percentage of the research on this population has focused on problems; however, a number of researchers have begun to challenge that perspective and to focus instead on resiliency, survival skills, prosocial behaviors, and strengths (Belgrave, 2009; Belgrave, Nguyen, Johnson, & Hood, 2011). Rather than limiting its research on aggressive behaviors among African American adolescents, the Belgrave et al. (2011) study focused on both prosocial and negative behaviors. This research study makes the following observation with regard to its sample of African American adolescents, many of whom lived in low-income communities where violence is prevalent:

> Youth in these communities may come to view aggression and violence as normative. However, many African American youth are resilient and not only survive but also thrive in spite of neighborhood disadvantage (Belgrave, 2009). Our analysis pointed to

a cluster of well-adjusted boys and girls. (Belgrave et al., 2011, p. 1020)

Promotive and Protective Factors

Various researchers have studied the crucial nature of protective or promotive factors in the resiliency of at-risk adolescents. As stated by Stoddard et al. (2013):

> Promotive [or protective] factors play a role in helping youth overcome the negative effects risk pose[s] on development and are important as they help compensate for or protect against the effects of risk on healthy development. Promotive factors may reduce the negative consequences of risk factors through direct effects (compensatory model) or through interaction effects (risk-protective model) (Fergus & Zimmerman, 2005). The compensatory model of resilience implies that promotive factors can compensate for exposure to risk factors (Garmezy, Masten, & Tellegen, 1984; Masten et al., 1988). The risk-protective model assumes that promotive factors buffer or moderate the negative influence of exposure to risk (Rutter, 1985). (p. 58)

Research on cumulative risk and promotive or protective factors found that greater levels of multiple risk factors were consistent with more youth violence and that greater levels of cumulative protective factors were consistent with less youth violence (Stoddard et al., 2013). Thus, clusters of cumulative protective factors can lessen the impact of cumulative risk factors among adolescents.

Individual Level Protective Factors

Research has shown that a number of protective factors exist on the individual level that can protect adolescents from many of the risk factors we have described. These include (1) negative beliefs about aggression, (2) self-efficacy, (3) self-control, (4) self-confidence, (5) lower impulsivity (McMahon et al., 2013), (6) intelligence, (7) academic achievement, (8) connections to school, (9) school engagement, (10) focus, (11) determination, and (12) sense of purpose (Stoddard et al., 2013). For youth living in areas where crime and community violence are prevalent, McMahon et al. (2013) found that high self-efficacy and low impulsivity were particularly strong protective factors. Stoddard et al. observed that hopefulness and optimism about the future led to less participation in violent activities among at-risk adolescents (Stoddard et al., 2013).

Empathy, defined as "a type of prosocial behavior . . . characterized [by] the ability to recognize, to take the perspective of, and to respond to another's emotion (Eisenberg, Fabes, Carlo, & Karbon, 1992)" (Belgrave et al., 2011, p. 1013), has also been recognized as a protective factor that can lead to more prosocial and fewer aggressive behaviors (Belgrave et al., 2011).

Beliefs about aggression are among the most important risk and protective factors. For example, on the one hand, many of the at-risk adolescents with whom we have worked felt that choosing not to fight when they considered themselves to be provoked would cause them to lose face among their peers and put themselves at greater risk for further acts of violence. Their firm belief that their only option was to fight put them at high risk for violence in their schools and communities. On the other hand, students whose families imparted the value that violence is wrong, shared that view themselves, had negative beliefs about violence, and were more likely to resist the provocation to fight. These beliefs can serve as protective factors even in schools or communities where youth violence is high (McMahon et al., 2013).

Anger management skills have been shown to correlate with less aggressive behavior and other antisocial behaviors (Sullivan, Helms, Kliewer, & Goodman, 2010). Adolescents with poor anger management ability may be more likely to respond aggressively to provocation by peers (Belgrave et al., 2011). Research has shown that greater knowledge and skills can lead to less aggressive behavior (McMahon et al., 2013).

Strong ethnic identity—pride and a sense of positive values and connection to members of one's cultural group—has been shown to lead to greater social competence (Belgrave et al., 2011) and has been identified in a number of research studies as a protective factor against violence and other negative risk factors for African American adolescents (Belgrave et al., 2011), even in areas with high rates of community violence and substance abuse. These protective factors have been shown to cluster. Belgrave et al. (2011) found that "well-adjusted [African American] boys and girls scored above average on positive attributes (e.g., anger management, ethnic identity, empathy) and below average on normative beliefs about aggression" (p. 1019).

Self-confidence and self-efficacy have been important factors in empowering adolescents to avoid peer pressure to engage in antisocial behaviors such as substance abuse, truancy, violence, and gangs (Henggeler et al., 2009). Self-efficacy—a belief in oneself and in the ability to achieve one's goals (Bandura, 1997)—can also play an important role in academic performance and success in school. McMahon et al. (2013), in finding that "high self-efficacy and low impulsivity protected youth from the negative effects of community violence exposure" (p. 415), have argued for programs that strengthen self-efficacy as well as self-confidence as a method by which adolescents may be protected from the impact of community violence. Low levels of impulsivity and more

self-control and self-regulation have been correlated with more prosocial behavior (Buckner, Mezzacappa, & Beardslee, 2009). Research has
also shown that self-efficacy for positive behaviors to reduce conflicts
can lead to more prosocial activities among adolescents (Belgrave et
al., 2011; McMahon et al., 2013). This research can provide hope for
adolescents, family members, teachers, counselors, mentors, and other
service providers by challenging the belief that adolescents from high-
crime areas with extensive community violence will inevitably become
involved in aggression and youth violence.

Parental and Familial Protective Factors

A number of research studies have documented the parental and familial
behaviors that can serve as protective factors for adolescents who are at
risk for a range of antisocial behaviors (Massetti et al., 2011). Gorman-
Smith et al. (2004) discovered that attentive parenting was a protective factor for adolescents in poor communities. As has been indicated,
research has consistently shown that parental monitoring and supervision are protective factors for at-risk youth (Dishion et al., 2003; Veronneau et al., 2016). Empowering parents and other caregivers to effectively monitor children has been a central component of evidence-based
multisystemic therapy (MST) interventions for at-risk or antisocial adolescents (Henggeler et al., 2009; Swenson et al., 2005). In cases where
parents are unable to perform sufficient monitoring due to long work
hours or other issues, MST therapists work with the family to identify
other social supports in the extended family, church, neighborhood, or
community (Henggeler et al., 2009). (See Chapter 7.)

In their research on high-risk youth, Resnick, Ireland, and Borowsky
(2004) found that parental monitoring, connectedness, and positive family relationships characterized by warmth can serve as protective factors.
In a study of adolescent boys and girls, high parent and family connectedness, in addition to parental expectation of academic achievement, helped
to protect at-risk high school adolescents against involvement in violence
(Resnick et al., 2004). Family connectedness and prosocial, antiviolence
messages by parents and family members were protective factors for at-
risk adolescent girls and resulted in lower levels of violence perpetration
and victimization (Shlafer, McMorris, Sieving, & Gower, 2013).

Peer Protective Factors

As indicated earlier, research has clearly documented the dangerous
role that association with delinquent peers can play in the lives of at-
risk adolescents (Dodge et al., 2006; Henggeler et al., 2009; Swenson et

al., 2005). Prosocial peers, however, can provide a protective factor for such adolescents through positive support and role modeling (Resnick et al., 2004). Research has demonstrated that involvement with prosocial peers can be one protective factor that can reduce the negative effects of cumulative risk factors (Stoddard et al., 2013). Youth engaged in positive activities, such as sports in school and the community; clubs in school and other recreational structured activities with prosocial peers in the community; and church-run, after-school programs, were perceived by a community sample of urban adults and adolescents as less likely to become involved in serious levels of youth violence, truancy from school, substance abuse, and community violence (Dodington et al., 2012).

Youth in the Dodington et al. study (2012) also identified the process of inviting other adolescents to visit and engage in activities in their homes as a potential protective factor. Henggeler et al. (2009) and Swenson et al. (2005), in their discussion of interventions with at-risk adolescents engaged in antisocial behaviors, have repeatedly raised the importance of parents reaching out to have contact with and meet the friends of their children, encouraging their children to bring prosocial peers to their homes, and becoming acquainted with the friends' parents.

School Protective Factors

A positive school climate has been identified as a major protective factor for adolescents. Components of this positive climate include (1) a focus on safety in an environment free of bullying, aggression, and drugs; (2) student engagement with teachers; (3) an atmosphere of connectedness in the school; (4) parental involvement; (5) a positive physical environment; (6) a principal who takes a positive leadership role; (7) clear rules and consequences; (8) order; and (9) an atmosphere that supports diversity (Bradshaw et al., 2014).

Universal anti-bullying programs have produced positive results in a range of schools. One example is the Olweus Bullying Prevention Program (OBPP) (Olweus, 1993), a universal, schoolwide program that has been implemented in elementary, middle, and high schools. Research conducted with both boys and girls (Limber, 2004; Massetti et al., 2011) has shown that this program has led to decreased bullying and victimization; improved social climate; and reduced negative behaviors, such as truancy and aggression.

In Chapter 10, the importance of school engagement as a protective factor is discussed in detail. Evidence-based programs such as Achievement Mentoring (described in Chapter 11) that engage students in their schools, build positive mentoring relationships with a supportive adult, and increase students' academic achievement can keep them engaged in the process of learning and can help to prevent at-risk students from dropping out of school.

Community Protective Factors

Community protective factors may come in many forms. Individuals may undertake leadership roles in the community, serving as facilitators between residents, schools, and mental health professionals. These informal leaders often surface over time as therapists and school personnel work in communities and get to know the residents. It is important to recognize these individuals and to encourage them to support positive programs and interventions for adolescents. In addition, they can be helpful in recruiting other adolescents, parents, and family members to become involved in prevention and intervention programs.

Swenson et al. (2005) described a model for neighborhood partnerships between mental health professionals and community leaders. A treatment intervention, MST, was offered to at-risk adolescents and their families who had been referred by schools, the police, the courts, and other community agencies. Clinicians strengthened the community and developed a network of protective factors by also meeting with key community members, such as ministers, youth recreational program directors, organizers of youth sports teams, along with parents and other interested adults, to develop opportunities for adolescents to be involved in prosocial activities. The Swenson et al. (2005) research also provided other examples of collaborative attempts to intervene in a positive and protective way for adolescents in the community, such as block associations and neighborhood crime watches. Through these interventions, individuals and organizations concerned about community violence, neighborhood crime, drug dealing, truancy, and substance abuse formed partnerships to amplify their voices and address these issues.

Throughout this book, we emphasize the cultural strengths of religion and spirituality for African American, Latino, and other ethnic minority families (Boyd-Franklin, 2003; Falicov, 2005, 2014; Garcia-Preto, 2005; Hines & Boyd-Franklin, 2005). Churches and other faith-based organizations can contribute to community protective factors for adolescents by providing prosocial opportunities and after-school, weekend, and summer activities in safe spaces in which adolescents can interact. Engaging in positive activities will "take them back from the streets" (Boyd-Franklin, Franklin, & Toussaint, 2001, p. 204) during times when parents are often working and unable to provide sufficient monitoring and supervision.

CHAPTER 3

Cultural, Racial, and Socioeconomic Issues

Throughout this book, we have encouraged practitioners to view clients and families in terms of their strengths. Because at-risk adolescents and families in trouble present with their problems, understanding their cultural, racial, and socioeconomic realities can enable therapists and school personnel to search for and identify strengths in difficult situations. In this chapter, we discuss the relevance of cultural, racial, and socioeconomic differences as they affect adolescents and families in need of help. The primary focus of this chapter is on groups with which we have had the most clinical experience—African American and Latino, and poor families from White as well as ethnic minority backgrounds (Boyd-Franklin & Bry, 2000; McGoldrick et al., 2005).

Excellent resources are available in the literature on many of these topics (Berg, 1994; Boyd-Franklin, 2003; Falicov, 2014; McGoldrick et al., 2005). The goal of this chapter is to address crucial areas of intervention with these adolescents and their families that are often not addressed in existing publications. Although socioeconomic issues are mentioned last in the title of this chapter, we begin with a brief discussion of this topic because so many of the families receiving home-based family interventions and other forms of outreach are poor. Many of these poor families from ethnic minority groups face racism and discrimination as well.

POOR FAMILIES

Families living in poverty include a wide spectrum of cultural and racial groups, and reside in rural and suburban, as well as urban settings. The literature has tended to equate families living in poverty with "ethnic minority" inner-city families. This is a serious error, for there are also many poor and working-class White families struggling at subsistence levels in the United States. (See Chapter 13 for a case example involving an at-risk adolescent from a "working poor" White family.)

Poor families from all cultural and racial groups often perceive themselves as being at the mercy of the powerful systems with which they interact. As this perception can lead to frustration, anger, and possibly learned helplessness, clinicians must avoid "doing for" these families and should instead empower them to take control of their own lives as a major treatment goal. A transformation from passivity to empowerment is often a gradual process. For example, impoverished parents may regard their child's school as a hostile, unresponsive place. The clinician can first role-play interactions with the school in family sessions and then accompany the client to the first meeting with school personnel. Ultimately the goal is for the parent and other family caregivers to be able to make these school visits and interventions on their own.

Readers are cautioned against adopting a "culture of poverty" approach that stereotypes all poor families. Practitioners should be aware of the many "working poor" families of all ethnic and racial groups whose only employment options are full-time minimum-wage or low-wage jobs; multiple part-time jobs; or even multiple full-time jobs. Most of these jobs provide no health care or other benefits. These individuals may have large or extended families to support on incomes of less than $20,000 a year. Serious illness, such as cancer, can devastate such a family emotionally, physically, and financially. Important preventative medical interventions, such as prenatal and well-baby care, dentistry, and annual checkups, are often neglected. Since the passage of Medicaid in 1965, many advances have been made to enable poor and working poor families to obtain health insurance for themselves and their children. In 1997, the Children's Health Insurance Program (CHIP) expanded low-cost health coverage to children in families with earnings that exceeded the Medicaid minimum, and the Patient Protection and Affordable Care Act (PPACA), also known as the Affordable Care Act (ACA) and "Obamacare," was enacted in 2010 to enable individuals and families to purchase health insurance on an income-adjusted basis. Many individuals and families are very concerned that the benefits of the ACA will be lost during the current administration.

Poverty should not be viewed as an independent variable. Race, culture, and socioeconomic level interact in complex ways that vary from family to family. Poverty is profoundly related to issues of homelessness, unemployment, underemployment, lack of access to good jobs, high school dropout rates, crime, dangerous streets, and communities with high levels of drug abuse and drug trafficking. These issues are exacerbated by the "double jeopardy" of racism and discrimination in the case of minority families. For some families, the interaction between poverty and racism may result in extremely negative situations.

AFRICAN AMERICAN CLIENTS AND FAMILIES

An important consequence of the history of racism and discrimination in the United States is that many African American families have developed "healthy cultural suspicion" (Boyd-Franklin, 2003; Boyd-Franklin & Bry, 2000; Boyd-Franklin et al., 2013; Hines & Boyd-Franklin, 2005). This suspicion is often the first response encountered by clinicians and school personnel working with these adolescents and their families, particularly in mandated home-based interventions. In addition, for many poor African American families particularly, multigenerational experiences with racism, rejection, and the perceived intrusion of schools and agencies have helped to engender the view that family dynamics are "nobody's business but our own" (Boyd-Franklin, 2003). Thus, their instinctual reaction to outside interventions is often to protect their families from intrusion by being secretive and sometimes unresponsive.

Too often, if a therapist or school personnel are unaware of this cultural pattern, an African American family may be dismissed as "resistant," or the practitioner may take such a response personally and attribute it to his or her race, ethnicity, or ability and withdraw from the family. It is extremely important for a home-based family therapist, other clinician, school counselor or teacher, achievement mentor, or representative of a community agency to be prepared for this reaction and be able to reframe it as the family's attempt to protect its members.

A supervisor needs to be especially vigilant in helping a clinician to recognize that this initial response is merely the beginning of a chess game of engagement between the therapist and the African American family, and not a checkmate or the end of therapy. "Healthy cultural suspicion" is a factor to be overcome when working with African Americans in both cross-race and same-race treatment. African American therapists are often surprised when this suspicion extends to them, as well as to teachers and therapists from other cultures.

It is also important for clinicians to be cognizant of the cultural strengths of African Americans, such as (1) the roles played by extended family members; (2) the common practice of kinship care or informal adoption; (3) spirituality or religious beliefs; (4) the desire for an education for their children, regardless of their feelings about the school system; (5) love of their children and the desire to be good parents; and (6) survival skills. These themes are illustrated throughout this book in case examples. For a comprehensive description of these strengths, see *Black Families in Therapy: Understanding the African American Experience* (Boyd-Franklin, 2003). Addressed in this chapter are the issues that are essential for professionals to understand when they are working with African American adolescents and their families: (1) knowing who has the power in a family; (2) spirituality and religion; (3) expressions of anger; (4) parenting styles, including physical punishment and the issue of respect for parents or elders; (5) issues confronting young Black males and females; and (6) messages about violence.

Knowing Who Has the Power in a Family

When African American families are suspicious of outside agencies and systems, they may hide key family members from clinicians until trust is established. In addition, the concept of therapy is new to many African American families, who view it as appropriate only for "sick people, rich people, or White people" (Boyd-Franklin, 2003). As is universal across cultures, the most commonly presenting family group consists of a mother and one or more children. However, fathers and boyfriends play key roles in Black families, as do extended family members (Hines & Boyd-Franklin, 2005) such as grandmothers, grandfathers, aunts, and uncles. When family therapists who treat the mother/children constellation in an office find themselves conducting endless family therapy sessions that do not produce change, it is often because the individuals attending sessions may be the least powerful members of their families. Other family members with real power may need to be engaged in the treatment process for change to occur.

Family therapists conducting sessions in a client's or family's home are in the advantageous position of being more likely to encounter powerful family members in their own environment. It is very important to reach out to these individuals and to greet them, even if they are not participating in the family sessions and only passing through to go to another room. As trust develops, it is perfectly acceptable to say to a nonparticipant (e.g., father, boyfriend, mother, grandmother, grandfather, older son or daughter) "I hope that you will feel more comfortable joining sessions as you get to know me better. Come anytime."

For example, a team of therapists had been doing home-based family interventions with an African American blended family, in which the father and his son (age 15) had been living with his girlfriend and her two children (ages 12 and 13). Initially, when the therapists came to the home, the father would get up out of his chair in the living room and disappear into the back of the house for the entire session. (This was a metaphor for his role and behavior in the family.) After a careful discussion with their supervisor, the family therapists decided that they would take a proactive approach by greeting the father at the beginning of the next session and inviting him to stay whenever he was ready because he was "so important to this family." He resisted for a number of sessions until his son was suspended from school. The family therapists were able to utilize this crisis to insist on his involvement in helping them to help his son. Because the therapists had laid the groundwork earlier, this time he responded positively. He was greeted enthusiastically by the family and the therapists when he joined the session.

Spirituality and Religion

Different Meanings of Spirituality and Religion

Although the distinction between spirituality and religion in the lives of African Americans has been addressed in detail in a number of sources (Billingsley, 1992; Boyd-Franklin, 2003, 2010; Boyd-Franklin & Lockwood, 1999, 2009; Hines & Boyd-Franklin, 2005), many clinicians are still confused about how to utilize these strengths and resources in work with African American families. Certain individuals, particularly older female members, may be very involved in church attendance and have an active and supportive "church family." Others, including some males and adolescents of both genders, may be in rebellion against what they perceive as the excessively strict religious practices of some family members. Although resistant to religion as such, these same family members may have a "crisis spirituality," in which their early training or belief in God becomes activated when they are in trouble or in a crisis (Boyd-Franklin, 2010; Boyd-Franklin & Lockwood, 1999, 2009). Therefore, although religion and spirituality are tremendous strengths for many African Americans, it is important for the practitioner not to assume that they are present in all families or family members.

Differences related to religion, spirituality, or their expression may cause intergenerational conflicts among African Americans. When such a conflict peaks—for example, when a religious African American mother or grandmother is overwhelmed by problems caused by a rebellious child or grandchild—it is common for the religious family member to state, "I have turned him [or her] over to God." It is important for a therapist to assess whether this is a positive act of faith in which the parent or grandparent is praying for the child while continuing "parental" functions, or whether it represents a sense of giving up on the child.

Religion and spiritual beliefs were often central to life in many African cultures (Boyd-Franklin, 2003; Hines & Boyd-Franklin, 2005; Mbiti, 1990; Nobles, 2004). Thus, religion and spirituality—essential components in the lives of many African Americans throughout their history in the United States—can be traced to the tradition of African religions.

African American clients are likely to reveal their particular uses of spirituality and religion as coping mechanisms during the assessment process, often using phrases such as "God will solve my problems," or "I am being punished for having sinned." Because of this intense spiritual connection, spiritual reframing may be a very useful technique in treating some Black families. Examples of such spiritual reframing are as follows: "God will know what your needs are and will supply," and "He gives you no more than you can carry" (Mitchell & Lewter, 1986, p. 2; see also Boyd-Franklin, 2003).

Many different denominations and distinct religious groups, both Christian and non-Christian, are represented in Black communities within the United States, including Baptists, the African Methodist Episcopal (AME) church, AME Zion churches, Jehovah's Witnesses, the Church of God in Christ, Seventh-Day Adventists, Pentecostal churches, Apostolic churches, Presbyterians, Lutherans, Episcopalians, and Roman Catholics. Of these groups, the largest numbers of Black people are affiliated with Baptist and AME churches (Boyd-Franklin, 2010). In addition, a smaller number of African Americans are Muslims (Sunni Muslims) or members of Islamic groups, such as the Nation of Islam (Boyd-Franklin, 2003). McAdams-Mahmoud (2005) has provided extensive clinical examples of family therapy with different types of African American Muslim families. It is noteworthy that individuals who convert to Islam may experience conflicts with other members of their families who have retained Christian beliefs (Boyd-Franklin, 2003; McAdams-Mahmoud, 2005).

The Role of the Black Church, Ministers, and the "Church Family"

Throughout history, Black churches have provided an escape for Black people from their painful life experiences, serving what Frazier (1963) in his early classic work described as "a refuge in a hostile . . . world" (p. 44). Black churches have historically been among the most viable institutions in African American communities (Billingsley, 1992; Boyd-Franklin, 2003; Hines & Boyd-Franklin, 2005). They were and often still are among the few places where Black men and women can feel that they are respected for their own talents and abilities (Billingsley, 1992; Boyd-Franklin, 2003, 2010; Boyd-Franklin & Lockwood, 1999, 2009). Among the first priorities for many African American families who relocate is to find a church in their new location so that they can become connected to a faith-based community.

Black churches often function as surrogate families for isolated and overburdened single mothers. Many Black single-parent mothers will tell therapists, "I raised my children in the church," or "He was brought up in the church," as a testament to the unique value provided by the Black church. Because of the need for services in many Black communities and the deep concerns about the education of Black children, many churches have begun to provide day care centers, after-school tutoring programs, and schools. Therapists, who are aware of these services, can help isolated Black families to obtain help for their children and to build new support networks. In some cases, these services may be available to families that are not members of the church congregation.

In many parts of the United States and for many African American (and Latino) families, ministers often have a great deal of influence both within the congregations and within the community. Ministers often serve multiple roles as spiritual leaders, pastoral counselors, community advocates, and political activists. The minister is usually a central figure in the life of a family and often may be sought out for pastoral counseling in times of trouble, pain, or loss. A Black church may have a board of deacons and deaconesses who assist the pastor in carrying out the duties of the church. Holding this position is clearly a strength and a sign of leadership ability.

After the nuclear and extended family, the church is the most common source of help among Black people. For many African American families, the Black church functions essentially as another extended family—the "church family." In addition, Black churches also serve a social function. Meals are often served after Sunday services, providing an opportunity for families to become acquainted and develop friendships.

One of the most important "family" functions that a Black church serves is that of providing a large number of opportunities and role models for young people, both male and female. Black churches often provide nonchurch-related activities as well, such as boy scouts, girl scouts, basketball teams, youth groups, and tutoring and mentoring programs. Churches also offer programs and services oriented toward every stage of life, from toddlers to senior citizens, such as Sunday school, vacation Bible school, and Bible study classes. Therapists should be aware of all of these resources and supports offered by churches in the community. They can help the families of at-risk adolescents, even those that are not church members, to access these services.

Expressions of Anger in African American Families

In keeping with the "healthy cultural suspicion" (Boyd-Franklin, 2003) discussed earlier, many African American families present initially with anger directed at racism, schools, outside systems and agencies, and practitioners. Although families of all races and cultures express anger in treatment, it is often more difficult for clinicians to deal with these issues with African Americans because of the dynamics of race and racism. An angry Black mother or father often elicits a fear response, particularly in cross-racial treatment (Boyd-Franklin, 2003; Boyd-Franklin & Bry, 2000). Another dynamic is that African Americans are often very emotionally expressive. Therapists from cultures more reticent about displaying emotions, particularly anger, may find this dynamic frightening. An additional aspect to be considered is that emotions may be exaggerated to test clinicians; that is, is the clinician able to tolerate such demonstration of emotion, or will he or she withdraw from treatment and abandon the family? It is essential for therapists to be aware of their own response to clients' anger and to seek advice from supervisors on understanding the basis of their clients' anger and not run away from it.

Parenting Styles of African Americans

There is considerable variability in parenting styles among African Americans, inasmuch as these styles are often a function of socioeconomic level, parents' degree of educational attainment, region of the country, religious practices, and age. Certain common themes, however, may present challenges to the clinician, especially "preaching," physical punishment, and the emphasis on "respect" for parents and elders (Boyd-Franklin, 2003; Hines & Boyd-Franklin, 2005).

Preaching

African American culture is a very verbal one. When parents become frustrated by their children's and adolescents' continued misbehavior, they may resort to "preaching" to them, often accompanied by threats of extreme consequences. These threats may be a reflection of anger and desperation, and their fear for the adolescent, rather than serious intentions. When parents do not follow through in a consistent fashion, however, children learn to "tune them out," leading to an even more problematic situation.

In treatment, "preaching" may manifest as parents who cannot stop talking. This issue is especially challenging for young or inexperienced therapists. Paradoxically, the way to get the monologue to abate is to

allow the parent some time to "vent" in the family session or in an individual session. The therapist should actively reframe the parents' vent-
ing of frustration and anger as expressions of the parents' love for their
children and their desperate efforts to find a way to help them. Since
parents often feel guilty about the problems of their children and are
anticipating blame from therapists, it may be very helpful for clinicians,
schools, courts, police and probation officers to offer them validating
messages, such as "You have tried very hard," "You have tried to do the
best you can," or "You really love him [or her] and underneath all of
your anger is your fear for him." Another reframe that we have found
very helpful with many African American parents or caregivers is "You
are a survivor and now we need to work together to help this child learn
how to survive." This can be used with any African American parent or
caregiver irrespective of their life circumstances or problems. If it is difficult for a therapist to find something positive in parents' actions, he or
she may need the opportunity for feedback from supervisors, coworkers,
or team members.

Physical Punishment

One of the most difficult areas for clinicians, whether from Black,
White, or other ethnic groups, in working with African American families relates to disciplinary practices involving physical punishment, such
as spanking. Many African American parents and grandparents have
adopted a "spare the rod, spoil the child" approach to child rearing,
often in response to fears of far more serious consequences that others may impose for the adolescent's misbehavior (Boyd-Franklin, 2003;
Hines & Boyd-Franklin, 2005). For example, some Black parents have
said, "If I don't discipline him, the police will." Memories and stories
of lynchings, beatings, false imprisonment, and more recent experiences
of racial profiling and police shootings are part of African American
parental testimony and have sparked their fears for generations.

Clinicians treating families where discipline is problematic should
acknowledge both the cultural parenting practices and the fact that the
law requires clinicians to report incidents of child abuse. A therapist
must evaluate whether a "spanking" is within cultural norms or whether
it constitutes child abuse. Careful questioning of the children and the
parents about what actually occurred is necessary before a clinician can
make this determination, as children or other family members may have
exaggerated the degree of discipline by using cultural terms and calling
a "spanking" a "beating." Also, children, particularly adolescents, may
manipulate parents by threatening to call child welfare or child protective services. Therapists from other cultures may have more difficulty in

ascertaining when an incident has crossed the line from a cultural prac- tice to a case of abuse. In such circumstances, seeking help and advice from a supervisor or an African American coworker, who can act as a "cultural consultant," may be indicated.

Therapists should not deny their responsibility to report serious child abuse when it occurs, nor should they collude with families to keep it a secret from child protective services. Therapists may need to communicate to parents that serious consequences may ensue if they engage in physical punishment, while at the same time communicating their concern for the family. For example, a therapist may say, "Yes, I know you and I respect your cultural practices, but I'm concerned that if you continue to spank them, your children may be taken away from you. I care about you and your family, and I don't want to see you lose your children. Let's explore other ways of getting them to listen to you without resorting to hitting."

When a parent does need to be reported to child protective services, it is often helpful for a supervisor or administrator to do the reporting. This allows the family therapist or clinician to continue to support the family through the process (Boyd-Franklin & Bry, 2000).

Respect for Parents and Elders

Given the lack of respect with which they are treated by the rest of soci- ety, African Americans often insist that their children show respect for them. Sometimes a parent's or older caregiver's definition of "respect" may be so comprehensive as to preclude any expression of angry or nega- tive feelings. For these parents, adolescents' typical expressions of oppo- sition (e.g., rolling their eyes, sucking their teeth, turning their backs, or cursing) can often be met with intense anger and physical retribution. Before these issues can be addressed in a joint family session, a therapist may need to work with a parent or caregiver and the adolescent individ- ually. The therapist negotiates with the parent(s) to allow the adolescent to express anger on the grounds that it will not be allowed to fester and thus be acted out in school or in the community. Once an adolescent has an individual alliance with the therapist, he or she can be helped to see that anger can be expressed to the parents "respectfully" (i.e., without cursing, eye rolling, or "getting loud"). The goal of the initial individual work is to join with the parent(s) and the adolescent, validate each party, and empathize with each. This process presents a challenge that often taxes the therapist's conflict resolution skills. All of these issues are par- ticularly intense when they involve Black male adolescents.

It is also important for family therapists to remember that many African Americans are very sensitive about how therapists address them.

This is particularly true of older family members. It is often best to start with "Mr." or "Ms." or "Mrs." or to ask "What name would you like me to call you?" before taking liberties with first names. In some of the case examples in the book, we have followed the family members' preference as to how they would like to be addressed. Younger parents may sometimes prefer first names.

Issues Confronting Young Black Males and Females in Schools and Communities

Many Black parents fear that they will lose their children (girls and boys) to violence, drugs, incarceration, or early death. African Americans are especially concerned about the survival of their male children given the punitive ways in which mainstream society reacts to Black males. The process can begin when Black boys are as young as 5 or 6, starting a course that often results in a failure syndrome for these boys in their schools. They are disproportionately labeled as "hyperactive," "aggressive," "distractible," "emotionally disturbed," "maladjusted," or "conduct-disordered," leading to their placement in special education classes, particularly in urban systems. These disparities exist with Latinos as well. African American and Latino boys are classified in special education in disproportionally large numbers (Skiba, Michael, Nardo, & Peterson, 2002), and researchers have found that African American and Latino males are disproportionally disciplined in terms of receiving in- and out-of-school suspension, expulsions from school, placements into alternative schools, or placements outside of the school district, ultimately leading to juvenile justice placements and the school-to-prison pipeline (Gregory, Skiba, & Noguera, 2010).

Some efforts have been made to improve the lives and educational trajectory of Black and Latino boys. Fergus, Noguera, and Martin (2014) identified schools that have been able to foster resilience in these adolescents and to produce positive educational outcomes for them. What each of these schools had in common was the commitment by all teachers, staff members, and administrators that every student could achieve, be academically successful, graduate high school, and go on to college. These high expectations were consistently communicated to the adolescents within the school and reinforced by parents and other family members.

Unfortunately, holding positive views and communicating encouraging messages to all students are often rarely evidenced in the schools that most African Americans and Latinos attend. Given the disparities we have discussed, Black parents are often extremely suspicious that racial motives underlie the acts of school authorities, police, juvenile justice officials, courts, and probation officers. In an attempt to protect their children, they may adopt a "not my child" position even when their children are in the wrong.

For example, parents with multigenerational experiences of problems with a school system may automatically take an adversarial position in response to a call from their adolescent's school or feel that the only way to defend their adolescent is to become angry at school conferences or when meeting with individuals associated with the police and courts. Unfortunately, these may be self-defeating strategies as they often worsen a family's relationship with those institutions and cause authorities to dismiss parental input or to adopt a self-fulfilling prophecy of "like parent, like child."

Teachers, other school staff, and therapists are often surprised by and unprepared when parents react to school and other authorities in a hostile and/or suspicious manner that may prevent their children from receiving the help and services that might reorient them toward a more positive path or lead to a better educational outcome. A family therapist or other clinician often has to intervene by joining first with the parent(s) and with the school separately before bringing them together.

African American parents are all too often correct in identifying situations in which their adolescents are discriminated against. It is not helpful for family therapists to deny this and to enter into a power struggle with these families. A "both–and" approach is indicated—one in which racism is acknowledged, *and* the parents' help is sought in teaching their children how to deal with racism when it occurs and not be defeated (or feel victimized) by it.

Once a strong bond with a parent has been established, the therapist can engage the parent in role play before parent–teacher conferences or Child Study Team meetings. For example, the therapist can say, "Many parents have told me that they want the school to take them seriously so that they can get what they want for their child. If they go in there and get very angry, the school will dismiss them and take action against their child. Let's rehearse how you can handle this teacher or principal and get the result you want for your son [or daughter]" (Boyd-Franklin & Bry, 2000).

When negative encounters have occurred between parents and school authorities previously, and the parent and an adolescent have a "rep" (i.e., a negative reputation), a therapist may have to first allow school personnel to vent their frustrations before the therapist can persuade them to give the family "another chance" and schedule a meeting. The therapist must work very hard to reframe to the school authorities small positive changes and outcomes that the family has accomplished, and to encourage the family by emphasizing the importance of the fact that the meeting is taking place.

Some parents, however, are at the opposite extreme and become passive and resigned in the face of authority figures who are involved in their adolescents' lives. For example, an adolescent girl had received repeated suspensions from school. During a home-based family session, when the therapist asked the mother whether she was aware of the suspensions, the parent responded that she was "fed up." She went to a nearby drawer and pulled out 15 unopened letters from the school as the stunned therapist looked on.

Gender Roles in African American Families

Gender roles in African American families are often complicated because of the racism and discrimination against and "invisibility" (Franklin, 2004; Franklin, Boyd-Franklin, & Kelly, 2006) of African American males in society. African American families have a great deal of love for all of their children (girls and boys). There is a saying, however, that some Black mothers "raise their daughters and love their sons" (Boyd-Franklin, 2003, p. 90). This does not imply that daughters are loved less; rather, it indicates the sense of fear, anxiety, and helplessness that many Black families feel about their inability to protect their male children in this country (Boyd-Franklin, 2003; Boyd-Franklin et al., 2001). Some African American families try to compensate for this reality of discrimination and danger by attempting to protect their male children within the family (Boyd-Franklin, 2003). Although well-intentioned, these sexist messages can have serious multigenerational consequences for couple relationships in some African American families (see Boyd-Franklin, 2003, for a more complete discussion of these complex issues).

This saying about gender differences in child rearing also indicates the burdens that young Black women often have to assume. In some African American families, girls and young women are raised to be strong and to take on major family responsibilities from a young age. As a consequence, some girls, who have been raised by struggling single-parent mothers, are given the message, "God bless the child who has her own," meaning that young women must be able to take care of themselves. In some Black families, they are raised with an understanding that they may be required to take care of and raise their families alone in the future, rather than expect that their Black male partners, who may be invisible in society and denied economic opportunity, will be able to contribute to this undertaking (Boyd-Franklin, 2003; Hines & Boyd-Franklin, 2005).

Both older girls and boys in some Black families are expected to function responsibly as "parental children" (Boyd-Franklin, 2003; Minuchin, 1974; Nichols, 2011), caring for their younger siblings. As they have often assumed adult responsibility since childhood, they are consequently less likely to accept adult direction and limit setting in adolescence. Parents and grandparents often complain that "they think they are grown."

Community Violence

One of the problems faced by African American parents, particularly in inner-city areas, is the risk of violence against their children. Whitaker and Snell (2016) analyzed the "staggering statistics" that engender so much of the pain and fear that Black parents have for their sons:

> [Black males have] high rates of being victims and perpetrators of homicides (Fox & Swatt, 2008), declining rates of life expectancy (Anderson, 2006), and growing rates of suicide (Poussaint & Alexander, 2000). The rates of incarceration, conviction, and arrest are the highest for African American males compared to every other demographic group in the nation (Gilgoff, 2007). These young men are in fact "playing for keeps," without the societal safety nets, just the attempts of their parents to keep them alive. (p. 306)

Black parents are haunted by stories of adolescents whose altercations ended with their being killed by someone with a gun (Boyd-Franklin, 2003; Boyd-Franklin et al., 2001). Parents raised in the era of fistfights often caution their children that they should not start fights but should defend themselves and fight back if provoked. Messages supportive of retaliation may need to be reconsidered now that the use of guns has replaced fists.

Unlike adolescents of other cultures, African American youth frequently experience a sense of their own mortality. This point was vividly conveyed in a group therapy session in which African American adolescents (ages 12–14) were asked to project their future dreams and hopes for themselves in an "I have a dream" exercise. One of the most intelligent, articulate members responded that he was convinced that he would be killed before he turned 25. Given this pervasive fear of street violence, it is not surprising that so many young male and female adolescents are tempted to seek protection by joining gangs or, less formally, by aligning themselves with groups of other at-risk adolescents (Thornberry & Krohn, 2003). This troubling trend is often ignored by parents, school officials, and juvenile authorities alike, particularly in gentrified urban neighborhoods, small cities, suburban, and rural areas, who may be in denial that there is a "gang problem" in their communities.

Racial Profiling and Encounters with the Police

Throughout history, African American parents have used racial socialization messages to prepare their children, especially their sons, for the realities of a world that can be racially hostile and dangerous to them (Burt, Simons, & Gibbons, 2012). Whitaker and Snell (2016) have described this process as an "essential rite of passage in African American homes and a cultural legacy that has been practiced for generations" (p. 304). It is particularly painful for many of these parents to recognize their own powerlessness to protect their children (Amber, 2013) and to face the reality that

> the same rules that apply to White children do not apply to their children (Burnett, 2012; Cooper, 2014; Fine & Johnson, 2013; Jamieson, 2014). These different rules are often unspoken but largely understood in the African American community. The most obvious unstated concern is that African American children will have different consequences for the same behavior. (Whitaker & Snell, 2016, pp. 303–304)

Media images of Black male adolescents and adults often contribute to the stereotype of them as violent. Racial profiling, a response to the media-driven perception that Black males are to be feared, is often a component of encounters with the police that may have a very negative outcome for Black males. Many African American parents, of all socioeconomic and educational levels, feel the need to prepare their adolescent children for this possibility in a discussion which many Black scholars and families alike have labeled "The Talk" (Whitaker & Snell, 2016). Parents, motivated by the desire to protect their children from all hurt, harm, and danger, are delivering what is essentially a very pessimistic message to their children—they may be negatively prejudged based on their skin color, and they may be feared. Yet, at the same time, they face the challenge of building their children's self-esteem, self-efficacy, and empowerment, all of which will help them to believe they can succeed in life (Whitaker & Snell, 2016). Some White therapists have expressed surprise when they discover that African American middle- and upper-class parents share these fears. Many Black parents realize that their professional degrees, financial security, higher paying jobs and homes in predominantly White upper-middle-class suburbs will not protect their children, particularly their sons, from this type of risk.

One example of the impact of racial profiling on all Black adolescents, irrespective of social class, is found in the aftermath of a reported crime, when the police target *all* African Americans of that gender in that age range, but particularly Black male adolescents or young adults, in an effort to identify the perpetrator. Whether the crime has occurred in an inner-city or a middle-class or an upper-middle-class community, young people who live in and attend schools in the community may be stopped and interrogated by the police and treated as suspects. Racial profiling can occur during any activity of daily life (Whitaker & Snell, 2016). Black families often prepare their children, especially their sons for "DWB," that is, driving while Black, which has often been the situation in which racial profiling can lead to deadly consequences (Boyd-Franklin et al., 2001). Sometimes Black adolescents and young adults from middle-class families may be even more at risk if they are driving the family car in a predominantly White neighborhood. Another illustration of racial profiling is the notorious incident in which a Neighborhood Watch coordinator in a middle-class gated community shot and killed Trayvon Martin, a 17-year-old unarmed African American adolescent, in Sanford, Florida, in 2012.

It is important for clinicians to be sensitive to a family's reality-based fears. If an African American parent has not had "The Talk" about how to deal with police and other authorities, a family therapist can empower parents to teach their children how to respond in a way that may help to avoid problems and to protect their children. Boyd-Franklin et al. (2001) and Gardere (1999) have offered helpful suggestions as to how parents might educate their children on the challenging subjects of the reality of racism and racial profiling, and how skin color may lead to encounters with the police, so that adolescents in these often dangerous situations may proceed with the least risk to themselves. Providing an adolescent with a cell phone is advised, so that parents can be contacted when their assistance is needed (Boyd-Franklin et al., 2001). Dr. Jeffrey Gardere (1999) has offered the following guidelines for parents to instruct their adolescents regarding encounters with the police:

- Do not try to run away.
- Do not make any sudden moves.
- Keep [your] hands visible or raised in the air.
- Say, "I am not armed."
- Respond to directives from the police.
- Do not resist arrest or resist being searched.
- Do not act smart or back talk. This can make [you] a target.
- Say "yes sir" and "no sir."
- As soon as possible, ask to make a phone call to [your] parents or family for help.
- Ask for a lawyer to be present before [you say] anything. (Gardere, 1999; cited in Boyd-Franklin et al., 2001, pp. 185–186)

Sadly, while observing these guidelines may help to defuse a danger-ous interaction with a police officer and prevent a negative outcome, they unfortunately may not always protect African American adolescents in racially charged, life-threatening situations (Whitaker & Snell, 2016), as cell phone videos of a number of police shootings have revealed.

SHOOTINGS OF AFRICAN AMERICAN MALES BY THE POLICE

These concerns of African American parents are underscored by the increase in the number of shootings of Black male adolescents and adults by the police throughout the United States within the last 10 years (Whitaker & Snell, 2016). Researchers (Moore et al., 2016, p. 254) have shown that

> the chances of a young Black male being killed by the police are 21 times greater than their White counterpart. Furthermore, between 2010 and 2012, young Black males between 15 and 19 were killed by police at a rate of 31.17 per million, compared to only 1.47 per million White males in that same age range. (Harris, 2014)

Although violence directed at Black males has been a legacy of the racism and discrimination that has existed throughout the history of this country, the recent numbers of high-profile killings of unarmed Black men by the police have led to public outcry, demonstrations, and the birth of the Black Lives Matter movement (Hadden, Toliver, Snowden, & Brown-Manning, 2016). The police killings of Michael Brown in Fer-guson, Missouri; Eric Garner in Staten Island, New York; Tamir Rice in Cleveland, Ohio; Freddie Gray in Baltimore, Maryland; Philando Castile in St. Paul, Minnesota; and Alton Sterling in Baton Rouge, Louisiana, are only the tip of the iceberg. There are many more African American adolescents and young men killed by police whose deaths have never made national headlines. It is of even further concern that when the police officers responsible for these shootings are prosecuted, there is often no accountability—charges are often dismissed or the officers are exonerated in jury trials. This has resulted in more anger and outrage among Black Lives Matter and other social justice groups throughout this country.

BLACK WOMEN WHO HAVE DIED DURING ENCOUNTERS WITH THE POLICE

Although the reports in the media have emphasized the killing of Black men by the police and many Black parents have focused on preparing their sons for these encounters, it is important to remember that Black women have also been killed by the police in many parts of this country. News reports have identified 22 Black women killed during encounters with the police or while in police custody (NewsOne, 2017), and these numbers continue to increase. Some of these women were killed during encounters such as one involving Yvette Smith, 47, a Texas mother, who was shot twice after opening the door to a sheriff's deputy, who was responding to a 911 call on February 16, 2014. Darnesha Harris, age 16, was killed in 2012 when police fired shots into the car that she was driving. Others, such as Symone Marshall, Sandra Bland, and Gynnya McMillen died of questionable "medical conditions" while in police custody (NewsOne, 2017).

In summary, it is important for therapists to recognize that many Black parents, adolescents, and other family members constantly live with fears of police encounters. These fears are real and should not be underestimated. Therapists can help these parents to talk to their adolescents about these realities, particularly when family members raise concerns in reaction to media news reports or incidents in their own communities.

LATINO CLIENTS AND FAMILIES

The terms "Latino" and "Hispanic" are U.S. terms used to describe families from a wide range of Spanish-speaking countries, cultures, and sociopolitical histories (Bernal & Shapiro, 2005; Falicov, 2005; Garcia-Preto, 2005; McGoldrick et al., 2005), including the following cultural groups: "Cubans, Chicanos, Mexicans, Puerto Ricans, Argentineans, Colombians, Dominicans, Brazilians, Guatemalans, Costa Ricans, Nicaraguans, Salvadorians, and all other nationalities that comprise South America, Central America, and the [Spanish-speaking] Caribbean" (Garcia-Preto, 2005, p. 154). Although the countries collectively known as Latin America share Spanish as their common language (with the exception of Portuguese-speaking Brazil [Korin & Petry, 2005]), many differences exist in terms of the idiomatic use of language, customs, and traditions (Falicov, 2005; Garcia-Preto, 2005), and individuals often identify themselves by their place of origin—for example, "I am Puerto Rican," or "My family is from Cuba"—rather than as "Latino" or "Hispanic."

Latino families also include individual family members who are at different points along the immigration/acculturation continuum. Although developed as a result of research conducted with an Asian American population, Lee and Mock (2005) constructed a schema of the acculturation continuum that provides a useful framework for viewing many clients and families who have immigrated to the United States. Families along this continuum are classified as: "traditional" families, "cultural conflict" families, "bicultural" families, "Americanized" families, and "interracial" families.

For Latinos and many other immigrant groups, this continuum requires modification to include the category of *undocumented* families, whose members include individuals residing in the United States illegally. Many have braved hazardous conditions in order to enter this country and live with the constant fear of discovery and deportation (Falicov, 2005, 2014). As a result of such fears, often outsiders, including family therapists or other clinicians, are viewed with great suspicion. Undocumented "families" frequently do not meet the conventional definition of a family, but rather may comprise a unit of children and adults who may or may not be biologically related living in the same home, often in very crowded conditions—it is not uncommon for 10–20 people to share a three-bedroom house or apartment. Family members may be in possession of false identification (e.g., a Social Security card, driver's license, or "green card"), to allow them to live and work in the United States. Often these underground community families only come to the attention of authorities when their children have problems in school, are arrested, or when a family member is taken to a hospital. Individuals who are not American citizens are not eligible for many federal entitlement programs, including Medicaid, Medicare, and Social Security, and some states have enacted even further restrictions, such as Proposition 187, an initiative passed in California in 1994 (later overturned) that prohibited state aid to these families (Falicov, 2005).

Much of the literature on Latino families has focused on *traditional families* whose cultural traditions and language are the most different from those of the American mainstream (Bernal & Shapiro, 2005; Falicov, 2014; Garcia-Preto, 2005). For the purposes of this chapter, the term refers to families where all members were (1) born and raised in Spanish-speaking South and Central American, and Caribbean countries; (2) still practice traditional customs; and (3) often speak primarily in Spanish. Although Lee and Mock (2005) described Asian families, many traditional Latino families also seek mental health and social service interventions only when referred by a medical practitioner; for Latinos, it is more culturally acceptable and comfortable to conceptualize psychological or emotional pain or family problems as having a medical, rather than a mental health, derivation.

Cultural conflict families either have children who were born in America or immigrated with young children more than a decade earlier, and these children grew up in America. The cultural conflict arises between acculturated children and adolescents and the parents and grandparents who spent many years in the country of origin and maintain that country's values and traditions (Lee & Mock, 2005; see also Falicov, 2014). Conflicts with adolescent girls about dating and with boys around issues such as the choice of delinquent peers and gang involvement are common. In addition, if one spouse becomes acculturated more rapidly than the other, traditional gender role expectations may also be challenged (Garcia-Preto, 2005). This cultural conflict group is the one most frequently referred by schools and child welfare departments.

Bicultural families consist of well-acculturated parents who grew up in Latin American, Central American, or Caribbean cities, who were from middle- or upper-class, educated families in their country of origin (Bernal & Shapiro, 2005; Falicov, 2005, 2014; Garcia-Preto, 2005; Vazquez, 2005). These families are often composed of parents who have professional jobs; were fluent in English before coming to the United States; and may be living in well-off urban neighborhoods or in the suburbs of the United States. They are frequently bilingual and bicultural and have begun to modify traditional cultural expectations. Lee and Mock (2005) point out that many of these families have modified the patriarchal gender roles of traditional families and now have a more egalitarian parental relationship. Some have extended family members living in the household; others, while still maintaining frequent contact with extended family members, live more as a nuclear family unit. Because of their higher socioeconomic status, many of these families do not face the challenges of poverty and basic survival that many poor immigrants experience.

In *Americanized families,* often both the children and their parents have been born and have grown up in the United States (Lee & Mock, 2005). These families may also consist of members at different points in the acculturation continuum. In some of these families, individual members do not retain their ethnic identities, and family members communicate largely in English. Many children, adolescents, and young adults in these families do not speak Spanish. These families are frequently upwardly mobile. Adolescents often report being perceived as different from their high school peers, but they have no strong cultural identity with which to identify in order to reinforce their self-esteem and pride. Many of these youth act out this sense of loss in their adolescence. Sometimes young people in these families reconnect with their culture and language during their college years.

The last category, *interracial families* (Lee & Mock, 2005), might be more appropriately termed *cross-cultural* or *cross-racial* families because some Latino individuals are "interracial" in the technical sense of the word. Their backgrounds may incorporate White European, African, and indigenous Indian races and cultures (Garcia-Preto, 2005). Cross-cultural or cross-racial families are those in which a Latino has married an individual who is not of Latino origin. Some of these families raise their children to experience the best of both cultures. Others struggle with conflicts in values, religious beliefs, language and child-rearing issues, and expectations of extended family involvement.

Language Issues

There are many traditional and cultural conflict families in which all of the adults in the household (parents, grandparents, extended family members, and newly arrived friends or boarders) speak only Spanish. Often these older relatives live in *barrios,* or neighborhoods, where everyone speaks Spanish. Inevitably, children and adolescents in traditional families become more acculturated than their parents and grandparents by virtue of their education in American schools and contact with other children in their classes. Some parents, who were fully in charge of their families in their homelands, find that they cannot adequately fulfill key aspects of their parental responsibilities because of their lack of English fluency (Garcia-Preto, 2005). Their school-aged children may be the only members of the household sufficiently fluent in English to interact with the outside world (Falicov, 2005, 2014; Garcia-Preto, 2005; Vazquez, 2005), and they are called upon by family members to shop; fill out forms and applications; handle banking; and serve as translators for their parents in stores, schools, hospitals, courts, and mental health centers. This reversal of generational roles may give older children or adolescents an excessive amount of responsibility at a young age and expose them prematurely to adult concerns (Falicov, 2005, 2014; Garcia-Preto, 2005). Having assumed adult roles during childhood, some of these adolescents then become defiant when parents later attempt to set limits and impose parental control. They also may become resentful of family responsibilities in adolescence, feeling that they have been deprived of the more carefree childhoods enjoyed by some of their American friends. These clashes of values can lead to other generational conflicts as well.

It is important that English-speaking family therapists avoid using parentified children or adolescents as translators in family sessions. This totally reverses the generational hierarchy in the family. Agencies should be pushed to hire bilingual therapists or interpreters. If this is not possible, parents can be encouraged to bring a trusted relative or friend to translate for them (see Chapter 8).

Generational Issues and Parent/Adolescent Conflicts

As just indicated, differences in the level of acculturation can lead to generational conflicts between Latino parents and their children. At no time is this more pronounced than during adolescence (Falicov, 2005, 2014; Garcia-Preto, 2005). Part of the problem for these families, particularly those from an agrarian society, is that the life stage of "adolescence" was not thought of as a time for separation and individuation but, rather, as preparation for adulthood—that is, girls were expected to marry young, and boys were expected to start contributing financially to their families. The typical North American and western European concept of "adolescent rebellion" is very new for some of these families (Falicov, 2014), and families expect children at this age to demonstrate responsibility and maturity. In addition, because of the cultural value of *respeto,* traditional families are horrified when adolescents openly disrespect their parents.

In a desperate attempt to control their adolescents' behavior, some families resort to traditional punishments that leave them open to charges of child abuse. This drama may be enacted around a family's concerns about an adolescent daughter's behavior. Traditional Latino families in the United States often get into power struggles when daughters wish to start dating at the age when their more acculturated Latino friends and those from other cultures start (Falicov, 2005, 2014; Garcia-Preto, 2005). Since it is customary for young women to be heavily chaperoned in order to protect their virginity, dating in the American sense is simply not allowed, and a daughter's desire to engage in what is very ordinary behavior in this country may be perceived by traditional Latino parents as being "wild." This issue can become a major source of contention in the high school years when adolescents, not permitted to date, feel "left out" of participation in important activities, such as attending proms and other events. Many of these adolescents keep their dating and other social interactions secret from their families.

Parents, even those who are bicultural and more acculturated, may object to cross-cultural (particularly interracial) dating. This can be particularly problematic when the family lives in a community with few other Latino adolescents. More acculturated parents may also be faced with rebellious teens who resent the parents' lack of cultural identification. Some of these youth may begin to feel that they do not belong anywhere—they are different from their White peers and some Latino peers may reject them because they do not speak Spanish and are not aware of cultural practices.

Religion, Spirituality, and Native Healers in Latino Communities

In common with African American families, many Latinos have strong religious and spiritual beliefs. The Roman Catholic Church still has considerable influence in much of Latin America (Bernal & Shapiro, 2005;

Falicov, 2005, 2014; Garcia-Preto, 2005). In many Latino communities in the United States, Catholic churches are served by Latino or bilingual priests, incorporate Latino music, and are an integral part of community life. These churches often serve as a support system for families, particularly for newly arriving immigrants. Pentecostal, Evangelical, and Charismatic sects have experienced a tremendous growth in popularity among Latinos in the United States. Latino families may be drawn to Evangelical churches, particularly when some local Catholic churches in the United States conduct services only in English or these families do not feel welcomed.

Recent Latino immigrants to the United States are sometimes attracted to small storefront churches, particularly those of the Pentecostal sect. The ministers of these churches are commonly from the homeland of the congregants, speak fluent Spanish, and offer music alive with Latin rhythms. Other members of the church are seen as *la familia de la iglesia* (the "church family"). These churches often have a great deal in common with small neighborhood African American churches. Catholic priests and Pentecostal ministers alike are often beloved and respected in their communities and can be important resources for families and support or entry points for community interventions (see Chapter 8).

Clinicians should be aware that many Latino families may have other strong "spiritual" beliefs that are not necessarily connected to their formal religion or church affiliation. For example, some families from Puerto Rico and from other Latino Caribbean nations may believe in *espiritismo* (the spirit world). *Espiritistas* or "spiritists" may be sought out by members of the community for help with death, dying, and other loss issues, physical and mental illness, emotional problems, relationship issues, and parenting (Garcia-Preto, 2005). *Espiritistas* are also sought for "faith healing" by those who believe that illness is caused by evil spirits.

Santería, a blend of the African Yoruba religion and Catholicism, is practiced by some Cubans, Dominicans, and other Latinos in the United States (Bernal & Shapiro, 2005). Historically, *Santería* evolved when African slaves, forbidden to practice their own religious beliefs by Catholic slave masters, gave the Yoruba gods the names of Catholic saints. In Cuba (Bernal & Shapiro, 2005), this religion is known as *lucumi,* and in Brazil, it is called *macumba.* Clinicians should also be aware that natural herbs sold at local stores called *botanicas* are often utilized by Latinos when a family member is ill because of a belief in their healing properties. For example, families that have emigrated from Mexico will often seek the help of a local *curandero,* or herbalist, to recommend remedies when they are sick. For families that believe deeply in these practices, *espiritistas* and *santeros* (practitioners of *santería*) are respected as healers and may serve as important resources if they are consulted by family therapists, with the permission of the family (Bernal & Shapiro, 2005; Garcia-Preto, 2005).

Gender Issues

Family therapists, even Latino therapists, often struggle with the gender expectations in more traditional Latino families. Gender roles are changing for many Latinos in this country. Thirty years ago, traditional male gender roles were encompassed by the term *machismo,* which was associated with "sexual prowess and power over women, expressed in romanticism and a jealous guarding of a fiancée or wife or in premarital or extramarital relationships" (Comas-Díaz & Griffith, 1988, p. 208). More recently, Garcia-Preto (2005) has indicated that "the cultural expectations of machismo and marianismo [see description below] are in transition, both here and in Puerto Rico [and other Latin American countries], and that socioeconomic factors strongly influence the process. Machismo, which emphasizes self-respect and responsibility for protecting and providing for the family, continues to have a positive connotation except when it leads to possessive demands and an expectation that all decisions be made by the man" (p. 246). Family therapists with a different concept of gender equality are cautioned not to lose sight of the positive aspects of the male role in these families—as provider and protector—by focusing solely on patriarchal domination.

Some Latina women are socialized in the tradition of *marianismo,* based on emulating the model of the Virgin Mary (Garcia-Preto, 2005). In very traditional Latino families, women may be expected to be self-sacrificing and to remain virgins until they are married. This expectation has changed in some of the more acculturated families, though the role of motherhood and bearing children, particularly sons, is highly valued. These gender dynamics may cause problems in traditional families because in the United States immigrant women often seem to find employment more quickly than men. This reverses the traditional gender power balance, frequently leads to conflict, and, in extreme cases, can result in domestic violence (Garcia-Preto, 2005).

Traditional gender role expectations can also lead to cross-generational conflicts in some Latino families. Because of the high value placed on maintaining a girl's virginity, the practice in some traditional families in Latin America has been for girls to marry at a young age, often to older men (particularly in more rural areas). This practice can cause problems in the United States where marriage is not legal for girls in their early teen years, and a nonmarital intimate relationship with an older man or adolescent may be considered statutory rape according to some state laws. An especially problematic situation arises when a girl becomes pregnant in this country and is under extreme pressure by her family to marry the baby's father. If a therapist finds it difficult to work with family members who are pressuring a pregnant daughter to marry, it is important to seek supervision from a Latino clinician who understands traditional Latino cultural practices. These practices may be more common in very traditional families than in more acculturated Latino families.

Another way in which traditional gender roles can clash with mainstream American expectations relates to education, particularly for teenage girls. In some poor traditional families, higher education is not seen as important for young women because of the expectation that they will marry and become mothers at an early age. In addition, a traditional or newly immigrated Latino family may encourage an adolescent daughter to drop out of school to take care of the home and younger siblings while both parents are working. This role may be perceived as crucial for the family's survival. A family's need for their adolescent daughter to care for children at home often creates conflicts with school authorities.

Intense conflict can also occur when acculturated women marry traditional men (Garcia-Preto, 2005). A Latina who was born in this country, or who has spent the majority of her life in the United States, may have expectations of more egalitarian gender roles and the sharing of child rearing and other household responsibilities. These expectations may be in direct conflict with the more patriarchal expectations of her more traditional husband.

Family Difficulties Created by the Immigration Process

It is important to note that Puerto Ricans are citizens of the United States and are free to travel back and forth and to work in this country. Latino immigrants from all other countries are forced to deal with the United States's strict immigration laws. One common scenario for Latino immigrant families has been the experience of parents who are forced to leave children behind in the care of extended family members in their country of origin, and come to the United States on a travel visa or enter the country illegally. Sometimes parents enter together, but in some circumstances, a woman may precede her husband or partner because, as indicated earlier, women often find employment sooner than men do in the United States. The first priority is often to find employment and someone to sponsor the newly arrived immigrant, usually a family member or an employer, for a "green card" which will allow this individual to live and work in the United States. After obtaining a green card, a person can "sponsor" or bring other family members to the

United States. Unfortunately, this process can take 6–7 years (or more). At the end of this time period, even though it is now a legal possibility to bring the family to the United States, it may not be possible financially. More time may elapse before parents are in the position to bring over each child in the family.

Children left behind at a young age may well be teenagers before they are reunited with parents. Parents may remember a toddler and be abruptly confronted with a rebellious adolescent. Moreover, additional children may be born to the parents while they are living in the United States, and these children, who have been living with their parents for their entire lives, may have a closer or different relationship with the parents than children who have spent a good deal of their childhood with extended family in their country of origin. When family therapists work with such a family in treatment or when school officials encounter such a family in school, the therapists are often initially unaware of this complicated history.

Many immigrant parents harbor a great deal of guilt about the length of their separation from their children and other family members during the 6- to 7-year "green card" process. Their inability to leave the United States and visit their country of origin is particularly difficult when their children or other family members are ill, or when a member has died and they cannot attend the funeral. The following case example illustrates many of these points.

Case Example

The Martinez family consisted of Juan (age 16), Angelica (age 10), and their mother, Lourdes (age 32). The family was referred for treatment by Juan's probation officer. Juan was charged by the court with break-ing and entering after he ran away from home and broke into an office building in order to have a warm, safe place to sleep. He was sentenced to probation, with the strong threat of being sent to a juvenile detention facility if he violated his probation.

FAMILY HISTORY

The family was from Nicaragua. Lourdes had become pregnant with Juan as an adolescent and had given birth to him at age 16. Given the cultural belief in virginity until marriage (*marianismo*), her family was furious and even more so when they discovered that Juan's father was already married. Once she gave birth, her parents sent her to live with a cousin in New Jersey while they raised her baby in Nicaragua. Through her cousin, who was in the United States illegally, Lourdes was able to find employment as a live-in babysitter. This family later sponsored her for her "green card."

Every payday, Lourdes sent money back to her mother in Nicaragua for the care of her child. She often sent barrels containing food and gifts, and she always sent presents for Christmas and birthdays.

In the last year of her "green card" process, Lourdes became involved with a man who had immigrated from Colombia. Her babysitting job required her to stay with her employer's family during the week, but during weekends she lived with her boyfriend. This man was abusive to her, and she soon found out that he was employed by a drug cartel and sold drugs. She ended her relationship with him after discovering that she was pregnant. Her second child, Angelica, was born just as she completed her "green card" process. Lourdes continued her live-in job and was allowed to keep her child with her. She bonded closely with her baby but felt very lost without Juan.

When the child she was caring for reached an age where he no longer needed a live-in babysitter, her employer let her go. The family she subsequently found work with would not permit her to bring Angelica to live with her. When Lourdes flew home to Nicaragua to leave Angelica with her mother, she saw Juan for the first time in almost 9 years. She told the family therapist that the years she spent waiting for the green card process to be completed were very difficult for her. Not only had she missed 9 years of her son's life, she had not been able to see her father before he died or attend his funeral.

Because of Lourdes's hard work and frugality, within 4 years of receiving her green card she was able to afford her own apartment and to bring both children to live with her. By this time, Juan was 13 and Angelica was 7. Lourdes was quickly overwhelmed by the demands of working full time and raising two children. She connected well with Angelica, as they had bonded when Angelica lived with her for a number of years after her birth. Her relationship with Juan, however, was problematic from the start.

Whereas his sister was bright and cute, quickly made friends, and began learning English in school, Juan experienced many more adjustment difficulties. Angelica was close to her mother, but Juan longed for his grandmother, Julia, whom he considered his "Mama." He grieved for her loss, became increasingly depressed and angry, and withdrew from his mother and his sister.

Juan also experienced many difficulties in junior high school. He had attended a rural school in Nicaragua and had never been exposed to a challenging curriculum. In addition, he was having a great deal of trouble learning English. He began acting out and had behavior problems both at home and in school. He failed his first year of school in this country and was forced to repeat the grade. He was transferred to a school with an English as a Second Language (ESL) program. He was much more successful in this new school than he had been in his previous school, helped by a committed teacher with whom he developed a good relationship, and was promoted to high school.

His transition to high school was very difficult. He was sent to a large, impersonal school without an ESL program. He missed his teacher from junior high school who was able to give him the individual attention he needed to do well. He became more and more angry. He was acting out at home, and in school he started to hang out with a group of other at-risk boys and got involved in an increasing number of fights.

By the time of the referral, the relationship between Juan and his mother was fraught with difficulty. He refused to accept discipline or limit setting from her, telling her that she was not his "real mother" and that she did not know him. Lourdes felt extremely guilty about having left him behind and was overwhelmed by his behavior.

TREATMENT PROCESS

The family therapist engaged both Lourdes and Juan. He found that he had to do this individually at first because they were so deeply alienated from each other. Gradually, he was able to have a number of home-based family sessions that included Lourdes, Juan, and Angelica.

One weekend Juan "destroyed" the couch in the living room and broke a number of lamps after an angry argument with his mother. In a session soon after this incident, Juan angrily accused his mother of not loving him and only caring about Angelica. The therapist moved Juan and Lourdes as close together as they could tolerate and asked her to talk to Juan about this argument. She sobbed as she told Juan that she did love him very much, but that he seemed like a stranger whom she did not understand. Juan in turn told his mother that she also seemed like a stranger to him. Lourdes was able to say that she wanted desperately to love him, to help him, and to be close to him. She also told him that she felt very guilty about having left him behind in Nicaragua.

The therapist asked Juan whether he had ever heard the story of why his mother left him with his grandparents. Both mother and son seemed surprised by this question and reported that they had never talked about it. With some help from the therapist, Lourdes shared with Juan that she had been very young when she had him (in fact, his current age of 16), and because her family had been so embarrassed about her pregnancy and so furious with her, they had sent her to live with a cousin in the United States. Mother and son cried while she described how hard it had been for her to leave him and how she had cried every night for many years. Juan seemed surprised by this revelation. They then held each other for a brief moment as tears spilled down both of their faces. This session proved a turning point in their relationship.

The therapist then worked closely with Lourdes on effective parenting skills. Her guilt was so overwhelming that she was unable to adhere to any limits she set for Juan. When he misbehaved, she would tell him he could not leave the home for a month, only to relent by the next day and revoke his punishment. His probation officer, a White male, was very supportive of Juan and encouraged his interest in sports. Lourdes, buoyed by the officer's interest in Juan, then invited him to a session so that she could ask for his help in working with Juan. To her surprise, he offered to "take him out sometimes to play baseball," and eventually he became a male role model for Juan.

Juan's performance in school remained problematic, however. He still had trouble with English and was failing many courses. The family therapist explained to Lourdes the process of requesting psychological testing and a Child Study Team evaluation. At first, Lourdes was very resistant to the suggestion that she meet with school personnel. In fact, the school had persistently requested meetings with her to discuss Juan's difficulties, but she was too intimidated by her lack of English fluency and the immense size of the school to respond to any of the letters sent by the school.

Understanding Lourdes's discomfort over her lack of English fluency, the family therapist asked her whether she had a friend or relative whom she could ask to serve as an interpreter at the meeting. She responded that she had a friend who would do it. The family therapist and this friend accompanied Lourdes to a meeting at the school. Lourdes was able to request the evaluation, and the therapist requested that Juan be given the psychological tests in Spanish and that a bilingual examiner be provided. The therapist also requested that the school consider transferring Juan to a smaller alternative school that had an ESL program. After the testing was complete, the Child Study Team agreed to this request.

After this change, things began to improve for Juan. He was placed in a smaller class in the new school, and the ESL teacher worked with him on his language skills. He was also away from the acting-out peer group that he had been drawn to in his former school. His behavior improved at home as Lourdes became more consistent in her parenting. At this point, his probation officer advocated for the end of his probation. When this request was granted, the probation officer continued to be a male figure in his life, taking him to baseball games. Treatment with this family was completed, and the family therapist checked in once a month for a "booster" session for the first 2 months.

CONCLUSION

Clinicians, school personnel, and mentors are encouraged to use their knowledge of cultural, racial, and socioeconomic issues as a lens through which to view their clients and families. In order to avoid stereotyping, this lens must be adjusted for each new client and family. Clinicians and mentors must bear in mind that there is considerable diversity among poor families, Black families, Latino and other immigrant families, and must carefully assess each family's needs and resources.

CHAPTER 4

Working with Kinship Care Families

Many at-risk adolescents are living in kinship care families in which they are being raised by a relative other than their birth parent. Because of stringent licensing requirements, many African American and Latino families cannot qualify to become formal kinship care providers. Thus, they do not receive stipends or financial compensation and so are living at or below the poverty level. As a result, many of these kinship care arrangements are made informally. Although these informal systems of care have a strong cultural foundation, functioning for generations in these families, they may not come to the attention of outside authorities such as child protective services.

This chapter explores many important aspects of kinship care. The first section discusses the cultural roots of kinship care and the reasons children are removed from their birth parents, including parental substance abuse and incarceration. Given the particular problems faced by caregivers of these children, we describe these challenges in greater detail. We then discuss different forms of care for children outside of their birth families, including licensed formal foster care, licensed formal kinship care, and informal kinship care, as well as the related legal issues of permanency planning, family reunification, termination of parental rights, adoption, and legal guardianship. The benefits and challenges of kinship care are then explored, with a particular focus on the unique challenges faced by grandparents and other older kinship caregivers, as they provide the greatest amount of kinship care. The special role of family systems interventions such as home-based family therapy, multiple family groups, and support groups for the kinship caregivers are also discussed. Finally, through a case example, we illustrate the complexities of home-based family therapy with a kinship care family involving a substance-abusing parent.

EXTENDED FAMILY INVOLVEMENT AND KINSHIP CARE

African American Families

Boyd-Franklin (2003) and Hines and Boyd-Franklin (2005) have described the central role of extended family members for many African American families. In these informal arrangements, child rearing is shared among a wide range of relatives not necessarily living in the same household. These family members may include older siblings, grandparents, aunts, uncles, or cousins. Nonblood relatives are also considered members of the extended family, including godparents, close family friends, neighbors, and church family members.

This informal system of kinship care has functioned for generations within the African American community, particularly among poor families. During difficult times, it is often customary for parents to utilize this underground network of care in which extended family members "take in" children and absorb them into their household. When this pattern persists for a longer period of time, these children may be informally adopted by these caregivers. Given that these nonblood kin may be an important source of help and support for their child and adolescent clients, it is essential that clinicians, family therapists, school counselors, teachers, school authorities, and child protective service agencies are aware of these informal arrangements. Despite their prevalence, these informal arrangements often remain unknown unless a crisis occurs.

Latino Families

As indicated in Chapter 3, Latino or Hispanic families encompass many different cultural groups and ethnicities. One common feature across these various groups is the value placed on family and extended family involvement. While living in their native countries, many immigrant Latino clients grew up interacting daily with extended family members, which might include parents, grandparents, siblings, aunts, uncles, and cousins. Nonblood relatives and close friends are also often considered part of the extended family, including *compadres* (godparents) and *hijos de crianza* (children who are formally or informally adopted). Garcia-Preto (2005), described an extensive informal kinship system among Latino families.

Compadrazco (godparenthood) is a system of ritual kinship with binding mutual obligations for economic assistance, encouragement, and even personal correction. *Hijos de crianza* refers to the practice of transferring children from one nuclear family to another within the extended system in times of crisis. The relatives assume responsibility, as if the children were their own, and do not view the practice as neglectful (Garcia-Preto, 2005, pp. 162–163). Although some recent immigrants can seek support from family members living in the United States, many must adapt to and mourn the loss of the supportive extended family network left behind in their country of origin. For those who have lived in the United States for a while, particularly when living in large immigrant communities, nonblood *compadres,* close friends, and neighbors may substitute for blood relatives. These extended family members become a part of an informal kinship system, as described earlier, and may take in children during times of crisis.

REASONS FOR PLACEMENT OF CHILDREN IN KINSHIP CARE

Children may be placed in kinship care, whether formal or informal, for many reasons. Like licensed foster care, formal kinship care often results from a report to child protective services with regard to physical, sexual, or emotional abuse; neglect; parental substance abuse, including placement in a substance abuse rehabilitation program; parental incarceration; parental hospitalization for mental health or medical reasons; parent(s) with a serious mental illness; or homelessness (Font, 2015; Gleeson et al., 2009). Informal kinship care, which accounts for the majority of children living with relatives, often arises from similar concerns (Gleeson, 2007). Many of these difficult realities may coexist simultaneously and are often interconnected. For example, parents with serious mental illness may abuse drugs to self-medicate, and sell drugs to provide for their family, which may lead to incarceration. In addition, economic realities, particularly during periods of recession, may lead to unemployment, foreclosure, or eviction. Resulting homelessness may leave families dependent on relatives to provide a place to live or to take in children while the distressed parents "get back on their feet." A parent who must relocate to another state to find employment might leave his or her children in the care of relatives or close friends until they are able to set up a household and reunite the family. Kinship care may also result from the death or serious illness of birth parents. Among these many overlapping issues, one of the most common and problematic involves parents who abuse or are addicted to drugs and/or alcohol.

Parental Substance Abuse and Kinship Care

Parental substance abuse is the most common reason for the separation of children from a biological parent and placement with a relative

(Gleeson, 2007; Kroll, 2007; National AIA Resource Center, 2004). Substance abuse was a factor in as many as 80% of kinship placements in the United States (Kroll, 2007). Many researchers have found that the disorganized and chaotic lifestyle of many substance-abusing parents can have an even greater negative impact on their children than the substance use itself (Kroll, 2007). For example, neglect of children due to parental substance use is often a major factor leading to placement with kinship caregivers (Howe, 2005; Walker & Glasgow, 2005). These parents may be very inconsistent in the care of their children, often leaving them alone for long periods of time and/or leaving them with many different, randomly selected caregivers (Howe, 2005), in a "revolving door" scenario. When substance-abusing parents also engage in domestic violence and/or have mental health problems, the home environment may be even more chaotic, exposing children to additional dangers, including physical, sexual, and emotional abuse (Woodcock & Sheppard, 2002).

Grandparents whose adult children are substance abusers face complicated issues. Upon learning of their adult children's substance abuse, some may express shock and surprise, and others may be in denial and choose to ignore the signs. Some grandparents may be among the many caregivers included in the revolving door scenario, stepping in whenever their adult children encounter problems related to their substance abuse. When these grandparents become kinship caregivers, their responses and level of prior involvement often complicate parenting of their grandchildren.

Incarcerated Parents with Substance Abuse Problems

The number of incarcerated women, particularly those of color, has increased significantly in the last 20 years in the United States (Engstrom, 2008). Many of these incarcerated women also have a history of substance abuse, as well as mental health problems, including posttraumatic stress disorder (PTSD) (Green, Miranda, Daroowalla, & Siddique, 2005), which left them unable to care for their children prior to their incarceration. As a result, other family members, particularly grandmothers, who already have had to assume responsibility for the children for many years prior, continue to care for them during their mother's incarceration (Mumola, 2000). These grandparents were listed as caregivers for their children by 45–53% of incarcerated mothers (Mumola, 2000). The realities for these grandparents are complex. Simmons and Dye (2003) reported that more than 85% of grandmothers providing kinship care for their grandchildren were between the ages of 40 and 69. Many, however, were older and presented with age-related physical and medical concerns, but neglected them owing to the overwhelming demands of raising multiple grandchildren. Although many of these grandparents report satisfaction, pride, and enjoyment in caring for a grandchild (Ruiz, 2004), when a large number of grandchildren are involved, they are more likely to report many strains and demands (Kropf & Yoon, 2006). Among these strains are coping with the incarceration and substance abuse of the parent, as well as the demands of raising grandchildren who may have experienced trauma (Engstrom, 2008).

Impact of Parental Substance Abuse on Children and Insecure Attachment

Some scholars and researchers have utilized attachment theory to explain the complex problems with emotional connection that these children develop as a result of parental substance abuse. For substance abusers, drugs and alcohol function as their primary attachment, a substitution that can seriously hinder their ability to form attachment relationships with their children and other family members (Flores, 2001; Kroll & Taylor, 2003). In addition, parents who are using drugs or alcohol may be psychologically unavailable and/or physically absent for periods of time, inconsistent in their emotional connection, and less responsive to their children's physical and emotional needs, welfare, and well-being. This disorganized lifestyle and resulting lack of consistent emotional and physical support can lead to problematic early attachment, insecure attachment, and even an attachment disorder in some children (Howe, 2005; Kroll, 2007).

Children of substance-abusing parents are often left feeling as if they are alone in the world (Howe, 2005; Kroll, 2007). They may feel that they are helpless and vulnerable, and that they have no control over their lives. To them, the world is a frightening and troubled place, where they cannot rely on their parents for stability and love. Children often blame themselves when parents reject them or are angry or abusive toward them, and as a result, may view themselves as unlovable (Kroll, 2007). It is no wonder that many of these children present at our clinics and schools with attentional difficulties, inability to focus on school-work, poor cognitive development, and difficulties with social relation-ships (Kroll, 2007).

Children often experience conflicting emotions when they are removed from the parental home and placed in kinship care with rela-tives or close family friends. On the one hand, they may feel relieved to be removed from an environment of neglect, abuse, chaos, violence, and/or unpredictability. On the other hand, they may feel guilt, concern, and excessive worry or anxiety about their biological parents.

In addition, family conflicts may arise when parental children are placed in kinship care (Kroll, 2007). Inconsistent parenting in their original households has caused these children, at a very young age, to assume the responsibility of primary caregiver for both their siblings and their substance-abusing parent (Boyd-Franklin, 2003). These children may have not been monitored by their parents and may be accustomed to a greater degree of freedom than they are allowed in their kinship placement. Despite the burden that the responsibility entails, parental children have a powerful role in the family system and may resist allowing adults to assume the role of decision maker once placed in kinship care.

Extended Family Dynamics with Children of a Substance-Abusing Parent

Many grandparents and other kinship caregivers offer to care for children of substance-abusing parents out of love, cultural values, and the desire to keep these children out of foster care and the child welfare system. However, they are often unprepared for the behavioral and emotional problems that some children may manifest as a result of their prior chaotic home environment. Depending on the degree of abuse or neglect, children may feel grief, loss, trauma, and fear of abandonment resulting from insecure or disorganized attachment—making it very difficult for them to love or attach to another family member (Kroll, 2007). When these children respond to their caregivers by rejecting them, pushing them away, and refusing to trust their offer of love and caring, caregivers may understandably feel shocked. They may also feel guilty about their own feelings of hurt, anger, and resentment when faced with this unexpected reality. It may take a very long time and a great deal of patience and dedication for a caregiver to establish trust and form a strong attachment bond with these children.

An insecurely attached child or adolescent can have an extremely negative impact on household dynamics when he or she enters a family placement. The impact is further complicated when kinship caregivers take in sibling groups. In this common scenario, each child may present with distinct attachment difficulties and problems. For example, the caregiver may have a good relationship with other children, but one insecurely attached child may pull for reactions from the caregiver that are not helpful to the child. This child may become the family scapegoat and the focus of a treatment referral (Minuchin, 1974; Nichols, 2011).

Therapists, clinicians, social workers, counselors, school counselors, and family case workers can play an important role in helping these grandparents and other family caregivers to understand these attachment-related dynamics. These professionals would benefit from adopting a family systems perspective and from joining with the kinship caregivers, parent(s), and children or adolescents alike, in order to help them through the difficult process of connecting or reconnecting. The following observation by Kroll (2007) may be very helpful to these caregivers and the professionals who work with them: "Just because there is a biological link, it does not mean that this phenomenon will not occur and [caregivers] may need considerable support and skilled help in order to enable the child to re-attach in a safe way" (p. 90).

DIFFERENT FORMS OF CARE FOR CHILDREN AND ADOLESCENTS OUTSIDE OF THEIR BIRTH FAMILIES

Approximately 5% of children and adolescents in the United States each year are estimated to reside in homes other than those of their original nuclear families (Font, 2015). These children are typically placed in one of three different forms of care: licensed formal foster care, licensed formal kinship care, or informal kinship care.

Licensed Formal Foster Care

When the removal from birth parents is at the direction of state or local child protection services, the majority of these children are placed with nonrelatives in licensed formal foster care placements. Pursuant to Title IV-E of the Social Security Act, nonrelative licensed foster parents, under the supervision of a child welfare agency, receive payments ranging from $226 to $869 per month for each foster child placed in their care (Ayon, Aisenberg, & Cimino, 2012). There is considerable variability across the states in the amount provided.

Licensed Formal Kinship Care

Approximately one-quarter of children in foster care are placed with relatives in licensed formal kinship care placements. Formal kinship care placements gradually increased in many states in the 1980s and 1990s (Boots & Geen, 1999), and in 1997, the Adoption and Safe Families Act (ASFA) officially recognized kinship care as a form of foster placement (Geen & Berrick, 2002). However, the states were given authority to determine their own guidelines regarding who qualifies as kin, the amount of monetary allowances for formal licensed kinship care providers, and licensure regulations—leading to disparities across states (Boots & Geen, 1999). In 2002, subsequent federal legislation eliminated these disparities by making licensure requirements for kinship care providers more consistent with those for nonkinship care providers. These caregivers receive "the same oversight and compensation as a foster parent caring for non-kin children" (National AIA Resource Center, 2004, p. 1).

Barriers to Providing Formal Kinship Care

Although the 2002 legislation addressed the lack of uniformity for licensure, it imposed increasingly restrictive requirements on formal kinship care providers for receiving funding, furthering the disparate impact experienced by many ethnic minority and poor kinship care families (Geen & Berrick, 2002; National AIA Resource Center, 2004). Many researchers have indicated that child welfare system licensing requirements devised with White middle-class families in mind do not serve people of color appropriately (Ayon et al., 2012). Many poor kinship caregivers are unable to meet the stringent regulations for formal foster care licensure (National AIA Resource Center, 2004). For example, caregivers with homes too small to meet licensure requirements may encounter a Catch-22: they may not be able to afford a larger living space until they receive compensation for providing foster care.

In addition, some caregivers may encounter obstacles when everyone in their household is required to provide valid photo identification and submit to a background check and fingerprint testing (Ayon et al., 2012). Disqualification for licensure may result if any involvement with the law or the juvenile justice authorities is found, or if anyone in their home is undocumented (i.e., does not have legal immigration status). Ayon et al. (2012) noted that 62% of Latino children in the United States live in households with a mixed status; that is, some family members have legal status, and others are undocumented. Families with undocumented members may avoid applying for licensure out of fear that a family member(s) will be deported, particularly in states that require child welfare workers to report any undocumented residents (Ayon et al., 2012). Ayon et al. have argued that the immigration status of the child or the child's family members should not prevent that child from receiving necessary services.

Although it is common in both African American and Latino families to include important nonblood relatives, states often do not recognize these relationships as kin, disqualifying them for licensure. States vary considerably in how they interpret "kinship," and many limit it to marriage, blood relatives, or relationships resulting from formal adoption (Ayon et al., 2012). Leos-Urbel, Bess, and Geen (2000) found that only 21 states accept a broader definition of kinship that includes nonblood relatives. For Latino families, not only would such an inclusive interpretation be consistent with cultural values, but it would increase the likelihood that these children would maintain a connection to their parents and extended families, as well as retain their own language.

To qualify as a formal licensed kinship care provider, caregivers often need to navigate an extensive child welfare bureaucracy, which can be challenging for caregivers who are not well educated. Leos-Urbel, Bess, and Geen (2002) have characterized the licensing process as lengthy and difficult to understand, with child welfare workers often providing little help and information about the process. The consequences to kinship care families of not understanding the child welfare system may include longer waits for services (Suleiman Gonzalez, 2004), prevention of the identification of appropriate kinship care placements, and problems in permanency planning (Gomez, Cardoso, & Thompson, 2009).

These consequences are far more likely when there are language barriers, as is often the case with Latino families, preventing them from acquiring the necessary information to successfully navigate the child welfare system. Although Title VI of the Civil Rights Act of 1964 required states to provide culturally competent service delivery (Ayon et al., 2012), language barriers continue to persist. Community-based organizations, mental health clinics, and social service agencies can be critically important in providing culturally competent and linguistically appropriate services to these families (Cordero-Guzmán, 2005). Such agencies that employ staff who are bilingual or who come from similar cultures can provide a sense of comfort and trust, thereby facilitating engagement with these families. Home-based family therapy services are another valuable avenue for reaching important family members who may feel uncomfortable visiting a clinic or agency.

Ayon et al. (2012) have indicated that there is a critical need for culturally appropriate services in Spanish, stating that

> the number of Latino children involved with the child welfare system has more than doubled in the past 15 years, currently representing 21 percent of known cases of child maltreatment (U.S. Department of Health and Human Services, Administration on Children, Youth and Families, HHS, ACYF, 1997, 2009). (p. 91)

Ayon et al. (2012) have also reported that there are 86,581 Latino children in foster care, many of whom have family members willing to provide kinship care but are prevented by the presence of undocumented members, language barriers, and the complex bureaucracy.

The imbalance of power that exists between these families and the child welfare bureaucracy can lead to a sense of disempowerment and frustration (Chipman, Wells, & Johnson, 2002). Power imbalances may be particularly stark with Latino families, who may feel further impeded by language barriers (Ayon et al., 2012). Ironically, a similar sense of disempowerment is sometimes experienced by child welfare workers, who are aware of the systemic inequities in treatment, but feel powerless to change the complex bureaucracy. This overall imbalance of power can affect the ability of families to advocate effectively for their needs.

Too often families feel that the ability to make decisions is taken away from them by child welfare workers or by the system. As a result, many African American and immigrant Latino families, who may already have a "healthy cultural suspicion" of government agencies (Boyd-Franklin, 2003), may resort to withholding information or keeping secrets about the realities of their lives in a desperate attempt to maintain a sense of control. Chipman et al. (2002) have argued that the early involvement of all parties in decision making may lead to more agreement, giving families more control in the process. In order for child welfare workers to increase their ability to facilitate planning meetings involving the child, biological parents, and potential kinship caregivers early in the process, their training in the home-based family systems approaches discussed in this book is recommended.

Informal Kinship Care

Given the myriad barriers to formal kinship care, it is not surprising that informal kinship care is much more common. The National Survey of American Families (NSAF) indicated that the number of "informal kinship care placements is approximately one and a half times greater than the number of formalized kin care placements (Ehrle & Geen, 2002; Ehrle, Geen, & Clark, 2001)" (National AIA Resource Center, 2004, p. 1). Although experts estimate that "over 2 million children" are in informal kinship care with relatives (Font, 2015, p. 20; Gleeson et al., 2009), an exact number is difficult to determine, as these arrangements are outside of the jurisdiction of the child welfare system (National AIA Resource Center, 2004).

Many of these families often care for multiple children (including siblings) but receive no compensation or support from the state, such as funds for clothing, child health insurance, and referrals for medical, mental health, and school-related services (Geen & Berrick, 2002). Although these caregivers may be eligible for stipends under Temporary Assistance to Needy Families (TANF), these payments—sometimes as little as $66 per month—are significantly less than formal foster care payments (Leos-Urbel et al., 2002; National AIA Resource Center, 2004). Poor African American and Latino families who may not even qualify for this minimal assistance are forced to subsist at or below the poverty level, placing additional burdens on those who, consistent with their cultural values, take in the children of relatives. Given the significant burdens faced by these well-meaning caregivers, changes in public policy are needed so that informal kinship caregivers, who are often from lower socioeconomic backgrounds, are eligible to receive compensation. In recent years, another option—legal guardianship—has become another possible choice for families providing kinship care (National AIA Resource Center, 2004).

PERMANENCY PLANNING: REUNIFICATION VERSUS TERMINATION OF PARENTAL RIGHTS

Prior to the enactment of the Adoption and Safe Families Act (ASFA), which prioritized kinship care placements, children were often automatically placed in nonrelative foster care without any consideration for family or extended family members who might take them in. In addition, these children often moved from one foster home to the next throughout their childhood until they aged out of foster care at 18. As a result, many of these children lost contact with their birth families and extended families. ASFA addressed this problem by emphasizing permanency planning, with the goal of establishing as early as possible whether reunification with birth parents was viable. If reunification did not occur within approximately 2 years from initial placement, child protection services were authorized to request the "termination of parental rights" by the courts, making the child eligible for adoption (Boyd-Franklin, 2003). The intent of the law was to allow children to be adopted at a young enough age so that they could experience a more stable home and family environment early on.

During the 2-year period between placement and the determination to terminate parental rights, the child welfare system was mandated to first offer services to parents to help them prepare for reunification. In most cases, parents were required to attend family therapy—often home-based treatment including the child (escorted by the child welfare worker) and parent(s). Many parents were often also mandated to take parenting or parent training classes. When children were removed because of abuse, parents were subject to additional requirements such as therapy, anger management, or, in the case of drug or alcohol involvement, attendance in a rehabilitation program.

Once parents fulfilled court mandates, they could petition the court for reunification. If it was clear that reunification was unlikely given the child's best interests, child protective services would petition the courts for a termination of parental rights. These cases, however, are often complex and not straightforward, particularly when substance abuse is involved, as the cycle of relapse and drug rehabilitation may be repeated many times over many years.

Adoption and Legal Guardianship

Federal policy favoring permanency planning, and the resulting pressure to terminate parental rights, presented many problems for kinship caregivers. Many of these ethnic minority families had been providing informal kinship care for generations without the loss of parental rights, and the concept of the termination of parental rights contradicted their cultural beliefs (Boyd-Franklin, 2003). Research has shown that kinship care providers were less likely to pursue formal adoption because it required termination of parental rights (Gleeson, 2007). Although very willing to raise these children to adulthood, many adamantly refused to adopt them and usurp parental rights. In addition, some kinship caregivers felt pressured by child welfare workers who threatened to remove the children from their home and place them in nonkinship foster care unless they adopted the children themselves (Gleeson, 2007).

Due to changes in federal and state policies resulting from these issues regarding termination of parental rights, another viable option, legal guardianship, has emerged for some kinship care providers. When the kinship caregiver becomes the legal guardian, parental rights are not terminated, but the caregiver is granted authority to act as the parent in certain areas, including school issues, medical care, and therapy (Gleeson, 2007). In some states, such as Illinois, legal guardians can become licensed and receive subsidies (Gleeson, 2007). Testa and Rolock (2001) have indicated that subsidizing guardianship with financial compensation has made it a more feasible alternative for some kinship families. Legal guardianship provides protection for children in situations where birth parents demand return of the children despite being unable to care for them, owing to their active substance abuse and/or serious mental illness. Many kinship families, however, feel conflicted about legal guardianship because it may run counter to cultural values. It may also be confusing to children when a relative has been granted legal authority to act on their behalf instead of the parent (National AIA Resource Center, 2004).

BENEFITS OF KINSHIP CARE

Kinship placements allow African American and Latino children and children from other ethnic groups an opportunity to preserve their ethnic identity and maintain biological family connections, especially with their parents (Kroll, 2007). Siblings are more likely to be placed together in kinship care, which can be arranged more quickly in an emergency, especially when there is more than one child in the family (Winokur, Rozen, Thompson, Green, & Valentine, 2005). Children in kinship care

are less likely to reenter the foster care system (Cuddeback, 2004) and remain in longer-term placements with fewer moves to new homes. Kinship care, therefore, provides greater stability, consistency, and permanency of care (Gleeson, 2007).

Some child protective service workers have expressed concerns that older kinship care providers may engage in harsh disciplinary practices, such as spanking or corporal punishment (Gleeson, 2007). However, research has shown that children in kinship care are as protected (Kroll, 2007) and as safe as children placed in other forms of foster care (Gleeson, 2007). Additionally, the National Survey of Child and Adolescent Well-Being found that only "a very small percentage of children in care are exposed to harsh discipline, and no differences were detected between kin and nonrelated foster care" (Gleeson, 2007, p. 9).

CHALLENGES OF KINSHIP CARE

Kinship care providers can face many challenges, particularly when the arrangements are informal and child protective services are not involved. Among these challenges are conflicts with birth parents, especially those who abuse drugs or alcohol and/or suffer with serious mental illness (Gleeson, 2007; Kroll, 2007). Many birth parents, despite their problems, love their children and want to fulfill their role as parents. Initially, they may feel relieved that a kinship caregiver is willing to take in their children when they have been arrested, incarcerated, or admitted to substance abuse rehabilitation or psychiatric inpatient treatment. However, they may have close relationships with their children, and over time they may feel guilty or conflicted about a relative raising them. When conflict arises between the birth parent and the kinship caregiver, each side may criticize the other in order to gain the children's allegiance, leaving the children in the middle of an angry battle. As with divorced families, children caught in these triangles can experience loyalty conflicts, leading to acting-out behavior, and creating challenges for the kinship caregiver. Adolescents are at particularly high risk, often resorting to abusing substances and running away in these situations.

Another challenge for kinship caregivers arises over the issue of visitation. In informal kinship care, without monitoring by outside child protective services, relatives often find it stressful to monitor visits between biological parents and their children (Gleeson, 2007). In formal kinship care situations or in nonrelative foster care, the child welfare workers can often arrange in-office visitation for birth parents and children, thereby avoiding some of the friction that may arise between kinship caregivers and birth parents. In cases of serious parental abuse, birth parent visitation may be forbidden by court order or child protective services. However, some kinship caregivers may feel torn, and so they secretly allow visitation in violation of the mandate.

Challenges for Grandparents and Other Older Kinship Caregivers

Grandparents provide a great deal of the kinship care in this country and, along with other kinship relatives and supportive friends, play a significant role in the lives of children who can no longer live with their birth parents. Motivated by a sense of obligation to their family members, love for their children and grandchildren, cultural values, and the desire to keep their grandchildren in the family, grandmothers are statistically more likely to serve as kinship caregivers than grandfathers and other relatives (Gleeson, 2007). Many of these kinship caregivers are able to provide for their grandchildren in ways their parents could not, by offering emotional support and love as well as a more consistent living environment in which they can be more closely monitored. Additionally, these kinship caregivers often provide protection for those children whose parents have had a chaotic lifestyle, preventing the dangerous and harmful circumstances that are often a consequence of neglectful and/or abusive parenting (Kroll, 2007).

Grandparents and older caregivers such as aunts and uncles often experience conflictual feelings about caring for the next generation. While they love their grandchildren or nieces and nephews, and do not want to see them in foster care, many may have looked forward to a more restful or enjoyable retirement. After years of hard work and sacrifice, they may have anticipated that their child-rearing years were behind them. They may perceive the birth parents as abandoning their responsibilities, resulting in feelings of resentment at the sacrifice involved in raising young children. This resentment can increase the conflict between grandparents and their adult children.

Relationship difficulties with their adult children are common when grandparents are kinship caregivers (Gleeson, 2007). Although many of these parents, particularly those with substance abuse problems, feel relieved that grandparents are raising their child(ren), they often experience guilt over neglecting their parental responsibilities (Kroll, 2007). In many families, grandparents have provided a stable refuge for their grandchildren for many years. Sometimes a "revolving door" scenario develops, however, in which parents attempt to regain custody of their children after each repeated instance of substance abuse treatment.

It is important for mental health, child welfare, and social service providers to recognize that these older kinship caregivers, particularly grandmothers, may have many additional stressors owing to competing demands and responsibilities. Along with caring for their grandchildren, some may still work full time, have other grandchildren and/or adult children living in their homes, or provide care for aging parents and/or other older relatives. Given these stressors and the age-related challenges older adults often face, it is not surprising that many experience declining health and functioning (Engstrom, 2008; Kropf & Yoon, 2006; Ruiz, 2004; Simmons & Dye, 2003). According to Gleeson (2007), grandparents who take on a parenting role with their grandchildren face particular challenges. As older adults, many already suffer from poor health, and the demands of caretaking often cause them to neglect their own health. Additionally, when more than one grandchild is involved, grandparents report poorer health and greater parenting challenges and stress (Gleeson, 2007). Children and adolescents may feel both relieved about being in a stable home and very upset about being removed from their parents, causing them to act out. Adolescents' acting-out behaviors can result in increased distress for their grandparents, including depression and feelings of being overwhelmed. Some employed caregivers are forced to resign from their jobs in order to care for multiple grandchildren in their homes.

The burden of raising children and adolescents can lead to a decrease in social support, due to serious marital problems or the loss of intimate relationships with adults (Gleeson, 2007). In addition, caregivers often do not have time to connect with their friends, church networks, and the like and may become very isolated. Social support is an extremely important need for these caregivers, as it can help reduce mental health issues such as depression and anxiety. Support groups provided by social services, community agencies, churches or other faith-based organizations, and/or mental health clinics can be very helpful to these caregivers. (See Support Groups for Kinship Caregivers below.)

As indicated in Chapter 3, spirituality and/or church involvement is an important support for many African Americans and Latinos raising their grandchildren. Their spiritual beliefs impact their resilience, survival, and coping skills. Some rely heavily on prayer and their personal relationship with God to sustain them through difficult times. In response to the needs of these families, some churches have established support groups for these senior caregivers, as well as provide transportation to church events, and, in some cases, home visits or respite care (Boyd-Franklin, 2003). In addition, some churches provide other services caregivers can utilize for help and support in raising children, such as day care centers, schools, after-school programs, tutoring and mentoring programs, vacation Bible school, and Sunday school.

CHALLENGES IN PROVIDING MENTAL
HEALTH SERVICES TO KINSHIP CARE FAMILIES

Although children in kinship care often have more positive mental health outcomes than children in formal foster care (Cuddleback, 2004), compared to the overall population of children in the United States, they have more emotional and behavioral problems (Smithgall, Yang, & Weiner, 2013). In addition, studies have shown that children in kinship care have many unmet mental health needs (Ehrle & Geen, 2002; Villagrana, 2010). Kinship caregivers are also at risk for mental health issues, and their mental health needs also often go unmet. The degree of unmet needs varies depending on race, socioeconomic status, geographic area, insurance, and household composition (Smithgall et al., 2013). Numerous studies have documented that kinship caregivers are more likely to be "older, single, less educated, unemployed, and of lower socioeconomic status" (Smithgall et al., 2013, p. 465). In addition, many kinship caregivers report health and mental health conditions such as "hypertension, arthritis, cardiac conditions, diabetes, asthma, and clinical depression" (Smithgall et al., 2013, p. 465). Many, however, do not receive the care they need: kinship caregivers receive "fewer services [including mental health services], supports, and caseworker visits" (p. 465).

A healthy cultural suspicion of outside systems, particularly in African American and other ethnic minority communities, may also contribute to the lack of utilization of these services, as kinship care providers often serve as gatekeepers when seeking mental health services for children (Burns et al., 2004). Informal kinship caregivers may also be hesitant to seek help for fear that if the degree of substance abuse, abuse, or neglect by the birth parents becomes known by the authorities, the children will be removed from the home (Smithgall et al., 2013). As a result, some kinship caregivers may feel compelled to hide the degree of parental substance abuse from outsiders, and, in some cases, from other family members and the children as well.

Children and adolescents who cause higher degrees of caregiver stress have been shown to receive more mental health services (Villagrana, 2010). Not surprisingly, children who internalize their stress, such as those who are depressed or anxious, often do not receive mental health services to the same degree as children who have externalizing or acting-out problems (Smithgall et al., 2013). Boys with externalizing behaviors are more likely to be referred than girls (Smithgall et al., 2013). In addition, children who experience physical or sexual abuse are more likely to receive mental health services than children who are victims of parental neglect (Burns et al., 2004).

Researchers have emphasized the importance of actively engaging families in therapy and of reaching out to engage all family members

(Schneiderman & Villagrana, 2010). Because many of these families are reluctant to seek treatment, it is important that clinicians be well trained in cultural competence, establishing therapeutic rapport and joining, and that they also be willing to provide outreach services and home-based family therapy.

THE VALUE OF HOME-BASED FAMILY THERAPY WITH KINSHIP CARE FAMILIES

At-risk children and adolescents living with family or extended family members often have complex living situations. They may live with their grandmother, but other family members may also reside in the home. For example, a child's mother who is abusing drugs and/or alcohol may come to stay with the family for periods of time, despite living elsewhere. In addition, other adult children and their families may move back into the grandmother's home during times of separation or divorce, finan-cial strain, loss of employment, eviction, homelessness, substance abuse rehabilitation programs, incarceration, and other forms of family disrup-tion. Home-based family therapy allows the therapist to experience the family's living situation firsthand, so as to better understand the chang-ing constellation of family members in the home. In addition, for many families, especially those with older kinship caregivers, home-based fam-ily sessions remove the overwhelming demands and expenses involved in attending an appointment, such as transporting the entire family or paying for child care, if younger children are not included in treatment.

Despite the many benefits of home-based family therapy, many eth-nic minority families may have a "healthy cultural suspicion" of therapy (Boyd-Franklin, 2003), making them hesitant to allow outsiders to enter their homes. It is important for therapists to be respectful of these feel-ings and to join or establish therapeutic rapport before proceeding to address the "business" of the session. This may be particularly true in families with a substance-abusing family member. Some of these families may deny the substance abuse in order to keep it a secret from children in the family, as well as outsiders. This may result in the "elephant in the room" scenario in which no one in the family openly acknowledges the substance abuse and other related behaviors.

THE VALUE OF GROUP INTERVENTIONS
Multiple Family Groups

Multiple family groups are another intervention that has proved help-ful in providing direct therapeutic support for grandmothers and other kinship caregivers. Kinship caregivers who understand the demands and pressures facing their families are in an ideal position to provide support for one other. Numerous research studies have documented the benefits gained by grandmothers who receive support through multiple family groups and other forms of support groups. One study of multiple family groups included a true multigenerational constellation involving grandmothers, mothers, and children (Dressel & Barnhill, 1994). Following the intervention, the grandmothers demonstrated gains in self-care and a decrease in symptoms of depression. In addition, they showed improvement in their relationships with their adult daughters and the grandchildren in their care. Engstrom (2008) described the use of multiple family groups as a support for caregiving grandmothers raising grandchildren whose mothers had substance abuse problems and were incarcerated. These groups can be particularly helpful in providing support for women who are reentering the community after their release from prison (Engstrom, 2008); this transitional period can be stressful for both the mothers and grandmothers who have been caring for their children during their incarceration. It can also be a difficult adjustment for the children, who may experience role confusion regarding parenting. Multiple family groups can address these intergenerational concerns and support positive outcomes for all family members (Engstrom, 2008).

Boyd-Franklin, Steiner, and Boland (1995) described a multiple family group that was designed for kinship caregivers raising children and adolescents whose parents had died of AIDS. Many of their parents had contracted HIV through intravenous drug use and needle sharing, and some of the children had been infected perinatally with the HIV virus. Caregiving grandmothers, grieving and mourning the loss of their adult children, were left to raise these children, some of whom might be very sick.

A psychology intern working in a community clinic initiated a support group for kinship caregivers who were raising their grandchildren after their adult children's death. This group was conducted while the HIV-infected grandchildren received treatment in the pediatric AIDS clinic, a process that could last 2 hours or more. When many of the uninfected, usually older, children and adolescent siblings in these kinship families exhibited significant amounts of conduct-disordered behavior both at home and at school, a community mental health center became involved. In order to address the issues of the conduct-disordered siblings, whose acting-out behavior was often found to have coincided with the mother's death, it was decided to combine siblings and caregivers in a multiple family group. By including this multigenerational element in the support group, adolescents and grandmothers were able to discuss their overwhelming feelings of grief together, sometimes for the first time.

Support Groups for Kinship Caregivers

When multiple family groups are not possible because of the family's circumstances (e.g., incarcerated mothers unable to participate), support groups for grandmothers and other kinship caregivers can be very helpful. When planning these groups, therapists and counselors should keep in mind the challenges these families face. Many older caregivers have health concerns and limited financial resources, so public transportation to and from a group may be difficult, interfering with participation. To facilitate transportation, a number of programs provide a van or medical transportation services. Alternatively, travel vouchers for the cost of public transportation can be provided. In addition, many of these caregivers also have young children in their care. As such, it can be helpful if child care services can be provided on-site to enable caregivers to relax and participate in the group, knowing their children are well cared for. Food can also be an important component of these groups, contributing to a more relaxed atmosphere.

We have also found that it is helpful to confirm the appointment by phone approximately two days before the meeting, as is done with many doctor's offices. Location is also extremely important. Because of healthy cultural suspicion, some African American kinship caregivers may be hesitant to come into a clinic, a mental health center, or a hospital. We have had success in locating these groups in convenient settings such as in the school that the children attend or in other local schools. Schools are convenient because they are familiar to the families and are often located in their communities. Principals, school social workers, psychologists, and guidance counselors should reach out to grandmothers and other caregivers and involve them in the planning process prior to starting a group. Daytime meetings may be preferable for caregivers who do not work outside the home.

It has also been helpful to locate group meetings in a local church or community center. As indicated earlier, in African American and Latino communities, churches can often serve a social service function and provide support for these families. To meet this common need, some African American churches have initiated support groups for kinship caregivers within their congregations and from the surrounding communities (Boyd-Franklin, 2003; Boyd-Franklin & Lockwood, 1999, 2009).

Schools, churches, and other community settings may be less threatening for those who attach a cultural stigma to obtaining therapy. Using the term "support groups" rather than "therapy groups" may also help counteract stigma.

THE VALUE OF A MULTISYSTEMS APPROACH

In Chapters 1 and 6, we advocate for a Multisystems Model (Boyd-Franklin, 2003) in working with families of at-risk adolescents. This systemic approach is essential for treating kinship care families (Ziminski, 2007) because these children, whether they are in formal or informal kinship care, are often involved with many systems, including child protective services, the courts, schools, substance abuse rehabilitation programs, the police, medical services, and the mental health system. It is therefore important for mental health providers to be aware of the various systems impacting the family; understand the relevant federal and state laws; and when necessary, contact or meet with representatives of other systems with the client or family members.

In addition, many conflicts between birth parents and kinship care-givers can be addressed, negotiated, and resolved in family therapy sessions. Therefore, it is important that providers adopt a family systems framework and intervene with key family members when appropriate. In addition, multisystemic case conferences to discuss options and to problem-solve may be very helpful when making difficult permanency planning decisions. These case conferences may include child protective service workers, therapists, birth parents, kinship caregivers, legal guardians for the children and adolescents, and, in some cases, lawyers. Similarly, when children in kinship care act out in school, which often occurs because of the pressures and conflicts that they experience, it may be helpful for therapists and family members and children, particularly at-risk adolescents, to meet with school staff to discuss plans and services. The following case illustrates the use of the Multisystems Model in providing a home-based family therapy intervention to a kinship care family.

Kinship Care Case Example

Michelle, a 15-year-old African American adolescent, was referred to a home-based family therapy program by child protective services. Michelle lived with her maternal grandmother, Mrs. B. (age 70), and her younger sister, Louise (age 6). The school social worker had been seeing her for individual counseling because of her fights with other students leading to repeated school suspensions, angry outbursts toward teachers, and poor academic performance, putting her at risk for failure. The school social worker was also concerned about the conflicts and tensions in the family. Michelle's mother, Mary (age 30), who had a history of substance abuse, recently completed a yearlong incarceration for drug dealing and was currently in a court-ordered drug rehabilitation program for heroin abuse. The child protective services worker informed the family therapist that if Mary did not successfully complete the drug rehabilitation program, termination of parental rights would be recommended.

Because of her drug abuse, Mary's parenting had been inconsistent, and Michelle's home life had been chaotic. Throughout her childhood and early adolescence, Michelle had been a "parental child" to her younger sister and, at times, a caretaker for her mother. On numerous occasions, when her mother was unable to care for Michelle and her sister, they had lived with her grandmother. All of these arrangements were made informally, without the supervision of child protective services, until Mary was arrested for drug dealing, when child protective services were contacted and the children were removed from their mother's home and placed with Mrs. B.

Although Mrs. B. had been working at the time of the children's placement, she was laid off shortly thereafter. Because Mrs. B. was not a licensed kinship care provider, she received no funding from child protective services. As a result, the family was living in poverty, supported only by her social security payments. When the family therapist visited their home, Mrs. B. reported that she loved her grandchildren and did not want to see them placed in foster care, but that she was overwhelmed with the responsibility of caring for them. In addition, Mrs. B. was overweight and had diabetes and high blood pressure. It had been Mrs. B.'s expectation that she would be retiring by age 67, and she resented that her daughter's substance abuse and incarceration had placed parenting demands on her at this late stage in her life. She reported that she had no trouble with Louise but that Michelle "thought that she was grown." Michelle had assumed parental responsibility within her mother's home and would not listen to her grandmother or follow her rules.

In an individual session with Michelle at her school, the therapist learned that she was a very bright, articulate adolescent who was very angry about her life circumstances. In particular, she was very angry about her mother's incarceration, which left her feeling abandoned. She and her sister talked with Mary by phone only about twice a year during her incarceration. When Michelle was younger, she had been close with her grandmother and enjoyed the times that she and her sister had lived with her. Now, since her mother's incarceration, she felt that her grandmother was always yelling at her and forcing her to do chores at home.

Michelle's mother had been involved in drug dealing both to support her drug habit and to provide for her family. Michelle reported that when she lived with her mother, she was able to dress nicely and get her hair done regularly. Since she moved in with her grandmother, she had "no money" and was forced to wear old clothes to school. She hated school, reporting that it was "boring" and school work was "too hard," so she could not "keep up." Also, although she had her own group of friends, some of the other adolescents were "mean," making fun of her because of the way she dressed. She felt that she had no choice but to fight, to "put them in their place."

The first family session took place in the living room of the grandmother's apartment with Michelle, her younger sister Louise, and Mrs. B. Mrs. B reported that Michelle thought she was "grown" and wanted to stay out late with her friends, but Mrs. B. expected her in the house by 6 P.M. on school nights in order to eat dinner and do her homework at a reasonable time. Michelle reported that when she lived with her mother, she was allowed to come home whenever she wanted, and she resented her grandmother trying to tell her what to do.

The therapist asked what occurred when Michelle stayed out late. Mrs. B. said that when Michelle stayed out late on Thursday night, coming home at 11 P.M., her grandmother yelled at her and asked her why she was late. Michelle became angry, yelled back, and stormed off to her bedroom. During the family session, Michelle and her grandmother were able to talk about their concerns. At the end of the session, Mrs. B. told Michelle that she would always love her no matter what happened. Michelle cried and told her grandmother that although she did not like her restrictions, she was very grateful to her for taking them into her home.

During the next few home-based sessions, the therapist did some problem solving with Michelle and her grandmother about the curfew time during the week. Mrs. B. expressed her concerns that Michelle was not getting her homework done and that she was in danger of being left back in school. She told Michelle that they would need to agree on a time that would allow her to get her homework done and also get to bed at a reasonable time. Michelle proposed 10:00 P.M., indicating that all of her friends came home much later, but Mrs. B. was clear that she would not allow such a late curfew on a weeknight. The therapist explored whether Mrs. B. would consider a later time on the weekend if Michelle came home on time and completed her homework during the week. After some negotiation, they agreed: Michelle would come home by 7:00 P.M. on weekdays and complete her homework before bedtime. Mrs. B. agreed that Michelle would then be allowed to stay out with her friends until 10:00 P.M. on Saturday night as a reward for completing her homework and keeping a weeknight curfew. Mrs. B. agreed with this arrangement as long as Michelle would inform her of where she would be and who she would be with on those Saturday nights.

The relationship between Michelle and Mrs. B. began to improve, enabling the family therapist to then begin to address the school fights and suspensions. In a very emotional session, Michelle explained that it was well known in the community and among her classmates that her mother had been arrested for drug dealing and that she did it to support her heroin habit. She also explained that her classmates teased her about her old clothes and how bad her hair always looked because she could not afford to get it done. Mrs. B. was devastated and told Michelle how badly she felt that since she had lost her job, they were living on only her social security. The therapist helped them to problem-solve the situation. Mrs. B. reported that she was considering getting a part-time job but was unsure whether she could trust Michelle to be responsible while she was at work. Michelle volunteered that one of their neighbors had offered to pay her to babysit her children on weekends. The therapist praised them for coming up with good ideas and encouraged them to pursue their plans. In addition, she offered to help Mrs. B. to apply for TANF funds, an extra $250 per month for each child, which would help with their dire financial situation.

A month later when the therapist arrived at their home, Michelle opened the door with a big smile on her face. She and her grandmother had both earned some money. Her grandmother was working part-time at a friend's beauty salon, and her friend had done Michelle's hair. Michelle reported that she had also earned some money babysitting. With their new combined earnings, Mrs. B. was able to take Michelle shopping for a few new clothes for school. Mrs. B. was also pleased that the babysitting now occupied Michelle's time on the weekends, and as a result, she was coming home earlier.

Although Michelle's report card in March showed improvement, she was still in danger of failing algebra. Utilizing a multisystems approach, the therapist asked Mrs. B. to contact the school social worker to arrange a meeting that would include the therapist, Michelle, and Mrs. B. During the meeting, the school social worker first praised Michelle for the improvement in her grades, then explored Michelle's issues with algebra. Michelle explained that she had always had difficulty with math in school. The school social worker suggested that Michelle enroll in an in-school program in which college students tutored and mentored high school students. Michelle agreed reluctantly but expressed concern that her classmates would tease her. The social worker therefore helped her arrange to participate in the program after school, so that she could get the help without her peers knowing.

By May, Michelle's grades in algebra had begun to improve. During a home-based session, the therapist praised both Michelle and Mrs. B. for their ability to cooperate and their willingness to seek the help they needed. Later that month, however, disaster struck, as the family learned that Mary had left the drug rehab program and had returned to the streets, abusing drugs. On numerous occasions she unexpectedly visited their home under the influence and engaged in angry arguments with Mrs. B. and Michelle. The therapist attempted to include Mary in several home-based family sessions. Although she participated briefly in one session, she stormed out of the house and refused to attend future sessions. During the last week of May, Mrs. B. called the therapist, crying hysterically: Mary had died of a heroin overdose.

During an emergency in-home session with Mrs. B., Michelle, and Louise, the therapist witnessed their clear devastation and grief over Mary's death. Mrs. B. and Michelle both felt extremely guilty, as they had said some angry things to Mary during her last unexpected visit, and the therapist helped them to express and understand their complex and conflictual feelings. Mrs. B. asked the therapist if she would attend Mary's funeral with the family. Although initially conflicted about whether to accept the invitation, the therapist ultimately decided to attend the funeral to support the family. During and after the funeral, it became clear that the therapist's relationship with Mrs. B., Michelle, and Louise had become stronger because of her support.

Family therapy sessions over the next two months focused on their grief and loss. During those sessions, Michelle and Louise shared numerous painful memories of abandonment by their mother from earlier in their childhood. They expressed how relieved they were when their grandmother would intervene and take them to her house. They also admitted feeling guilty about that relief, but Mrs. B. and the therapist helped normalize their feelings.

Although painful for the whole family, this time taken to process their loss led to greater closeness and a stronger bond among them. During a meeting at the school at the end of June, school administrators revealed that Michelle had passed all of her courses and had not been suspended for fighting in months. Michelle also decided she would continue participating in the tutoring and mentoring program during the following school year. The family completed therapy at the end of August. During a follow-up session three months later, the therapist learned that the family was doing well and that Michelle and Louise were both performing well in school.

CHAPTER 5

Multigenerational Patterns in Families of At-Risk Adolescents

Families of at-risk adolescents referred for home-based family therapy or problems in school often present with a history of many serious issues, such as homelessness; medical crises; sexual abuse, physical abuse, and/or neglect; drug and alcohol abuse; suicide attempts; and arrest or incarceration. Often, these same issues were present in the lives of the parents, grandparents, and other relatives of the families being treated. In a unique study comparing 17 families with multiple problems through a Bowenian perspective, Hurst, Sawatzky, and Pare (1996) documented the multigenerational nature of problems such as physical, emotional, and sexual abuse; drug and alcohol abuse; mental illness and suicidal ideation; out-of-home foster placement; and serious teenage acting out. Treating these families often proves daunting for even the most experienced therapists, as very little change seems to occur over time, despite the array of services offered to these families through schools, government agencies, child protective services, social welfare departments, and other agencies.

In addition to the multigenerational aspect, another common feature of some of these families is that they may have become habituated to functioning in crisis mode. One function of a crisis is that it often precipitates actions from others to help the at-risk adolescents and the family (Boyd-Franklin & Bry, 2000; Minuchin, 1974; Nichols, 2011). When behaviors, often those of the "identified patient" in a family, lead to interventions, the family's feelings of powerlessness may be replaced by relief as individuals such as therapists, school personnel, and child

welfare workers, or members of other systems, such as the police department or courts, take control (Boyd-Franklin & Bry, 2000; Kagan, 2017;
Kagan & Schlossberg, 1989).

There are families, however, that seem predisposed to crisis, not in
order to be "rescued" by others, but because the crisis serves a function
in its own right. Researchers and clinical scholars (Kagan, 2012; Kagan
& Schlossberg, 1989), exploring multigenerational histories of trauma—
that is, violence, abuse, and neglect—suggested that crisis, rather than a
state to be avoided by such troubled families, often served a purpose for
them by providing a counterpoint to the hopelessness and despair that
otherwise surrounded them. As described by Kagan and Schlossberg
(1989) in their classic book *Families in Perpetual Crisis*: "Living in a
crisis oriented family is like riding a roller coaster 24 hours/day; terrify-
ing, energizing and addicting" (pp. 2–3).

MULTIGENERATIONAL CRISES AND "TOXIC SECRETS"

Crises brought on by such events as death, serious illness, hospitalization,
loss of a job, or divorce cannot be avoided even in the most functional
families. What distinguishes these events in the lives of crisis-oriented
families of some at-risk adolescents is that there is no progression toward
recovery—recovery is the unknown, crisis is the familiar (Kagan, 2017;
Kagan & Schlossberg, 1989). For example, any family experiencing a
crisis may feel acute grief; families that operate in continual crisis mode,
however, have become inured to loss and block the further pain.

Thus, crises become a pattern for some families and the method by
which they deal with painful experiences, memories, and past traumas.
Buried pain may rise to the surface on certain occasions. For some at-
risk youth and their families, a particularly painful event, loss, or trauma
that is left unresolved can trigger a reaction (often an unconscious one)
as the time of year or anniversary of the occurrence approaches, that is,
an "anniversary reaction" (Boyd-Franklin et al., 2013; Pollack, 1970).
These traumatic memories can then lead to repetitive acting out in an
attempt to master the pain of the earlier experience or to avoid it. Many
family members report being "in crisis" or feeling "out of control" during these periods.

This chapter discusses six serious issues in the families of at-risk
adolescents that often have their roots in a family's multigenerational
patterns (Boyd-Franklin, 2003; Imber-Black, 1993): (1) teenage pregnancy, (2) domestic violence and physical abuse, (3) child sexual abuse,
(4) juvenile delinquency and criminal behavior, (5) gang involvement,
and (6) alcohol or drug abuse. These multigenerational patterns may
be secrets to some family members. Paradoxically, secrets are often

"known," albeit on an unconscious level in some families, although one or more generations may attempt to avoid the pain of the earlier trauma by never discussing it openly. An at-risk adolescent's acting out in response to a trauma may be a repetition of how a parent responded to a similar trauma as a child. Ironically, the action most feared by a family—open discussion of the secret—is often the very thing that leads to a decrease in repetitive crises.

EMPHASIZING STRENGTHS AND RESILIENCE IN TREATMENT

At-risk adolescents and their families often present first with their problems. When starting treatment with a family having a history of complicated multigenerational crises, even experienced therapists can feel overwhelmed. One normal instinct in the face of such long-term entrenched difficulties that seemingly have never been addressed is to blame the families for their problems. Therefore, it is important for therapists to actively assess the strengths as well as the problems of the families they treat. Supervisors, particularly those who are working with relatively new therapists, must be prepared to help clinicians with this difficult process. Walsh, in her books *Normal Family Processes* (2012) and *Strengthening Family Resilience* (2016), has pointed out that there has been a tendency to overpathologize the types of families discussed in this chapter based on a standard of functioning that is not realistic for any family—that is, "the erroneous assumption that healthy families are problem free" (p. ix).

Many families with a multigenerational history of trauma have developed personal and cultural survival and coping skills that have helped them to rebound from crises and hold their families together. Our challenge as therapists is to recognize their strengths and resilience—qualities that can be found even in the families discussed in this chapter in the midst of complicated, multigenerational crises—and to validate them (Boyd-Franklin, 2003; Boyd-Franklin et al., 2013; Walsh, 2016). Walsh (2016) defines resilience as "the ability to withstand and rebound from crisis and prolonged adversity" (p. vi). Resilience theory formed the basis of the strengths-based approach that each of the therapists incorporated with the troubled families discussed in this chapter.

TEENAGE PREGNANCY: A MULTIGENERATIONAL PATTERN

Teenage pregnancy may be a multigenerational pattern in some families of at-risk adolescents, particularly in inner-city areas. Although this is clearly not true of all families in which a teenage pregnancy occurs, it is very relevant for some of these families. In these cases, there may be a family history, going back to a great-grandmother, of a young woman becoming pregnant at about the age of 15 or 16. If a mother and a grandmother both became pregnant in their teenage years, they often become hypervigilant and anxious as their adolescent daughter/granddaughter approaches this stage. If this issue is not discussed, addressed, and resolved, it can be "acted out" both by the family and by the adolescent (Boyd-Franklin, 2003; Boyd-Franklin & Bry, 2000; Tatum, Moseley, Boyd-Franklin, & Herzog 1995).

Family members act out this anxiety in one of two ways: (1) they become overly strict, restrictive, and punitive toward the adolescent at the onset of puberty in order to prevent pregnancy; or (2) they seem to give up control of the adolescent girl, treat her as if she is "grown," and wait for the inevitable pregnancy to occur. Unfortunately, either of these scenarios can set in motion a self-fulfilling prophecy in which still another generation is caught in the trap of early pregnancy and parenting.

The following case example* of teenage pregnancy illustrates the multigenerational family transmission process (Bowen, 1978; Nichols, 2011).

Case Example

Sharon Smith, a 17-year-old at-risk African American adolescent, was referred for home-based family therapy during her last trimester of pregnancy. A genogram or family tree was constructed with the family. (See the Multisystems Model case example in Chapter 8 for an example of a genogram.) At the time of referral, Sharon was living with her maternal grandparents, Bob (54) and Margaret Smith (51), together with other extended family members, in an inner-city apartment. Prior to her pregnancy and for the first 5 months of her pregnancy, she had lived with her mother, Susan Smith (33); Susan's boyfriend, Fred (24); and her half-sister, Dawn (12), in a nearby town. Conflict between Sharon and her mother had become so intense that she had moved to her grandmother's apartment, as she had at various other difficult times in her life. The grandmother was a powerful figure who dominated the lives of many generations of her family. The grandfather was severely disabled and uninvolved with Sharon's care and with the subsequent therapy (Boyd-Franklin & Bry, 2000).

Although Sharon was enrolled in an alternative educational program, her attendance had been inconsistent, both because of her unstable living situation and medical issues related to her pregnancy. This

---

*Sections of this case are adapted from Tatum et al. (1995). Copyright © 1995 by ZERO TO THREE. Adapted by permission.

pregnancy was Sharon's third. At age 14 she had had an elective abortion, and at 16 she had given birth to a stillborn baby at 6 months' gestation. Her current pregnancy was considered high risk because of her health history and toxemia. The father of Sharon's baby, Chris (age 20), was still involved with Sharon, although he was disliked by both her mother and her grandmother and was consistently discouraged from seeing Sharon or from being involved with his child.

The intergenerational themes regarding adolescent parenting and role confusion were immediately evident in this family. Sharon's mother had also been a teenage parent—Susan had given birth to Sharon at 16. Susan had wanted to terminate her pregnancy with Sharon, but her mother had discouraged this option and had been very involved in Sharon's care for the early years of her life. Thus, Sharon had initially been cared for primarily by her grandmother while her mother finished school and worked. Although Sharon lived with her mother once Susan was financially able to establish her own household, Sharon had frequently retreated to her grandmother's home in times of family conflict.

Treatment During Pregnancy

The first home-based session included two cotherapists, Sharon, Mrs. Smith, and a cousin who was emotionally supportive of Sharon. Sharon was often intimidated by her grandmother, an extremely talkative and forceful individual. In this first session, Sharon and her grandmother agreed that there were many conflicts in the family and that it would be helpful to meet with the therapists once each week to discuss family problems and to prepare for the infant's arrival. Sharon was very nervous, afraid that she would lose another baby. The grandmother was able to share that she had had several miscarriages herself and understood Sharon's concern. Thus, from the first session, the therapists facilitated more open and affect-laden communication between Sharon and her grandmother.

Sharon agreed to allow the therapists to refer her to a high-risk prenatal program and to assist her in keeping her appointments there. For the next few months, the treatment had two functions. The first was to help Sharon and her family understand and resolve some of their recurring conflicts so that a more stable and supportive environment could be established for Sharon and her baby. The second function was to ensure that Sharon received the specialized prenatal care she needed. The focus of the present discussion is on the family therapy, which addressed the first function of treatment. However, it should be understood that the therapists' efforts to support Sharon's medical care were viewed so positively by both Sharon and her family that these efforts were critical in developing the trust needed to do the family therapy.

In the first weeks of treatment, which primarily involved Sharon and her grandmother, Mrs. Smith, some of the patterns and difficulties in this family became apparent. Sharon's mother, though invited, failed to come to any sessions, demonstrating her reluctance to meet with her mother and daughter. Not surprisingly, Mrs. Smith, accustomed to telling her family what to do and how to behave, dominated the sessions, barely allowing Sharon a chance to talk. Mrs. Smith did not know how to listen. One of the main foci of her discourse was extensive criticism of Sharon's boyfriend. Mrs. Smith had "no use" for Chris. She accused him of not being able or willing to support Sharon. She talked of how the situation reminded her of Susan's pregnancy with Sharon. This opinion alerted the therapists to an intergenerational or multigenerational family transmission process: Mrs. Smith had had "no use" for Sharon's father, either. Sharon acknowledged never knowing her father and having no idea where he was now. With feeling, she said that she wanted her child to have a father, and so she wanted to keep Chris in her life.

In the second month of treatment, the therapists conducted more home-based family therapy sessions. Sharon and her grandmother began to acknowledge somewhat improved communication. Mrs. Smith was beginning to listen to Sharon, although she still insisted that Sharon did not listen to her—which really meant that Sharon did not always do what Mrs. Smith wanted her to do. For a few sessions, one therapist talked with Mrs. Smith while the other talked alone with Sharon. This strategy gave each an opportunity to tell her own story fully and was particularly helpful for Sharon, who began to talk more about her mother. It was clear by now that it was difficult for Sharon to say positive things about her mother in front of her grandmother because the two women sometimes competed for the role of chief parent.

Over the next few sessions, Sharon continued to share that she had recently had some positive contact with her mother and wished to repair that relationship. Although Susan still did not attend therapy sessions, she and Sharon saw each other more often and with less accompanying conflict. However, Sharon told of being uncomfortable with her mother's present boyfriend, who was in his early 20s. The issue of her mother's relationships with men still troubled Sharon greatly.

By the end of the third month of treatment, Sharon was ready to deliver her baby and was planning to move back in with her mother after the birth. Although she and her grandmother were much more able to talk and listen to each other, there was some continuing conflict, especially over Chris. Sharon's mother had managed to avoid joining the treatment except in regard to practical issues, such as planning medical appointments. Finally, in early January, Sharon delivered a healthy full-term baby girl, Christine, and returned home to her mother's apartment.

Sharon Becomes a Mother

Living with Susan, Sharon, and Christine were Sharon's 12-year-old half-sister, Dawn, and Susan's 24-year-old boyfriend, Fred. Although sessions continued at Susan's apartment, Susan herself was seldom there. Despite efforts to accommodate her work schedule, Susan continued to be reluctant to join the treatment.

As in the past, conflict erupted in the living situation, and Sharon again returned to her grandmother's home. For the next few months of treatment, Sharon alternated between these two residences, with her mother caring for the baby when Sharon needed a break. Both her mother and her grandmother still objected to Chris. Sharon wanted to be her child's primary caretaker and did not want to relinquish the care of Christine to either her mother or her grandmother, but with these two strong women so firmly present in her life, Sharon felt she was losing control of her baby. Finding a balance between taking advantage of the support these two offered with regard to the baby's care and maintaining her own role as a mother became a focus of treatment, and Sharon, who was now close to 18 years of age, began to consider setting up her own household with Christine.

Although much of the therapy during this interim period was carried out with Sharon alone, the focus of the work was on intergenerational family patterns. These patterns included women relinquishing their roles as mothers to their own mothers and women expelling male figures from relationships with their young children. Sharon, who was still involved with Chris, began to acknowledge that there were some problems with the relationship, primarily concerning her doubts about his sense of responsibility. During this period, Sharon was working on her GED while attending the alternative educational program, but she felt that Chris was not as strongly motivated as she to finish his education, nor was he employed. She wanted to continue to give him a chance and to encourage him to get serious about his education and job training. The positive aspects of the relationship (he treated her respectfully and was an active presence in their child's life) outweighed the negative. Sharon and Chris began to consider moving in together with their daughter so that they could be independent from Sharon's mother and grandmother.

A Crisis

A period of crisis finally brought all the family issues into clearer focus for everyone. After a call from Mrs. Smith reporting great conflict in her home over Sharon and Chris, an emergency session was held. Mrs.

Smith shared that she felt the current situation with Sharon and Chris was causing her to reexperience what she had gone through with her daughter. Mrs. Smith was reliving the anger and hurt she had undergone when her daughter then, as Sharon now, would not "listen" to her and continued in relationships with men who were "dogs." The therapist pointed out to Mrs. Smith that this was an example of the intergenerational projection process regarding men.

As a result of Mrs. Smith's conflicts with Chris, Sharon and Christine had once again moved in with her mother, Susan. As Susan began to feel more stress caring for her daughter and her granddaughter, she finally agreed to participate in the family sessions. A few sessions still included Mrs. Smith, but most involved Susan with her two daughters, Sharon and Dawn. It was interesting that Mrs. Smith's continued conflictual relationship with her daughter could be seen in how reluctant each was to be an active participant in home-based family therapy when sessions were not held in her own home. During sessions at Susan's home, Susan revealed a family secret: She had always felt that her parents favored her siblings. As an adult, she learned that the man she thought of as her father, who raised her, was not her biological father, although he did father the other children in the family. She recalled having visited a man as a young child who she now suspected was her biological father, but his identity had not been disclosed and this matter subsequently had never been discussed. So Susan and Sharon actually shared the experience of not knowing their fathers and of feeling left out in their families. Acknowledging this history helped Susan accept Sharon's wish to keep Chris involved in her baby's life.

Another critical issue for this family was Susan's relationship with Fred (24), a much younger man. Sharon and Dawn were both highly critical of him and felt that Susan was trying to be an adolescent like them. As Susan began to mourn her own lost adolescence, she also recognized the effect her behavior had on her daughters. She began to become more responsive to Dawn's emerging adolescent needs, and their communication grew more open and effective. Susan expressed her commitment to parent Dawn in such a way that the intergenerational repetition of an adolescent pregnancy in this family would no longer be a self-fulfilling prophecy.

Mother and Grandmother

Another important issue for Susan and Sharon to work on was the role of mother. Although Susan felt that her ability to apply what she learned in treatment was very helpful to her relationship with Dawn, Dawn was already an adolescent. Susan wanted the experience of finally being a successful parent and thus often wanted to take over the care of Christine. At the same time, however, she felt resentful of the responsibility as she also wanted to get on with her own life. Ways in which she could support and assist Sharon without taking over were explored. Susan also came to understand that if she took over care of Christine, the family cycle would repeat itself, leading to parenting problems in future generations. She was proud of the way Sharon was functioning in the role of mother to Christine, and as Susan was able to let Sharon separate and be a mother, she began to enjoy her role as supportive grandmother.

At the conclusion of treatment, many of these intergenerational issues had been resolved. Role conflicts and communication issues had been addressed. Chris had frequent contact with Christine, who was attached to both her parents and was developing well. With her family's encouragement and support, Sharon was living on her own and attending school. Susan, Sharon, and Dawn were communicating openly, and both young women were doing well in school and with their peers. Although Mrs. Smith was not actively involved in the treatment, Sharon, with the encouragement of the therapists, maintained her relationship with her grandmother and visited her regularly with Christine so that she was also bonded with the baby.

Discussion

The Smith family illustrates many of the intergenerational themes presented by families with teenage parents. The home-based family therapy approach used in this treatment involved many of the key family and extended family members, and allowed the multigenerational themes to be addressed directly. Many of the family therapy sessions focused on the relationships among the grandmother, mother, and both daughters. It was clear that Sharon's pregnancy had evoked memories of prior adolescent pregnancies in the two previous generations of this family. As these issues were discussed openly in the family, communication between the generations was enhanced, role conflicts regarding the parenting and care of the baby were discussed, and the guilt and angry feelings of the past were separated from present events. The multigenerational family cycle of the exclusion of fathers was broken, as the multiple generations of adult women in the family were helped to see that they were projecting their anger toward men in their past onto the baby's teenage father. The father was encouraged to maintain an active role in his child's life. Through this family therapy intervention, the teenage mother was supported by her family in becoming a competent parent, living on her own, and completing her education.

Summary

The Smith family can be seen as a prototype of many families with a history of intergenerational adolescent pregnancy. Their case illustrates the power of the home-based family therapy approach to build trust with families, to address multigenerational issues directly, and to produce positive change for teenage parents and their children.

DOMESTIC VIOLENCE AND PHYSICAL ABUSE

Family violence—which includes domestic violence, partner abuse, physical abuse of children and elder abuse—has been shown to be the most common form of violence in the United States (Tolan & Gorman-Smith, 2002). It may be a "secret" or hidden issue in the families of some at-risk adolescents. Researchers have recognized a pattern of multigenerational transmission of family violence. Findings indicate that (1) exposure to domestic violence modeled by parents may contribute to partner abuse in relationships of older adolescents (Widom, 2000); (2) physical abuse and observing domestic violence may convey the message to children that violence is acceptable (Tolan, Gorman-Smith, & Henry, 2006); (3) parents who were victims of child abuse are at high risk for abusing their children (Widom, 2000); and (4) over the course of a lifetime, the same family member might be a perpetrator at one time and a victim in another situation (Tolan et al., 2006).

These multigenerational patterns can also affect behaviors such as mate selection and partner violence. Women who saw their mothers abused may choose mates who abuse them (Tolan et al., 2006). Tolan et al. (2006) provided an extensive review of studies of risk factors, multigenerational patterns, and interventions in the many forms of family violence. Loseke, Gelles, and Cavanaugh (2005) have studied the social policy implications of these forms of family violence, particularly domestic violence perpetrated by men against women (Loseke & Kurz, 2005). It is interesting, however, that police departments and national studies have begun to report more instances of women abusing men or of mutual partner abuse, particularly in younger couples (Tolan et al., 2006). In addition, although domestic violence has been reported across all socioeconomic levels, Benson and Fox (2004) have shown that poor families experience higher levels. Research has shown that families that have experienced domestic or partner violence are at high risk of physical abuse of children (Cicchetti, Toth, & Maughan, 2000).

Tolan et al. (2006) have demonstrated a link between family violence, particularly maternal partner violence, and delinquency. They argued that in some of the families in their study, mothers who were violent toward their partners were also less likely to monitor their children effectively and to employ harsh disciplinary practices, factors that increased the likelihood of their son's involvement in delinquency. This multigenerational family transmission pattern (Bowen, 1978; Nichols, 2011) can be addressed effectively through couple and family therapy interventions, particularly those with a prevention component. Such treatment has been shown to have a positive effect and to reduce violence in relationships (Markman, Renick, Floyd, Stanley, & Clements, 1993).

Case Example

Kaylan (age 36) and Mathew (age 38), an unmarried African American couple with two adolescents, Mara (age 15) and Ben (age 13), were referred for couple and family therapy pursuant to a court order resulting from a charge of disturbing the peace. Neighbors had called the police to report a loud altercation and crashing noises emanating from their apartment. When the police arrived, the couple admitted to having an argument, cursing, and throwing dishes at one another. No physical abuse was involved. Neither had any interest in pressing charges against the other. Their adolescents had been present for the incident.

In light of their lack of health insurance and low income, they were referred to a university-based home-based family therapy program that charged a minimal fee on a sliding scale. In the first session, which took place in their home while their adolescents were involved in after-school activities, the family therapist joined with the couple and established therapeutic rapport. She explored the incident that had brought them to treatment and the issues that led up to it. The couple explained that their angry argument about money had escalated into loud threats, cursing, and throwing dishes. They were both very ashamed of their behavior, especially as it took place in front of their adolescents, mortified that their neighbors had called the police, and apologetic to everyone involved. They were not prepared for the consequences—the mandate for treatment—of what they considered to be a private matter. The therapist explored their feelings about being in therapy. They both expressed a sense of stigma regarding being in therapy and their lack of belief in its effectiveness, but agreed to be compliant with the judge's order and continue with the treatment process.

In the next session, the therapist explored their family histories. Both partners reported domestic violence as a commonplace occurrence in their households during their childhood. Kaylan reported that her mother and father often fought with each other. Although an incident usually began with a verbal altercation, it would often escalate into physical violence in which both parents hit each other.

Although Mathew did not grow up with his biological father, his mother's live-in boyfriend customarily abused her and "beat her up," often in front of the children. When Mathew became a teenager, he began trying to intercede to defend his mother, only to find himself engaged in physical fights with the man. He tearfully explained that he had sworn that his life and his relationships would be free of that kind of "drama." Even though his arguments with Kaylan had not involved physical abuse, he reported that he feared this eventuality in the future if he could not contain his rage. The therapist explored again whether there had ever been a history of physical violence between them or in prior relationships. Both Kaylan and Mathew denied this, but the therapist discussed how physical violence might occur in the future if they did not address their anger at each other and find more constructive ways to resolve it. At this suggestion, both of them began to cry.

In future sessions, the therapist helped them see that their volatile family histories had contributed to problematic attachment and anger management issues for both. This process created a cycle in their relationship in which anger could spiral out of control. The therapist added that their teenagers were watching these behaviors in their parents' relationship just as Kaylan and Mathew had observed these patterns in their homes when they were children. She added that unless these issues were addressed and resolved, Mathew and Kaylan were putting their own adolescents at risk for future relationships that would re-create this dynamic. Both of the partners were stunned by this warning, and they began to talk about additional traumatic experiences in their childhoods. Mathew shared that he never wanted things to get so out of control that his children would feel compelled to put their own safety at risk to intervene, as he had done as a young adolescent.

In future sessions, the therapist worked with the couple to explore the cycle of anger between them. Both had grown up in poor families where there was never enough money to meet the family's needs. As a result, money issues had always acted as a major trigger for each. Six months prior to the altercation that resulted in mandated treatment, the plant where Mathew worked closed suddenly and he had been laid off without notice. They were already living "paycheck to paycheck" before his job loss, and now the couple was deeply in debt. Kaylan was very concerned about their financial situation as she was the only one employed at the time.

Although Mathew was conducting an active job search and had had a few telephone and Skype interviews, he received no requests for a second interview or job offers. On the night the police were called by neighbors, Kaylan had found an eviction notice in her mailbox upon her return from work as a supermarket cashier. She explained that receiving an eviction notice was a major trigger for her. Her father's chronic unemployment during her childhood resulted in her family being evicted a number of times, forcing the family to stay in homeless shelters or move in with relatives. On one occasion, her family lived with an aunt who had five of her own children. Kaylan explained that her anger upon seeing the eviction notice turned into rage when she opened the door and found Mathew sitting on the couch watching television. She stated that she experienced a "flashback" when she saw Mathew idle while she worked all day—her mother had been the sole provider for the family for most of her childhood while her father's heavy drinking progressed into alcoholism.

The therapist helped the couple to share their feelings about these events with each other. It was clear that both partners loved each other; however, the dynamics in their families of origin served as triggers for each in their relationship. Mathew reported that he was so discouraged by his inability to find a job that he had become depressed and that it was hard to get motivated to keep looking when he had experienced nothing other than rejection. Because of Kaylan's family history, she was hesitant to move in with family members. She reported that they had already borrowed money from everyone they knew—relatives and friends—and she no longer felt that borrowing money was a realistic alternative.

The therapist helped them to problem-solve their options. As they explored employment possibilities for Mathew, the therapist asked whether they owned a car. As Mathew had a car, she asked him if he had considered becoming an Uber driver. This possibility had not occurred to him, but he agreed to investigate it right away. In the next session, both partners appeared happier and more positive. Mathew reported that he had just started driving for Uber. He had not been able to earn much money yet, but he was hopeful that it would work out for him. Kaylan reported that she had spoken to the landlord, informed him that her husband had just started working again, and asked him to reconsider the eviction. To her surprise, the landlord gave them until the end of the month to pay the current month's rent, and she agreed to try to pay a small amount each month toward the arrears.

With the immediate financial crisis and the threat of eviction averted, the couple was able to work with the therapist on learning communication skills, understanding their cycle of anger, exploring ways to defuse their anger, and devising techniques to recover from a trigger rooted in their past before unleashing their anger at each other. The couple continued in treatment for the remaining 3 months of the court mandate. At the end of that time, their relationship had improved significantly. Having begun to understand the multigenerational transmission process they each shared, they were committed to reversing that cycle for themselves and for their children.

SEXUAL ABUSE

In recent years, as the denial about sexual abuse has begun to change to knowledge, incidence studies have begun to reveal the extent of the problem. Many experts in this area believe that child and adolescent sexual abuse in the family is significantly underreported, with its prevalence far greater than statistics would indicate (Cohen, Mannarino, & Deblinger, 2006; Deblinger, Mannarino, Cohen, Runyon, & Heflin, 2015; Figley & Kiser, 2013; Finkelhor & Dziuba-Leatherman, 1994; Gil, 1995, 1996; Runyon, Deblinger, & Steer, 2014). Clinicians may discover a multigenerational pattern in some families of children and adolescents who have been sexually abused (Boyd-Franklin & Bry, 2000). For example, as an adolescent, a mother may have experienced a brutal rape by a family member. This incident was never discussed in the family and became a toxic secret. Her daughters were sexually abused by an older cousin when they became adolescents (Kagan, 2017; Kagan & Schlossberg, 1989). In order to prevent what may otherwise become a legacy of trauma, families need help to heal (Figley & Kiser, 2013). Clinicians should not automatically assume, however, that all cases of child or adolescent sexual abuse in families are multigenerational in nature (Deblinger et al., 2015; Tavkar & Hansen, 2011; Trepper & Barrett, 1986). For further discussions of clinical interventions in sexual abuse cases, therapists are referred to Deblinger et al. (2015), Gil (1995, 1996), Tavkar and Hansen (2011), and Trepper and Barrett's (1986) classic book on systemic approaches to incest.

The following case example illustrates some of the issues involved in multigenerational sexual abuse, including the need for both individual and family treatment (Boyd-Franklin & Bry, 2000).

Case Example

Mary was the 13-year-old only child of Alice Duffy, a 35-year-old single parent from an Irish American family. Mary's teacher, concerned when Mary became increasingly depressed and withdrawn, referred her to the school guidance counselor. In one of the early sessions with the counselor, Mary revealed that she was afraid of her mother's boyfriend, Paul Graham (age 36). The subject matter was so frightening to Mary that she refused to say anything more about it for the remainder of the session.

In Mary's next session, the guidance counselor tried to help Mary over-come her fears by telling her that many children and adolescents had let her know that they were afraid of someone, and usually it was because the youth had been hurt by this person and been warned not to tell anyone about it. Mary then told the counselor that Paul had hurt her "down there." She pointed to her vagina. When this was explored in more detail, it became clear that some form of sexual molestation had occurred.

There were far-reaching consequences once the counselor became aware of the sexual abuse of Mary:

1. The counselor was bound by law to report the sexual abuse to child protective services.
2. Alice was summoned to a meeting at the school with the guid-ance counselor, who informed Alice of the serious nature of her daughter's sexual abuse by Alice's boyfriend.
3. Alice told Paul he had to leave the home.
4. Mary received a medical exam.
5. Child protective services removed Mary from her home and placed her in a foster home while they conducted their investiga-tion.
6. The police were notified, and Paul was arrested, facing criminal charges.
7. Mary and Alice were referred to the sexual abuse treatment cen-ter.

The first home-based therapy session was with the mother alone while Mary was still in foster care. Alice tearfully reported that she was feeling very guilty for not having protected her daughter and then not having believed her when Mary had informed her of the incident after it occurred. Alice had "thrown Paul out," and after his arrest he was under the jurisdiction of the courts for his sexual abuse of Mary. As there was no longer a dangerous situation in the home, Alice had asked child protective services to return Mary to her home. After Alice's request to reunite with her daughter, the therapist obtained written permission from Alice to contact all of the agencies involved: Mary's school, child protective services, the foster family, the police, and the prosecutor's office. She sent a letter to each agency requesting information and then followed up with phone calls.

The therapist next met alone with Mary, who was brought to her office by the child protective services worker. (This session was held in the therapist's office as Mary's foster home could not offer the pri-vacy needed.) The therapist used this session to join with Mary and to begin to explore the sexual abuse. Mary reported that while her mother was out shopping, Paul came into Mary's room as she was napping and began touching her "down there." When asked to point to the area on an anatomically correct drawing of a female handed her by the therapist, Mary pointed to the vaginal area. She reported that he first touched her with his finger and then with his penis. When asked to point this out on an anatomically correct drawing of a male, she pointed to the penis. She stated that he pushed his penis in and it hurt. (This statement was consistent with the medical report the therapist had obtained.) When asked what happened next, Mary said she ran to the bathroom, locked the door, and stayed there until she heard her mother's voice. The therapist praised her for thinking to do this. Mary then told her mother that Paul had touched her "down there" and pointed to her vagina. Her mother then went into the bedroom with Paul. They had a loud argument, but this incident was never mentioned again.

The therapist continued home sessions with the mother while conducting office sessions with Mary. During one session, Alice told the therapist that the experience Mary had been through had stirred up many feelings and memories for her. As a teenage girl of 14, Alice had been sexually abused by her father. When she told her mother, her mother did not believe her. Alice cried and asked over and over, "How could I not believe my own daughter?" and "How could I let this happen?" The therapist asked Alice what the answers were to her questions. Alice cried and eventually said she "did not want to lose Paul." Both of her parents had died, Mary's father had abandoned her when she became pregnant, and she was afraid of being alone. In addition, Paul's financial contributions were crucial since he was the primary breadwinner for the household of three. The therapist told Alice that she understood her feelings and encouraged her to use some of their sessions to explore these issues further. The therapist also reinforced her decision to remove Paul from her home and to support her daughter on her own.

Mary was returned to her mother's home approximately a week later. As the relationship between mother and daughter was still tenuous, the family sessions were held in the office rather than the home. In addition, the office offered a greater degree of privacy to talk to each individually. During the initial family session, the therapist first met with them together and then gave Mary and Alice individual time. In the joint portion of the session, Mary seemed timid and withdrawn with her mother. The therapist sensed that they were holding back from each other.

Mary was seen alone first, and the therapist asked her how she felt being with her mother. She replied, "Scared," and then began to cry. When the therapist inquired about why she felt scared, Mary said that she thought her mother was "mad" at her because she had "told on Paul." When the therapist explored further why she felt this way, Mary said, "My mom did not believe me at first." The therapist asked what Mary hoped would happen now between her and her mother. She tearfully stated, "She'll love me again." The therapist told Mary that she sensed that Mary very much wanted her mother's love. Mary nodded. The therapist then asked whether Mary would accept some help from her in talking to her mother about her apprehensions and worries and Mary eagerly agreed. The therapist also asked her permission to share some of Mary's concerns with her mother individually before meeting with them together; Mary hesitated at first but then agreed.

While the therapist spoke with Alice alone, Mary sat in the waiting room. When the therapist asked Alice what she felt during the session with Mary, Alice reported, "It felt strange. We seem so far apart." She explained that this feeling was not new, as there had often been distance between them in the past. The therapist told Alice that Mary had felt that distance also and, having received Mary's permission, disclosed Mary's fear that her mother would be mad at her for making Paul go away. Alice cried and said that she was not angry with Mary at all. She was angry at herself for not having believed Mary, and she only wanted to help her daughter. The therapist asked whether Alice would be willing to talk with Mary about it. She agreed.

Mary was brought back into the session and took a chair closer to her mother. The therapist moved her chair close to both of them and told Mary that she had shared her concerns with her mother. The therapist next asked Alice to talk to her daughter about it. Alice blurted out, "I'm not mad at you, Mary." She then started crying. Mary began crying too. The therapist moved their chairs closer together and encouraged them to hold each other. Mary eagerly went into her mother's arms. The therapist quietly encouraged Alice to tell Mary of her love for her, and Alice did so. Mary then said, "I thought you would be mad at me." Alice replied hesitantly, "I was at first, but I'm not now." She added, "I just wish that I had believed you before." The therapist asked the mother whether she believed Mary now. The mother replied, "Absolutely." The therapist asked Alice to ask Mary's forgiveness for not believing her earlier.

The therapist asked that they continue to meet in her office. She said that in the next session she would give them each some time alone and then meet with them together. In the next few sessions, Mary discussed her anger at Paul, but she was not yet ready to address her anger at her mother for not believing her.

In a number of individual sessions, Alice's own sexual abuse experience and her anger at both her mother and her father were discussed. The family session during this period was used to explore bonding activities for Mary and Alice, one of which was Alice playing a game with Mary on her cell phone. As both sat rigidly in their chairs, the therapist encouraged them to try the "homework task" of reading together or watching a television show together before bedtime. This activity at home facilitated their seeming closer in the family part of the session.

Finally, after 2 months, Alice stated that she was ready to tell Mary what had happened to her as a child and to let her know how badly she felt that "history was repeating itself." Mary listened avidly as her mother described her experiences.

In the next session together, Alice shared with her daughter how angry she had been at her own father for abusing her. The therapist helped Alice to ask whether Mary had been angry at Paul. Mary nodded timidly. The therapist encouraged Alice to talk with Mary about the incident. Both of them expressed their anger at the men who had abused them. They both left the session closer together than the therapist had ever seen them.

It took much longer (3 months) for Mary to begin to address her anger at her mother. During this time, the therapist began to alternate weekly sessions between the office, which continued to follow the divided format between individual and "together time," and with home-based sessions where they worked on the bonding between Mary and her mother. In the home-based sessions, the therapist helped them to establish an activity just before bedtime, in which Alice would sit close to Mary on the couch and read to her. As this activity was role-played on the couch in the living room, they were at first awkward, but gradually they seemed more at ease.

In the individual sessions in the office, Mary continued to report feeling sad. Then the therapist encouraged her to draw pictures and tell stories about her drawings. She first drew a girl as a very small figure at the bottom of the page, relating that the girl was a "bad girl" because she let the "bad man" touch her. (This feeling that she was responsible for Paul's actions is a very common reaction among child and adolescent victims of sexual abuse.) The therapist asked Mary what she thought she did. Mary cried and said, "I smiled at him." The therapist told Mary that she had a beautiful smile and that her smile did not cause this to happen to her. The therapist explained that it was Paul's fault, not hers, and that any time an adult abuses a young person, it is never the young person's fault. In later sessions, Mary began to describe the ways in which Paul had threatened to hurt her if she ever talked to her mother about the incident again. (Intimidation is also quite common among perpetrators of child or adolescent sexual abuse.) The therapist helped Mary to see that she was just a scared girl who had done the best she could do at the time. In a later family session, Alice was able to reinforce for Mary that none of this was her fault and that Paul was to blame. Over the months, Mary's mood and affect began to change.

Eventually, in her individual sessions, Alice began addressing her own anger at her mother for not believing and protecting her. After a number of these sessions, Alice asked, "I wonder if Mary feels the same way toward me." In their next family session, Alice asked Mary whether she remembered the time when they discussed her experience of being sexually abused by her father. Mary nodded. Alice asked whether she remembered their talk about how angry she was at her father. Again Mary nodded. Alice then told her that she had also been very angry at her mother, who also did not believe her or protect her. With the therapist's help, Alice said to Mary, "I am sure that you had some angry feelings toward me." Mary was silent and looked fearfully at the therapist. With the therapist's prompting, Alice explained to Mary that if she did have those angry feelings, she (Alice) would not be mad at her (Mary). Mary nodded and cried. The mother spontaneously put her arms around Mary and told her that she understood her anger and wanted her to know that she loved her. Mary did not speak much in this session but continued to hold her mother.

This session was a turning point for Mary and Alice. Mary spontaneously asked her mother if they could do something special like go to the movies together that weekend. Their relationship continued to improve, and treatment was terminated 2 months later (Boyd-Franklin & Bry, 2000).

DISCUSSION

This case illustrates many lessons for family therapists and other clinicians. This family's situation clearly demonstrates how quickly outside agencies, such as child protective services, the school, medical authorities, the police, and the court system, can become involved in a crisis (Figley & Kiser, 2013).

The therapist flexibly utilized the Multisystems Model in her combination of treatment modalities. Individual work with the mother was necessary because of her own sexual abuse history. In order to allow both Mary and Alice the privacy to explore their issues individually, many sessions were conducted in the therapist's office rather than in the home. This privacy is important when a child or adolescent's natural sense of trust has been destroyed and needs to be rebuilt, as is often the case with sexual abuse.

The therapist began building the bond between the parent and the adolescent gradually through sessions in her office with both of them.

After preliminary work in this area had been done and more trust had been established, home-based sessions were resumed, although some office-based sessions continued to be held so that the individual work could be done with more privacy (Boyd-Franklin & Bry, 2000).

JUVENILE DELINQUENCY

As discussed throughout this chapter, a crisis involving an at-risk adolescent may be a repetition of a trauma suffered by a parent that has never been openly discussed. The following case illustrates the ways in which themes of secrets about father absence and delinquency or criminal behavior can be repeated through many crises in the family. It is also an excellent example of the ways in which prior losses or traumas can become "toxic secrets" (Boyd-Franklin, 2003; Boyd-Franklin & Bry, 2000; Imber-Black, 1993; Kagan, 2017; Kagan & Schlossberg, 1989).

Case Example

Aisha Simmons, a 30-year-old African American single mother, was referred for family treatment by the police following her 14-year-old son Malik's second arrest for juvenile delinquent activity. His first arrest, for defacing subway cars with graffiti, had also resulted in a referral for family therapy, but Malik had refused to return after his mother accompanied him to the first session. Malik's second arrest, approximately 1 month prior to the current referral, was for "joyriding" with two boys who had stolen a car. This pattern was becoming repetitive—both arrests had been triggered by Malik's following other adolescents into committing acts of serious delinquent behavior (Boyd-Franklin & Bry, 2000).

In the first session of mandated therapy following the second arrest, Aisha was extremely angry and critical of Malik. She stated that she was very "disappointed in him," described him repeatedly as "bad," and reported that he had hurt her so much that she was giving up on him and had therefore "shut him out." The therapist initially felt overwhelmed by Aisha. She was argumentative, often contradicting the therapist's statements. Her tone of voice and body language in the session often appeared angry or antagonistic. Aisha also talked incessantly, and it was difficult for the therapist to intervene. When the therapist did speak, Aisha engaged in hostile gestures, including rolling her eyes, sucking her teeth, and shaking her head. The therapist felt dismissed by the mother and felt that she scapegoated her son constantly. In addition, the therapist was troubled by the fact that each time she asked Aisha about the family's history or attempted to construct a family tree or genogram (Boyd-Franklin, 2003; McGoldrick, Gerson, & Petry, 2008), she either changed the topic or said, "That's the past. I leave it in the past." After the first session, the therapist attended supervision and was helped to process some of her own feelings of anger at the mother.

With the supervisor's help, the therapist was able to join with Aisha. During the first months of treatment, Aisha gradually began to share her history. She revealed that her mother had died when Aisha was 3 years old, after which she had been sent to live with her maternal grandmother and aunt. She felt abandoned by her father, who had quickly remarried and started another family with his second wife. She had little contact with her four half-brothers. Aisha also felt abandoned by Malik's father, who had been incarcerated since Malik was a year old. Aisha had kept this fact secret from Malik, who had been told that his father was dead. It now became clear that the repeated crises with Malik and the police reflected a pattern in the family and that Aisha was terrified that her son would "follow in his father's footsteps."

The therapist could now empathize with Aisha's response to Malik. Behind the facade of anger lay her intense fear that he would be sent to prison like his father had been. This fear corresponded to her own intense fears of abandonment: an imprisoned Malik would be the third "man" in her life to desert her. As these themes emerged, the therapist began to approach Aisha about sharing these secrets with Malik, a suggestion that she resisted. In addition to treatment with Aisha and Malik, the therapist also engaged the systems involved with the family; notably, she joined school counseling sessions with Malik and Aisha, met with Malik's probation officer, and accompanied the family to court.

Despite all of these efforts, Malik provoked yet another crisis. He was again caught joyriding in a stolen car. During the session following this event, Aisha was furious, not only at Malik, but also at the therapist for not "fixing" Malik. This incident proved the turning point for Aisha, however, showing her the need to listen to the therapist's view of the importance of discussing his father's history with Malik and how it influenced her fears for him.

In the first of a series of emotional sessions, Aisha told Malik about his father's incarceration. Malik was angry at first that he had been lied to and had been told his father was dead, but then began to ask questions about him. When Malik asked to contact his father, Aisha adamantly refused at first, but eventually, after many sessions, she relented and agreed that Malik could write his father a letter.

In a later session, the therapist helped Aisha share her genogram with Malik. Malik seemed fascinated when he learned of her father's large family. When he expressed a desire to contact them, Aisha, still feeling abandoned and fearful that her father's other family would judge her parenting of Malik, was reluctant to agree.

As the sessions continued, Aisha's earlier statement that when Malik began to get in trouble she had "shut him out" began to make sense. Through many painful experiences with men, and the prospect of nothing but pain in the future, she developed the view that "when they hurt, disappoint, or abandon you, you shut them out." Finally, she was able to listen to Malik's feelings about her habit of shutting him out following a crisis. His crises—the repeated run-ins with the police—had served the function of pulling her back into his life.

Aisha was able to make a firm contract with Malik about his continued attendance at family sessions, school performance, and adherence to the terms of his probation. She learned new communication and problem-solving skills, and she began to praise him even for small changes he made in his behavior. She developed consistent disciplinary measures for the first time, enforcing his curfew and establishing clear consequences for his behavior. As a result, Malik's behavior began to improve. The number of crises decreased and finally stopped; what is more, he passed all his courses and was promoted to the next grade. Regular family sessions ended once he successfully completed probation. The therapist conducted brief monthly "booster sessions" (Bry & Krinsley, 1992) by phone with Aisha and Malik for 3 months to make sure that the positive behavior continued (Boyd-Franklin & Bry, 2000).

MULTIGENERATIONAL GANG INVOLVEMENT

Similar to the multigenerational patterns in juvenile delinquency discussed earlier, research has shown that familial influences, particularly the gang involvement of parents, older siblings, and older relatives, significantly predicted gang membership of at-risk adolescents (Gilman, Hill, Hawkins, Howell, & Kosterman, 2014). Qualitative studies of gang members have shown that many of them grew up with influential family members, including parents, siblings, uncles, and cousins, who were actively involved in a gang lifestyle (Gilman et al., 2014).

An adolescent's involvement may be gradual. Younger brothers, sisters, or cousins may be recruited to be "lookouts" during a gang robbery or to serve as "runners" transporting drugs for dealers. As they become older, they often choose to associate more and more with delinquent peers, which has also been shown to be an additional pathway to gang membership (Esbensen, Peterson, Taylor, & Freng, 2009).

Much of the research on gangs has focused on boys because male gang members outnumber girl members by far (Gilman et al., 2014). But this is not to say that girls are not also at risk for gang involvement, particularly if they have family members who are gang involved (Gilman et al., 2014). In addition, the number of girl members of gangs has increased in the last 20 years (Howell, 2012). There has been some debate in the literature about the gender differences in the risk factors for gang involvement. While some studies have found that boys experience additional risk factors for more dangerous forms of delinquency than girls (Kroneman, Loeber, & Hipwell, 2004), others have found that risk factors for serious delinquency in boys are also present for girls (Penny, Lee, & Moretti, 2010).

A family gang connection has often offered protection in dangerous communities even when an at-risk adolescent has not been initiated into a gang. Receiving the protection of the gang without actual involvement is referred to as having been "blessed in." Some adolescents may be influenced to become gang involved themselves because of the "prestige" and protection that their connection to a gang member may grant them in the community.

Having family members who are involved in gangs not only puts adolescents at risk for gang involvement, but also may increase the risk of gang retaliation against the family. In some inner-city communities, when incidents or "beefs" occur between rival gangs, family members may be targeted and injured as a message to a gang member. The following case illustrates this process.

Case Example

Khalid was a tall, dark-skinned 13-year-old African American male in the eighth grade. He lived with his mother, Ms. C., his younger brother, Rob, age 10, and his older brother, Barak, age 20, in an apartment in an inner city, low-income housing project. Barak, who had been a member of the Bloods gang for a number of years, had been involved in a gang-related robbery of a store. This put the entire family at risk because the store owner was the uncle of a member of a rival gang. Shortly after the robbery, at a time when Barak was not at home, three members of the rival gang broke into the family's apartment while they were eating dinner, threatened them, and beat up Khalid when he tried to protect his mother. Khalid, angry and fearful, became more involved with his brother's gang, seeking protection from other attacks, and, although he had not been formally initiated into the gang, he began "hanging out with the gang members" in the projects. His grades began to decline. When his mother received his report card, she was alarmed that he was in danger of being left back to repeat the eighth grade, rather than being promoted to high school. She reached out to the middle school guidance counselor to try to obtain some help for her son.

The guidance counselor referred Khalid to a school-based program that provided counseling services in the school in conjunction with home-based family therapy. In addition, she arranged for a college student who volunteered as a tutor/mentor in the school to help him with his academic work. Khalid's family counselor treated him in the school with individual therapy and also reached out to conduct home-based sessions with his family. When the family counselor initially reached out to Khalid's mother by phone to explain the purpose of the program, Ms. C. was extremely responsive. She reported that she was "very scared for Khalid" and that she was afraid that he would "end up like his older brother."

In school, Khalid presented as a leader in his peer group and was well liked. He was well liked by his teachers as well, who reported that he was intelligent despite his poor school performance. His college student mentor/tutor, who met with his teachers and obtained weekly progress reports, also saw him as very bright.

At the first home-based session, Khalid, his mother, and his younger brother were present. Barak was not home and had refused to participate when asked. During the meeting, Khalid's mother recounted the rival gang members' attack on her family in their home and her fears for all of her sons. The family counselor helped Khalid's mother to talk directly to him about her concerns. She told him she knew that he was angry after the attack in their home, but the changes she saw in him since the incident worried her. The counselor emphasized his mother's fears and her love for him, and encouraged Khalid to respond. He told his mother that he loved her too, but that she did not understand life on the streets. His mother told him that she was praying for a miracle that would take Barak out of that life and that would protect Khalid and his little brother from becoming involved in the gang. She told him that her dream had always been for her sons to go to college and that she had been working for all of these years to try to get Khalid and his brothers to "make something of themselves." As she spoke of her wishes for her children, she began to cry. Khalid became uncomfortable and told her "don't cry, Ma." It was clear to the counselor at the end of the session that Khalid loved his mother and wanted to please her, but that the lure of gang life and the protection it offered was stronger than his mother's dream for him.

In the next 2 weeks, the counselor met with Khalid a number of times at school. He told the family counselor that when he was younger, he had done well in school. School work had come easily to him. and he cared about getting good grades. His mother and teachers had always talked to him about going to college. When the counselor asked whether he shared that dream, he reported that he used to, but now he was not sure. The counselor then asked if he would be willing to try to get his grades up enough to be promoted to go to high school, and Khalid agreed. His guidance counselor arranged for his family counselor and the tutor/mentor to meet with his teachers along with Khalid to discuss what he would need to do in each course to pass. Once all the input had been obtained and a plan had been formed, Khalid agreed to do his part.

In the next home-based family session, when the family counselor asked Khalid to share the results with his mother, even the counselor was surprised by his level of commitment. He explained that he did not want to be "left back" and have to stay with the "little kids" in middle school. The counselor praised him for his efforts and encouraged Khalid and Ms. C. to discuss how he could be supported at home to study and focus. They problem-solved and agreed on a plan for him to do home-work after school with his mother's help.

Over the next few months, the counselor discussed Barak's partici-pation in the family sessions. Ms. C. reported that Barak always claimed to be "too busy" when she asked him to attend. Three months later, Barak's leg was broken during a gang fight, which resulted in him being at home more than usual. The counselor asked Ms. C.'s and Khalid's permission to reach out to Barak. When she phoned and asked to come to the house to talk with him, he reluctantly agreed. She met with Barak while Khalid and his brother were in school, and asked for his help with his brother because Khalid looked up to him and wanted to be just like him. Barak looked pleased but somewhat uncomfortable and stated that he did not want Khalid "following after him." The counselor asked why, and Barak told her that in the gang fight in which he was injured, Duran, a good friend of his, had been killed, and he "did not want that" to hap-pen to his brothers. The counselor asked Barak if he would be willing to join them for a family session and discuss this with his brothers. Barak reluctantly agreed.

Barak participated in the next family session but was initially silent, listening as his mother talked to Khalid and Rob about her fears for them. As she began to cry, Barak appeared to be increasingly uncom-fortable, as did his brothers. The family counselor asked Barak what he thought about his mother's comments. He shared that he was also concerned for his brothers and did not want them to "get pulled into the streets." When the counselor asked Barak if he would be willing to talk with Khalid about that, he agreed. He told Khalid that "gang banging is no kind of life" for him and he did not want to see him killed like his friend. Khalid responded that it had worked for him. Barak became angry and told Khalid that all of his friends were in the gang, so he just followed them because he "didn't know any better." He added that there were many times when he had regretted this choice and wanted to get out. Khalid asked why he didn't, and Barak told him that the only way to get out was to avoid getting in the gang in the first place because once you were "jumped in" (initiated into the gang), it was very difficult to get out. He told Khalid that he did not want to see him or Rob "go that way." Khalid talked with him about the dangers of the streets and the need for protection. Barak told him that because of his involvement, Khalid and Rob would not need to join the gang themselves to receive protection. The counselor praised Barak for his willingness to talk with Khalid and his brother. When asked if he would participate in the next session, Barak agreed.

In the next session, which took place after a 3-week break due to the holidays, the counselor asked what Barak's hopes and dreams were for his brothers. He said he shared his mother's dream for them to graduate from high school and go on to college. Khalid laughed, and the counselor asked him to tell Barak why he was laughing. Khalid said he was just surprised because Barak had never seemed to want that for himself. Barak then became serious and said he was a young "knucklehead." He reminded Khalid that he got in trouble early in his life. He was arrested for his gang activities while still in high school and ended up in a juvenile detention center. He continued in that path because he didn't know any better, but he reiterated that he did not want that life for either Khalid or their younger brother. The counselor encouraged Khalid to talk directly with Barak about this and about what he was doing in school so that he could meet his mother and brother's expectations that he would have a better life. Khalid explained his efforts to get better grades so that he could go on to high school. His mother told Barak that Khalid had been trying very hard. Barak seemed surprised and told Khalid that he was proud of him for "being a man and taking care of his business." When Khalid responded that he wanted to be a man like him, Barak at first was quiet and then told Khalid that he did not want to see him "follow in my footsteps," risk being killed like Duran, or "doing time like so many of the other guys on the block." He asked Khalid to promise him that he would continue his education and try to get into college. Khalid seemed uncomfortable but agreed to try.

Three months later, when Khalid learned that he would graduate with his class and enter high school in the fall, the counselor met with the family in a home-based session and they all celebrated this news. In one of the last family therapy sessions just prior to Khalid's graduation, the counselor was informed that Barak, along with a number of members of his gang, was arrested for drug dealing. Khalid, his mother, and Rob all expressed how upset they were about this news. In the last session, Khalid reported that Barak had written him a letter from jail asking him to promise to stay away from the streets and gang life and to not end up in jail. In a very emotional family session, Khalid shared his feelings about Barak's advice with his mother and his younger brother, and told the counselor that he had made that promise in a letter he wrote to his brother. In the last session, the family acknowledged that family counseling had opened a way for Khalid to connect with Barak and listen to Barak's positive hopes and goals for his brother. The mother, crying throughout, was grateful that she could now be less afraid that all of her sons would lead dangerous lives.

DISCUSSION

This case is an example of the value of home-based family therapy. As Barak initially had refused to be a part of the family sessions, it is unlikely that he would ever have been willing to attend a session in the school or in a clinic. Because the family counselor had gained the trust of Khalid and his family, they were willing to share the serious nature of Barak's gang involvement. When Barak was home with an injury, the therapist succeeded in reaching out to him and thus learn of his concerns for his brother. This led to a series of family sessions in which Barak shared with Khalid that he did not want to see him "follow in my footsteps" and enter gang life. This input from his brother changed the course of the counseling and Khalid's life.

It is important first to meet alone with this family member and explore his attitudes concerning the future of his younger relatives, as Khalid's family counselor did. It is unfortunate that many family therapists feel reluctant to engage family members who participate in risky and/or dangerous behavior, such as drug or alcohol abuse and gang membership, or who have been incarcerated. These are precisely the family members who often can play a major role in reversing the multigenerational family transmission process. The message that they do not wish their young at-risk family member to pursue the same lifestyle may be very powerful. Family sessions can provide an opportunity for them to share their hopes and dreams for family members with their families. We have been continually impressed and surprised by the number of times family members have expressed a desire to reverse negative patterns. The next section illustrates a similar process in the family of an at-risk adolescent coping with multigenerational drug and alcohol abuse.

DRUG AND ALCOHOL ABUSE

Adolescent drug or alcohol abuse is a particularly disturbing presenting problem because it places adolescents at risk for many dangerous consequences, including overdoses, HIV/AIDS through needle sharing, crime, and violence (Boyd-Franklin & Bry, 2000). Moreover, adolescents often pay for their drug habits by shoplifting, prostitution, and dealing drugs, which put the adolescents even more at risk for incarceration. As is the case with gang activity, adolescents are often introduced to alcohol and drug use by "hanging around with the wrong crowd."

At-risk adolescents with family histories involving parental alcohol or drug abuse are often more vulnerable to addiction themselves. In addition, when parents are unable to care for their children properly, they are often raised by grandparents, and these grandparents may often be struggling with their own issues, such as guilt about their own substance abuse histories, feelings that they failed as parents because of their adult children's addiction, and doubts as to whether they can "save the grandchildren" from a similar pattern despite a strong desire to do so. For a more comprehensive discussion of grandparents and other relatives raising children with substance-abusing parents, see Chapter 4 on kinship care.

Many grandparents are awarded custody of their grandchildren when child protective services become involved. Even when removal of the children from the homes of their biological parents is pursuant to court mandate, the parents may still continue to be a presence in the grandparents' homes, which can prove disruptive. Older family members often have difficulty setting limits on their adult children's behavior. The following case illustrates the dynamics when grandchildren model their behavior on that of their parents (Boyd-Franklin & Bry, 2000).

Case Example

Ramon, a 16-year-old Puerto Rican adolescent, was referred for home-based family treatment by the court after his arrest for possession of marijuana and cocaine in school. The Ramos family consisted of Ms. Melinda Ramos (age 65), his paternal grandmother; his younger sister, Maria (age 12); his father, Arturo (age 40), who was in and out of the family and had a long history of drug abuse; and his young uncle, Pablo (age 25), who worked in a nearby car wash. Ramon's mother had died in a car crash when he was 5.

Ms. Ramos and Ramon were present for the first home-based family therapy session of court-mandated treatment, and Maria wandered in and out. The session was held in the kitchen (where all major family activities seemed to occur). Ms. Ramos chopped onions and garlic at the table during the session, and stirred pots on the stove throughout and yet was very engaged. This first session focused on Ramon's immediate issues, including his suspension from school and his pending court hearing. Ms. Ramos had been unaware of Ramon's drug involvement prior to his arrest and asked him many questions about his activities. At first, Ramon was surly and refused to talk about these issues, but eventually he began to cooperate.

Ms. Ramos was obviously the family spokesperson and the "switchboard" through which all communication occurred in the family. She was determined that Ramon succeed with his education. With the therapist's encouragement, Ms. Ramos contacted the school and helped to arrange for a postsuspension transfer to an alternative school where he would have more individualized attention.

During a later home-based session, Ramon's young uncle Pablo returned early from work, and the therapist invited him to sit at the table. As the session progressed, it was clear that Ramon really looked up to Pablo. The therapist asked Pablo to ask Ramon about how he had first gotten involved in drug use. Ramon explained that he had been recruited by drug dealers at age 11 to act as a "runner," selling "nickel bags" (small $5 packets) of marijuana and, later, cocaine to his friends at school. He did not use drugs himself at first, but as he got more involved in dealing, he began to smoke marijuana and later to snort cocaine. Once he developed a drug habit, his dealing accelerated to support his addiction. With his grandmother's encouragement, Pablo talked with Ramon about how he had been on a path similar to Ramon's, but how he had gotten help and he was forced to attend drug rehab. He spoke to a very resistant Ramon about getting drug treatment. The therapist learned for the first time of Ramon's father's drug history when Pablo revealed this information. Ms. Ramos appeared troubled by her oldest son's drug addiction and refused to talk about it initially.

In the meantime, Ramon presented another crisis: Ms. Ramos called the therapist in a panic because Ramon was again arrested for drug possession. He and his friends were hanging out in a house that had been raided by the police, and all of them were arrested. During the subsequent home visit, the therapist discovered that Ramon's father, Arturo, had returned from drug treatment and was now living with the family. The therapist spent a few minutes getting to know Arturo and asked whether he was aware of what was happening with Ramon. Arturo replied that he knew only that Ramon had been arrested. The therapist asked Ms. Ramos to share the details with Arturo. The therapist then told Arturo that he was one of the most important people in Ramon's life, and he asked for his support in helping his son. Arturo looked skeptical but agreed to participate in sessions.

In the next session, Arturo and Pablo supported Ms. Ramos's attempts to set limits for Ramon. They all agreed to a curfew and to clear consequences if it was violated. The next week, in a very moving session, Arturo shared with Ramon his own history of drug addiction and dealing. He told Ramon that he did not want him to turn out "like me." He also told Ramon about his drug treatment program. Ramon listened intently but refused to go.

Finally, a week later, Ramon created still another crisis: He was arrested again, and this time he was placed in a juvenile detention center. The therapist first met with Ramon at the center and then went to the home for a family session with Ms. Ramos, Arturo, and Pablo. She discussed with them the need for "tough love," in which they would request that the court mandate that Ramon attend drug treatment in a locked facility. Ms. Ramos was appalled at this suggestion. She repeated, "*No, el es mi bambino*" ("No, he is my baby"). Her preference was for the judge to release Ramon to her custody. The therapist asked Arturo and Pablo to discuss this alternative with Ms. Ramos. Arturo reminded her that she had bailed him out as an adolescent and repeatedly since. Ms. Ramos became a bit defensive and replied, "*Pero el es mi familia*" ("But he is my family"). This comment was true to her Latino culture; love of family was all-important to her. The therapist then asked the "miracle" question (Berg, 1994). That is, she asked what she would want to see happen for Ramon if a miracle occurred during the night. Ms. Ramos replied that she would like to see him "turn his life around." When the therapist asked her what she meant by that, she replied that she wanted him to "finish school, get a job, and lead a good life." The therapist asked whether Ms. Ramos knew someone who had "turned his life around." She thought for a long time and then turned to Pablo and said, "You did." He seemed surprised.

When the therapist asked Pablo what he thought about what his mother had said, he responded that he never thought of his life in that way. When explaining what she meant by Pablo having "turned his life around," Ms. Ramos described a time when Pablo was about 16 and was in and out of trouble with the law and drugs. He was arrested, and a judge ordered him to a drug detox program and a treatment facility. Pablo interjected that he worked with a counselor there and had been involved in a Twelve-Step program (Narcotics Anonymous) ever since. The therapist commended him for turning his life around and then asked him how Ms. Ramos and the family had supported him in this process. Pablo said, "She never gave up on me." Ms. Ramos was in tears.

The therapist faced two difficult decisions. She wanted to validate Ms. Ramos's love and caring, but she also sought to address her enabling and codependency. At the same time, the therapist did not want to leave Arturo out by artificially setting Pablo up as the "good son." The therapist therefore turned to Ms. Ramos and said, "So you went along with the judge and still continued to support your son. What stopped you from trying to get the judge to let him out?" She replied, "It was helping him."

The therapist then included Arturo and asked for his thoughts on what had been said. He hesitated and then turned to his mother and said, "I wish you had done that for me." He explained that his mother had always talked the judges, police, and school authorities out of punishing him. The therapist tried to reframe this comment by saying, "So you knew your mother loved you, but you wished she could have used more 'tough love.'" Arturo said, "Yes." The therapist asked Arturo what he wanted for his son. He said, "For him to be clean of drugs." The therapist asked him to talk to his mother about this wish. In a very passionate discussion, both Arturo and Pablo emphasized that Ms. Ramos was a loving mother and grandmother, and that they all needed to show "tough love" now in order to get Ramon the help he needed. Ms. Ramos tearfully agreed.

In the next session, the therapist discussed with Ms. Ramos, Arturo, and Pablo the possibility of doing an "intervention" (Morgan & Litzke, 2013) at the juvenile detention facility with Ramon. The therapist explained the process whereby each family member would tell Ramon of their love and each would express their fears for him if he continued on his present path. In order to empower Arturo, the therapist asked him to call the counselor at the juvenile detention center and Ramon's probation officer and ask for a meeting.

The family session held at the juvenile detention center included Ramon, Pablo, Arturo, Ms. Ramos, the therapist, the juvenile detention counselor, and the probation officer. All of the family members told Ramon of their love and stressed that he must get help. In a very large step, Ms. Ramos told him that, with his father and uncle's support, she was going to ask the judge to mandate drug treatment for him. Ramon initially was angry and resistant, but he also seemed quite surprised by this turn of events. Finally, the probation officer reported that Ramon's choices were few. If he did not agree to report for drug treatment, the judge might decide to sentence him as an adult, in which case Ramon would be sent to prison rather than a juvenile facility. Ramon looked frightened and was now willing to consider drug treatment. When Ramon asked the therapist what drug treatment entailed, the therapist asked his father to describe it to Ramon. After Arturo explained the process, Ramon acceded to his family's wishes and agreed to enter drug treatment.

The entire family supported the "tough love" position of mandated drug treatment when they appeared in court several days later. Ramon entered a residential drug treatment program and began working on his GED as part of the program (Boyd-Franklin & Bry, 2000).

DISCUSSION

As these case examples show, even families facing seemingly intractable multigenerational problems can be aided by trained family therapists to recognize the causes of their pain and to begin, with help, not to let their past dictate their future. The pitfall for family therapists is to ignore patterns of repetitive crises and attempt to "fix" each problem as it arises. This may, in fact, exacerbate a family's situation as the members unconsciously increase their acting-out behaviors.

This last case with its multigenerational issue of drug abuse and the central role of a grandmother serving as a kinship caregiver represents a particular type of family often seen in our work with at-risk adolescents. It illustrates the importance of recognizing the strengths that may lie in families when they present with serious problems (Boyd-Franklin & Bry, 2000).

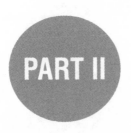

PART II

THE MULTISYSTEMS MODEL
AND HOME-BASED
FAMILY THERAPY

CHAPTER 6

An Overview of the Multisystems Model and Home-Based Family Therapy

M any therapists have been trained to work primarily with individuals. Even with their systems focus, many family therapists often confine their interventions to the nuclear family. This is unfortunate, since all of our clients are embedded in complex interactions with different systemic levels (e.g., individual, family, extended family, friends, peers, schools, churches, community) (Boyd-Franklin, 1989, 2003). This chapter presents an overview of the Multisystems Model, which has been the central theoretical model guiding our work with at-risk adolescents and their families (Boyd-Franklin, 1989, 2003; Boyd-Franklin & Bry, 2000; Boyd-Franklin et al., 2013; Hines & Boyd-Franklin, 2005). As indicated in Chapter 1, Boyd-Franklin introduced the Multisystems Model in her book, *Black Families in Therapy: A Multisystems Approach* (1989). This was the first book to provide a combination of a Multisystems Model with a multicultural approach to the treatment of African American families. This approach offers a conceptual framework that can empower the therapist to obtain and organize information about clients and their families and to intervene at different systems levels.

The Multisystems Model builds on the ecological framework of Bronfenbrenner (1979) and has features in common with the work of many prominent researchers and clinical scholars in the family therapy field (Aponte, 1995; Boyd-Franklin, 1989, 2003; Boyd-Franklin & Bry, 2000; Boyd-Franklin et al., 2013; Haley, 1976; Henggeler et al., 2009; Minuchin, 1974; Minuchin, Colapinto, & Minuchin, 2006). It represents a combination of structural family therapy (Minuchin, 1974; Nichols, 2011), strategic (Haley, 1976), and behavioral/family systems (Robin & Foster, 2002) approaches.

The first part of this chapter introduces this model and describes its value to families of at-risk adolescents, particularly poor families, who are involved with many systems. One essential aspect of the model involves reaching out to systems and individuals that will help to facilitate needed change. Within the framework of the Multisystems Model, we have found that home-based family therapy has many advantages when the therapist is working with families who might not be willing to participate in office-based treatment. This chapter begins with a discussion of the model. The second part of the chapter provides a framework for conducting home-based family therapy within the Multisystems Model, including (1) basic principles, (2) suggestions for meeting challenges often encountered when using this approach, (3) the four stages of the initial home-based therapy session, (4) the use of the genogram, and (5) problem-solving strategies that will enable families to resolve difficult issues. Imparting problem-solving skills is a key component of future sessions once the therapist has helped the family to clarify the immediate problems that need to be addressed and their overall goals.

THE MULTISYSTEMS MODEL

Poor clients and families are vulnerable to a wide range of outside systems, such as the schools, police, courts, juvenile justice system, and child welfare agencies, which may exercise a considerable amount of power in their lives (Boyd-Franklin et al., 2013). In addition, many of these clients and families are also vulnerable to societal stressors, such as poverty, homelessness, racism, discrimination, sexism, and homophobia (Boyd-Franklin, 2003; Boyd-Franklin & Bry, 2000; Boyd-Franklin et al., 2013). In accordance with this complexity, our Multisystems Model has nine levels, as listed below (see also Figure 6.1):

- Level I   Individual
- Level II   Family Subsystems
- Level III   Family Household
- Level IV   Extended Family
- Level V   Nonblood Kin and Friends, Including the Adolescent's Peers
- Level VI   Churches, Schools, and Community Resources
- Level VII   Social Service Agencies and Outside Systems (Child Welfare, Police, Courts, etc.)

- Level VIII Work
- Level IX   External Societal Forces (poverty, racism, discrimination, sexism, etc.).

Reaching Out in the Multisystems Model

Many of our clients and families have a history of negative experiences with schools, child protective services, the police, the courts, probation officers, and other systems. Coupled with the culturally based healthy cultural suspicion discussed in Chapter 3, it was often difficult to engage these families in office-based treatment. We discovered, however, that engagement of these families could often be facilitated by reaching out through home-based family interventions. In addition, given that the Multisystems Model recognizes that individuals and families are embedded within multiple systems and levels, the process of reaching out led us to connect with schools, the courts, and many of the other systems important in the lives of these clients and families.

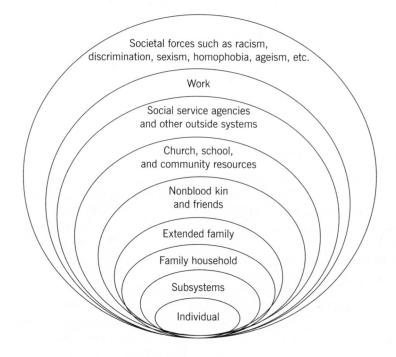

FIGURE 6.1. The multisystems model. Adapted from Boyd-Franklin (2003, p. 242). Copyright © 2003 The Guilford Press. Adapted by permission.

Reaching Out to Schools

One extremely important component of the Multisystems Model involves the process of reaching out to schools (Boyd-Franklin & Bry, 2000). Chapters 10 through 14 describe the process of reaching out to at-risk adolescents within schools through the Achievement Mentoring Program. Many clinicians, who provide home-based family therapy or office-based family therapy in clinics, agencies, and hospitals, have found that the presenting problems of their adolescent clients include serious academic and behavior problems in their schools. Therefore, it is important for these clinicians to reach out to the schools that their clients attend. In some cases, a school visit may be possible; in others, clinicians have found that it is helpful to call guidance counselors or to utilize technology and explore websites, email teachers or counselors, or arrange conferences by Skype or conference calls. As indicated in the next section, these conferences or conference calls may include representatives of other systems.

One of the challenges that therapists face in working with families involved with many systems is that each system may have a different and sometimes contradictory viewpoint and expectation. When attempting to navigate these systems on their own, clients are often left feeling confused, overwhelmed, frustrated, and angry. One strategy we have found particularly helpful in these situations has been to arrange a multisystems case conference or a conference call in which all stakeholders are invited to participate (see the Multisystems Model case example in Chapter 8) (Boyd-Franklin & Bry, 2000; Boyd-Franklin et al., 2013).

Multisystems Case Conference

The multisystems case conference or conference call gives the family the opportunity to collaborate and agree on the prioritization of specific problems, goals, and intervention strategies with the various systems impacting their lives (Boyd-Franklin, 2003; Boyd-Franklin & Bry, 2000; Boyd-Franklin et al., 2013). It is crucial that the therapist utilize this process to empower the family, particularly the parents or caregivers, to be a central part of calling the meeting, setting the agenda, and determining the goals to be achieved. In some cases, therapists have found it helpful to ask the parents or caregivers to make a list of the issues they would like to address in a session prior to the case conference. Some parents are further empowered by role-playing the issues with the therapist prior to the meeting so that they can take a major role in leading the meeting. For example, in the case example in Chapter 8, we discuss how the therapist involved the parents in contacting the school and the probation officer to participate in the multisystems case conference.

Identifying Family Strengths, Positive Prosocial Peers, and Social Supports

The strength-based approach presented throughout this book requires that the therapist both identify and validate the family's strengths. The approach allows the therapist to go beyond the nuclear family and to identify strengths and supports that may exist at many systems levels in the extended family; individuals who are very close to the family but not related by blood; friends; positive prosocial adolescent peers; the school; the church; the neighborhood; and the community (Boyd-Franklin, 2003; Boyd-Franklin et al., 2013). For example, in the Multisystems Model case example in Chapter 8, the therapist empowers the family to identify (1) an extended family member who can help with child care; (2) a member of the church family who can translate at school and court meetings for the Spanish-speaking parents; and (3) programs in the church for adolescents which can connect them to prosocial peers and keep them away from delinquent peers, after school, on weekends, and during the summer. Thus, by widening the lens of treatment beyond the individual and the family, the therapist can collaborate with the family to identify strengths and supports that can help the parents or caregivers to become more effective in parenting and monitoring their children. This process is helped by reaching out to the family through home-based family treatment.

A FRAMEWORK FOR HOME-BASED FAMILY THERAPY

Home-based family therapy offers a rare opportunity to observe family interactions *in vivo* and provides significant advantages over office-based family treatment. For example, office-based family therapists often struggle to engage key family members who are reluctant to come into an office. As shown in Chapter 3, reluctance to attend office treatment sessions is common among ethnic minority families, but it can be even more prevalent among immigrant families when some or all family members have an undocumented status (Falicov, 2005, 2014; Garcia-Preto, 2005). Family members who are residing illegally in the United States are often terrified of deportation and thus may avoid social service agencies and institutions, such as hospitals, clinics, and schools. Once a family therapist has established trust, these family members may feel safe enough to take part in sessions, particularly when they can be conducted in the home.

A further advantage of home-based sessions is that in many working poor households, parents or caregivers have to work long hours, sometimes at more than one job, in order to earn enough to survive. A home-based therapist may be of help to parents or caregivers by empowering them to negotiate times, particularly for school-based meetings (see Chapter 8), which may be more accommodating to their job situation. Unlike middle-class and professional families, these parents or caregivers often have jobs that do not permit them to take time off to attend important meetings in the school or to make court appearances. They risk losing their only means of financial support if they do so.

As introduced in Chapter 1, there are six key areas in which home-based treatment may be preferable to office-based treatment (Berg, 1994; Boyd-Franklin & Bry, 2000) as it provides the family therapist with the opportunity to:

- Meet important members of family, extended family, and friend support networks, most of whom would be unlikely to attend an office session.
- Engage the truly powerful figures in the family in the treatment process.
- Get a firsthand view of the family's living situation, especially of stressors such as poverty, substandard housing, drugs, overcrowding, crime, and an unsafe neighborhood.
- Be exposed to the culture of the family (the food, music, language, support system, religion, spirituality, etc.).
- Observe the family's child-rearing practices.
- Experience the home through the family members' eyes.

For family therapists who conduct in-office sessions, even one well-timed home visit may be crucial to a successful outcome in treatment.

Guidelines for Office-Based Therapists: Making One Important Home Visit

Many therapists who treat families in their clinic or agency office often face a dilemma when they have worked with a family (e.g., a mother and children) over a period of time, but nothing has changed. There often may be other family members who may live with the family or be involved on a regular (even daily) basis, such as the father of the children, the mother's boyfriend, the mother's girlfriend, a grandmother, grandfather, an aunt, or another extended family member, whose participation may be necessary for positive change to occur. In these instances, it may be helpful to construct a genogram (or family tree) with the family to identify these critical individuals. For example, in many African American and other ethnic minority families (see Chapter 3), these individuals may be very involved in child rearing and may even have more power in the household than the parent; however, they may be reluctant to come in to the office for therapy. With the parents' written permission, the therapist may contact such key individuals and invite them to join a session. If this does not lead to a positive result, the therapist might get the parent's permission to come to the home for a session and to invite the significant family member(s) to attend. This one home-based session can sometimes change the course of the treatment and, in ideal situations, may result in the key family member(s) agreeing to join the family sessions in the office. The following guiding principles can be helpful for therapists conducting home-based family therapy sessions, whether for one session or on a regular basis.

Principles of Home-Based Therapy

The guiding principles for conducting home-based family interventions, discussed later in this chapter in more detail, are as follows:

1. Remember your own "home training."
2. You are on the clients' "home turf."
3. When in doubt, join.
4. Never underestimate the power of praise.
5. The effective use of self is the most powerful technique.
6. Empowerment of the parents or caregivers is the goal, not helping (Boyd-Franklin & Bry, 2000).

Remember Your Own "Home Training"

It may be disorienting or difficult at first for family therapists who have been trained to conduct treatment in their offices to surrender that degree of control and treat clients and families in their homes. Clinicians who make this extra effort, however, will be amply rewarded when this intervention empowers clients and families to change. Family therapists can benefit greatly from the exercise of putting themselves in the family members' position and considering how they might feel if an uninvited stranger came into their home asking painful, difficult, and sometimes intrusive questions. Imagine further that the person is there at the behest of an outside authority, such as the school or the courts, and that family members are mandated to comply. Given this complex context, it is not unusual for family members to be guarded and uncomfortable in the first home-based session; however, family therapists can do a great deal to put family members at ease during this first contact. Never underestimate the value of a pleasant personality and personal warmth (Boyd-Franklin & Bry, 2000).

You Are on the Client's "Home Turf"

For family therapists or other clinicians used to structured office sessions, home-based interventions can present a number of challenges. Unlike an office environment in which the family comes into the therapist's domain, the therapist is entering the family's world in a home-based session (Boyd-Franklin, 2003; Boyd-Franklin & Bry, 2000). One rule for the first session is to learn to "go with the flow" of the family. Try to relax, fit in, and get to know all of those present. Do not be in a hurry on a first visit to impose rules or your own sense of order. An error sometimes made by beginning family therapists is to try to draw too rigid a boundary around the family in a first session. If visitors arrive during a session, greet them, and ask the parents or caregivers whether they are comfortable talking now or whether they would prefer for you to return later. Do not continue with an exploration of personal family matters without the consent of the parents or caregivers. Take your cues from them.

Even when the family members are expecting the therapist's visit, the therapist is likely to find them in the middle of their normal family activity. They may be eating, children may be watching television, adolescents may be listening to music or dancing, or parents with small children may be changing a baby's diaper or feeding a child. Be prepared for family members to be engaged in activities that therapists would not necessarily be doing when expecting a visitor. For example, one of our student family therapists was surprised to find a grandmother at the kitchen sink washing her hair. Another was told that the visit was limited to 15 minutes because that was all the time this African American mother had left before she needed to wash the relaxer out of her daughter's hair (Boyd-Franklin & Bry, 2000).

In some families, the tone may change dramatically if the father, boyfriend, or father figure is home. This is particularly true for families who are receiving TANF funds (see Chapter 4) for the care of their children and who may be afraid that the family therapist will jeopardize their financial support by reporting the presence of a man in the home. Even though it has been many years since this was the case legally in the former welfare system, some families may remember these fears from their own early years.

When in Doubt, Join

Sometimes eager family therapists make the mistake of "getting down to business" too quickly in the first session. We often tell family therapists in home-based work that their main task in the first session is to be allowed to return for a second session. This is particularly important when there is a mandate to work within a limited time frame. The first session may be utilized more beneficially by chatting in a friendly manner with all family members and getting to know them. Joining is one of the most important interventions, particularly with ethnic minority families (Berg, 1994; Boyd-Franklin, 2003; Boyd-Franklin & Bry, 2000). For example, some Latino families need to feel a sense of *personalismo* (Falicov, 2005, 2014; Garcia-Preto, 2005); that is, they need to feel comfortable with a person first before business can be done. Such a family may invite the therapist to join them for a meal if they are eating, or the family may prepare a special meal as a way to welcome the therapist. If food or a soft drink is offered, it is good manners to accept, especially in a first session (see Chapter 8). Although many of us were trained not to accept "gifts" from families, Latino families may feel rejected by a refusal to accept food or a small token, such as a handmade gift given at Christmas.

Young children will often offer an opportunity for joining and entry in a family session. If the therapist would not consider it too distracting, sitting down next to a child, playing with a toy, reaching out one's hand, or speaking with and engaging the child can be ways to "break the ice." It is important to observe the family members' interaction and to be actively engaging and speaking to all members (Berg, 1994; Boyd-Franklin, 2003; Boyd-Franklin & Bry, 2000).

Never Underestimate the Power of Praise

Parents or caregivers whose children are getting into trouble often feel that they are failures and that they are being blamed by others for their children's problems, particularly if families are not self-referred (Boyd-Franklin, 2003; Boyd-Franklin & Bry, 2000). This may well be the result of direct messages to that effect communicated by schools or outside agencies. Both in early joining sessions and throughout treatment, it can be beneficial to find something to praise in the behavior of parents or caregivers, especially when an adolescent's problems are the focus of treatment. Positive feedback, such as "It sounds like you have tried everything you could think of to help him," can be very helpful.

Families in which there are multiple problems often have trouble recognizing small gains (Berg, 1994). In such a family, the family therapist will often be the "container of the hope" (Boyd-Franklin et al., 2013) or belief in the possibility of change. Praising family members for small gains is an essential part of this treatment approach.

For example, a parent was complaining unrelentingly in a session about how far behind her daughter was in her homework assignments.

Not completing homework was a serious issue for the daughter, as she had passed tests in all her subjects but failed most of her courses in the previous marking period due to not handing in her homework. After trying and failing to help the mother see the progress her daughter was now making in catching up, the family therapist finally changed course to focus on the mother, rather than the daughter, and to praise the mother's efforts: "You know, I've noticed a change. Somehow you have encouraged Martha to do her homework every night this week. How did you do that?"

One rule to remember is that praise should be genuine and sincere (Berg, 1994; Boyd-Franklin & Bry, 2000). The case of a court-mandated therapy session in which the family members did not want to participate illustrates this point. The family therapist, acknowledging the one positive aspect in a father's otherwise resistant attitude, made the following statement to him: "Mr. Watson, I really admire you. You have been very honest with me about the fact that you didn't ask for this help and don't want it. I respect you a lot for coming today, even though you didn't want to, and for being here for your son."

Reframing or using positive connotation (Boyd-Franklin, 1989, 2003; Boyd-Franklin & Bry, 2000; Minuchin, 1974; Nichols, 2011) is another effective tool. For example, parents or caregivers who may be feeling very frustrated and saddened by an adolescent's misbehavior may cry during a session. These tears may be reframed as "tears of love" or "tears of strength," since some parents can view tears as a sign of weakness. An African American grandmother, who was considered a "tower of strength" by her entire family, described her fears that her grandson would become involved with drugs and "follow in his father's footsteps." She began to cry, and it was clear to the therapist that she was becoming increasingly upset and embarrassed by her inability to control her emotions. The therapist turned to her grandchild and asked, "How do you feel when you see your grandmother cry? Those are tears of strength and love that she's crying for you."

Family therapists should not be surprised or concerned if some family members resist their attempts at praise or positive reframing. Continue to do it anyway. Persistence in this approach will often eventually lead to a softening of the parental stance or attitude.

The Effective Use of Self Is the Most Powerful Technique

Aponte (1995), Aponte and Kissil (2016), and Boyd-Franklin (2003) have emphasized that the effective "use of self" is the most powerful technique family therapists can learn. Clearly, this is important in all forms of treatment, but it is essential in home-based family interventions. The effective use of self is based on a therapist's good understanding of herself or himself. The family therapist's own treatment can be helpful in facilitating this process. In training, we acquaint family therapists with genograms (McGoldrick, 2011; McGoldrick et al., 2008), and we ask each therapist to construct his or her own family's genogram. This process enables family therapists to experience for themselves the complexity of this tool and to recognize the multigenerational issues in their own families of origin. In the following case example, a consultation with her supervisor enabled a therapist to see how her own sensitive area affected her work with a family in treatment:

Janet was a beginning family therapist who was working with the Johnson family—a mother, father, and two children, ages 5 and 13—that had been referred because of the acting-out behavior of Patricia, the 13-year-old daughter. The father was authoritarian and judgmental, and often yelled at his daughter in sessions.

Janet acknowledged to her supervisor that she was frightened of the father and could not stop him or interrupt his "blaming" of his daughter. The supervisor explored with Janet what the father's behavior was evoking in her. Janet revealed that Mr. Johnson reminded her of her own father, who was also authoritarian and abusive. Janet also reported that she was working on these issues in her own treatment.

The supervisor was then able to help Janet to distinguish between Mr. Johnson and her own father. Through the technique of role-play sessions with her supervisor, Janet gradually learned to join effectively with the father in this family and to help him to connect more effectively with his daughter. She learned to use herself as a bridge to help Mr. Johnson talk to his daughter and listen to her concerns.

Empowerment of the Parents or Caregivers Is the Goal, Not Helping

Beginning family therapists, particularly when given referrals of families with many problems, often feel that they have to "fix" or "solve" these families' problems. Although this approach to addressing urgent problems may be an excellent joining technique in the initial treatment process, it should not constitute the only method by which the therapist engages with the family. As indicated earlier, it is important to impart to parents or caregivers the tools that will empower them to parent their adolescents successfully, to interact effectively with other systems, and to begin to find their own solutions (Boyd-Franklin, 2003; Boyd-Franklin & Bry, 2000; Henggeler et al., 2009) (see Chapter 8). With this in mind, family therapists must learn to give credit to parents or caregivers for the changes they make, and not to take the credit for themselves (Berg, 1994;

Boyd-Franklin & Bry, 2000; Minuchin, 1974). Helping, in the absence of empowerment, may create a dependency on the family therapist that is not healthy or beneficial to the family in the long run.

Challenges in Home-Based Family Therapy

The practice of home-based family therapy presents a number of challenges for family therapists—some similar to those faced by all family clinicians, others unique to, or exacerbated by, the nature of home-based work. This section explores a number of these challenges, including "resistance," angry clients, family conflict, and "multiproblem" families. Many clients and families, particularly those being treated by public agencies, present with one or more of these issues.

"Resistance"

We place the word "resistance" in quotation marks because client ambivalence must be viewed within the context of the nature of the referral. As discussed previously, many of the families described in this book are not self-referred but have been sent by schools, social welfare agencies, child protective services, the courts, or police authorities. Those under the court's jurisdiction have been mandated to participate. When the treatment decision is made by another party or agency, families may view it as a further intrusion into their lives (Berg, 1994; Boyd-Franklin, 2003; Boyd-Franklin & Bry, 2000; De Shazer & Dolan, 2007). Not surprisingly, families whose members did not ask for help may not be receptive to the services offered. These families and their referral sources are likely to view the need for treatment quite differently. When families feel they have been forced to participate, particularly those from ethnic minority families, they may view family therapists as part of that coercive process (Berg, 1994; Boyd-Franklin, 2003). Given this perspective, responses such as anger, resentment, and "resistance" to mandated or forced treatment should not be unexpected. A further difficulty may result if the family therapist's training has been limited to work with families whose members are self-referred and seek treatment for help with a particular problem.

Family members manifest their "resistance" in a number of ways. In an office visit, they may not arrive for their first appointment. In a home-based setting, they may not be home, or they may be home but refuse to open the door. They may also absent themselves from participating in the session by engaging in other activities (cooking, watching television, talking on the telephone, tending to a baby, etc.). Respectful persistence is vital for family therapists. Often the ability to establish rapport with such a family requires the flexibility to follow the pace and direction of the family. Such flexibility is a necessary part of training in home-based family treatment.

When families vent their anger at their sense of feeling "controlled" by others—a fairly common experience during a therapist's first encounter with them—it is important that clinicians accept and validate these feelings, and not feel obligated to defend their own or others' past actions. In fact, it is often helpful for family therapists or agency workers to distance themselves from past interventions (Berg, 1994; Boyd-Franklin, 2003; Boyd-Franklin & Bry, 2000).

It is important that family therapists be trained to expect initial "resistance" and anger from those family members who feel they are being forced to participate in treatment, and that they be prepared to work harder to engage these family members in the treatment process. Thus, they may be enabled to react more positively and will be less inclined to take negative responses personally (Boyd-Franklin & Bry, 2000; Boyd-Franklin et al., 2013).

Angry Clients

Anger Directed at Family Therapists

Clinicians should be trained to respect their clients' anger and to understand its causes and legitimacy. Anger is not only related to being forced into treatment; as shown in Chapter 3, it may also be related to culturally based trust–mistrust issues. Clients who have worked with a series of therapists and other workers from a multitude of agencies have often experienced loss, frustration, and disappointment. Anger forms a shield and serves a gatekeeping function to protect them from getting close to new therapists or child welfare workers, whom they fear will only disappoint or leave them (Berg, 1994; Boyd-Franklin, 2003; Boyd-Franklin & Bry, 2000).

Clients may also use anger as a test. This is especially relevant when working with African American families, as discussed in Chapter 3, who may need to be reassured that therapists can accept their anger over racism or other societal injustices. Family therapists' training should include role playing related to the issue of anger. It is legitimate for a family therapist to validate clients' feelings of initial distrust by asking them to discuss their experience and saying something like this: "I understand that you are very angry over the way you have been treated in the past. Can you tell me more about it?"

Another important guideline for family therapists is to avoid getting into shouting matches with clients (Berg, 1994; Boyd-Franklin & Bry,

2000). It is helpful for a therapist to demonstrate an ability to tolerate a client's anger without responding in kind. If family therapists feel anger coming on and are afraid of expressing this anger or insulting clients—a very normal reaction to an angry confrontation—they should respectfully tell the clients that they will return and resume the session at a later time. The therapists should then seek guidance from a supervisor or more experienced family therapist in order to process the anger so that it does not interfere with the therapeutic relationship.

In circumstances where a family therapist is continually embroiled in angry confrontations with a particular client or family, it may be helpful to try a cotherapy relationship in which a team of family therapists treat the family together. It also may be useful for the supervisor to accompany the therapist to a home session. After personally experiencing the client or family, the supervisor will be in a better position to offer suggestions as to how the family therapist might improve the relationship. When a family therapist feels that a relationship is so poor that it is unlikely to be improved or repaired, it may be helpful to have a case conference where a number of staff members work together to generate creative therapeutic suggestions. As agency directors and supervisors need to develop a creative, supportive learning environment for family therapists and other clinicians (Boyd-Franklin et al., 2013), comments should be framed in the most positive way.

If the suggested approaches have been tried and a relationship between a client and a therapist still has not improved, the therapist should be encouraged to discuss with his or her supervisor the possibility of transferring the case to another clinician. Although many agencies struggle with the realities of large caseloads, supervisors are encouraged to take great care to ensure, if at all possible, that no family therapist is given a disproportionate number of very difficult clients.

Anger Directed at Children and Adolescents

In addition to situations in which a client's or family's anger is directed at a therapist or agency, anger may even more commonly be manifested during a session as conflict between one or more family members, often children and adolescents. In particular, a mother, father, or caregiver, fearful of being blamed for being a "poor parent," may be very critical of an adolescent during a family session. The metamessage to the therapist is, "I am not a bad parent; he is a bad kid." Parents or caregivers who have tried everything may report giving up on an adolescent whom they describe as "no good."

Therapists often become very angry at parents who are highly critical of their adolescents or who seem to be scapegoating or rejecting them in the session. A common mistake made by family therapists is to become angry and judgmental of the parents and to side with or defend the adolescent. As a result, therapists may withdraw from these parents or caregivers, discontinue family sessions, and focus on individual treatment of the children or adolescents. This outcome is unfortunate because the essential relationship between the parents and adolescents and the nature of their communication style are not being addressed. In truth, many clinicians are afraid of parents' expression of anger.

Supervisors need to provide clinicians with a safe place in which they can address this anger so that they do not become judgmental and withdraw from or blame parents. It is helpful for clinicians to attempt to understand the parents' motivation for their anger. For many parents, particularly those living in inner-city areas, their anger masks their fears for their children. These fears include a feeling of "losing their kids to the streets," gang violence, random violence, drug and alcohol involvement, crime, trouble with the law, teenage pregnancy, and/or early death. Their anger may also reflect their feelings of powerlessness to protect their children from the enduring nature of racism. (See Chapter 3 for further discussion of these issues.)

One strategy clinicians can use in addressing this anger in parents is first to empathize with their anger and then to reframe it as fear for their adolescent. Here is an example: "I hear your anger at him for getting himself into this mess, but I also hear your fear for him. Tell me about that." When clinicians fail to reframe the words of these angry parents and thus jeopardize their ability to join with them, they are in danger of dismissing the parents' role by becoming "child rescuers" and ultimately losing these families from treatment. This potential problem should be avoided whenever possible, and it is important for supervisors to be vigilant about it.

Another strategy clinicians can use is praise. The following case example illustrates the process whereby a family therapist's persistent use of empathy, praise, and reframing was successful in softening a mother's extremely critical approach.

CASE EXAMPLE

Arlene, a 29-year-old African American single parent and mother of Tareek (age 15) and Duquan (age 10), was referred for family treatment by the courts. Tareek had been arrested during a fight on the local basketball court. Frustrated and angry, Arlene made very negative statements about her son in the first session.

ARLENE: I am sick of him. He is just no good. You want him; you take him. He can't live in my house if he's going to continue to do this crap.

THERAPIST: You really are feeling frustrated in your attempts to change his behavior. Tell me about what you have tried.

ARLENE: I'm sick of trying. I've had it.

THERAPIST: I hear you. You love him, you care about him, but you're sick of beating your head against the wall.

ARLENE: That's right, I'm tired.

THERAPIST: Yes, you've tried hard for a long time, and now you're tired.

ARLENE: I can't do it all alone any more. Take him—tell the judge to get him out of my house before he messes up his little brother.

THERAPIST: You know, Arlene, you and Tareek are not in this all alone any more. You've sought help. Now you have me. You and I are partners in figuring out how to help Tareek.

ARLENE: Partners?

THERAPIST: Yes, we're in this process together now. You two are not alone. We can work together. Are you willing to work with me to help him through this?

ARLENE: (*after a pause*) I'll try.

It is very important for a family therapist not to lose an adolescent in the process of talking to a parent or caregiver. Adolescents in these situations also feel judged or blamed and may appear angry, oppositional, and/or defiant in the session. The therapist in this case therefore made it a point to join with Tareek.

THERAPIST: Tareek, I get the sense that this has been a really hard time for you and your mom.

TAREEK: Yeah.

THERAPIST: Can you tell me about it?

TAREEK: Huh?

THERAPIST: Tell me about what this last week has been like for you.

TAREEK: Hell.

THERAPIST: What do you mean?

TAREEK: (*angrily*) It's been hell.

THERAPIST: So it's been real bad for you.

TAREEK: Yeah.

THERAPIST: I hear you. Can you describe it to me?

TAREEK: No.

THERAPIST: I understand. You don't want to talk about it right now.

TAREEK: (*shrugging*) Yeah.

THERAPIST: (*looking at Arlene and Tareek*) So the last week has been really rough for both of you. (*Both Arlene and Tareek nodded their heads.*)

Family therapists should not be offended by the monosyllabic, often angry tone of many at-risk adolescents. As we can see in this dialogue, the therapist did not try to talk Tareek out of his anger and frustration. He took whatever the adolescent told him, validated it, and moved forward. At the end, he generalized the frustration to both the parent and the adolescent. This began the process of drawing them together (Boyd-Franklin & Bry, 2000).

Families with Multiple Problems

A reality that must be acknowledged is that families referred for home-based treatment often present with many problems (see Chapter 5). When a therapist is faced with a family experiencing multiple problems, it is a normal reaction for the therapist to become overwhelmed and begin to view the situation as "hopeless" (Boyd-Franklin, 2003; Boyd-Franklin et al., 2013; Kagan & Schlossberg, 1989). Whether consciously or unconsciously, the therapist may begin to label the family pejoratively as "multiproblem" and assume that its members cannot be empowered to change.

Even the most experienced therapists may become overwhelmed by a family's problems and be tempted to "bring out the cavalry" (Berg, 1994, p. 198), pulling in many different agencies and services in an attempt to fix all of the problems. This cycle is very unfortunate and can lead to a multisystemic nightmare in which many agencies, all trying to help the client or family, give different and often conflicting solutions (Boyd-Franklin & Bry, 2000).

Berg (1994, p. 199) offered a truly elegant blueprint for charting a therapeutic course with families who present with many problems:

1. *Do Not Panic!* . . . be calm.
2. Ask the client what is the most urgent problem that he [*sic*] wants to solve first. Follow his direction, not yours. Be sure the goal is *small*, realistically achievable and simple.

3. Ask yourself who is most bothered by the problem. Make sure it is not you; you do not want to be the "customer" for your own services.
4. Get a good picture of how the client's life would change when that one goal is achieved. . . .
5. Stay focused on solving that one problem first. Do not let the fact that the client is overwhelmed affect you. . . .
6. Find out in detail how the client made things better in the past. . . .
7. Be sure to compliment the client on even the smallest progress and achievements. Always give the client the credit for successes.
8. When one problem is solved, review with the client how he solved it. What did he do that worked?

The first step begins within the family therapist. By remaining calm and not becoming swept up in the family's panic, the therapist can help to keep the family focused on one goal at a time. The first problem to be addressed should be small, manageable, and "do-able." By highlighting and validating the family's efforts, the therapist can build upon even the smallest success. The importance of good supervision in this process cannot be overestimated; the supervisor, consultant, or team of peers can help an overwhelmed therapist gain perspective on the problems and help the family to set priorities.

Stages of a Home-Based Family Session

To achieve the best results with home-based treatment, family therapists need to acquaint themselves with the protocol involved in such interventions. Jay Haley (1976), in a classic chapter on the initial interview, provides family therapists with a blueprint that can be applied to all family sessions. He divides the session as follows:

1. Joining or social stage
2. Problem stage
3. Interaction stage
4. Task setting and ending

Joining or Social Stage

The initial communication sets the tone. Family therapists should remember their own "home training" and exercise good manners by calling first, introducing themselves, and asking the family's permission to visit. Surprise visits should be avoided. When a family does not have a telephone, a note such as the following may be mailed to the home:

Hello, my name is _____. I am a counselor [or therapist] with [Name of Agency] and I would like to make a time to come and visit your family. I have time available on Tuesday evening at 5:00 P.M., June 14. Would this time be convenient for you? If not, please call me at _____ and I will be happy to schedule another time.

If I don't hear from you, I will see you on Tuesday at 5:00. I am looking forward to meeting you.

[Sign Your Name]

(Boyd-Franklin, 2003)

In some cases, it may be helpful for the family therapist to text the parent or caregiver. For agencies that provide home-based family therapy, it is very helpful to provide each therapist a work cell phone that can help to facilitate communications between family members and the therapist. If the arrangement has not been made by phone or text, however, it may take more than one visit to gain entry to the home. For example, difficulties with literacy (because of either an incomplete education or limited fluency in English) may preclude the family from reading the letter or the text. If parents or caregivers speak another language, it is often helpful to have the letter translated into their language (see Chapter 8). Even if a letter has been sent and read by a key family member or parent, other family members may not have consented to the visit.

When a therapist is visiting a family, a certain protocol is indicated. First, the therapist should introduce himself or herself at the door, ask for the parent or family member who was originally contacted by telephone, text, or letter, provide a reintroduction if necessary, and remind this person of the phone call, text, or letter. It should never be assumed that an open door is an invitation to come in. The therapist might ask, "May I come in for a short while to meet you and your family?" or "Is this a good time for a brief visit?" (Berg, 1994; Boyd-Franklin & Bry, 2000).

It is helpful to allow the client(s) to take the lead and decide where the meeting should take place. A therapist should not follow children into a home without a direct invitation from a parent or parental figure. Each person should be greeted upon entry. Some beginning family therapists are so focused on the person(s) they came to interview that they forget good manners and do not address other family members or visitors in the home directly. Saying, "Hi, how are you doing?" is often a way of acknowledging each person present. The therapist should always include children and elderly family members in the greetings. A simple "Hi, my name is _____," or "Hi, I'm [give your name], and you are . . . ?" can be helpful to put family members at their ease.

The first session should not include a great deal of note taking. This is the opportunity to try to get to know all family members and visitors, and to establish trust.

Problem Stage

In the problem stage (Haley, 1976), the therapist identifies and assesses the issue(s) with which the family needs help. With a family whose members are not self-referred, it is often beneficial to articulate the reason for their referral in a positive manner, such as the following: "Ms. _____, the counselor at the school felt that Johnny could do better in school. Many other adolescents and families have been helped by our program, and she recommended that I talk to you about it." Family therapists should be cautious, however, about aligning themselves too closely with the referral agency or school, particularly if a family has an adversarial relationship with that agency. If this is the case, family therapists might want to make it clear that they are not from the referral agency. For example, they may say, "I know that you were referred by your child welfare worker [school or other agency], but I am not from that agency and I am more interested in how you see the problem."

In the problem stage, it is important to get the opinion of all of those present about the problem. Frequently a parent, often the mother, has become the "expert" on the problem and the family spokesperson about it (Haley, 1976). This person can take over the session and not allow other family members to speak. The therapist may intervene and say, "Thank you. That was very helpful. You've given me a good idea of the problem. I'd like to go around the room now and hear everyone's opinion about this." The family therapist can then ask family members individually to describe their view of the problem. This should include the "identified patient" but should not begin with him or her. If family members interrupt, the therapist might initially not intervene in order to observe this process, but if the interruptions persist, the family therapist can say, "You have many good ideas, but I need to hear everyone's opinion. Please hold the thought, and I will come back to you a little later."

Interaction Stage

The interaction stage is a unique aspect of the structural family therapy approach (Boyd-Franklin, 1989, 2003; Boyd-Franklin & Bry, 2000; Haley, 1976; Minuchin, 1974; Nichols, 2011) that can be particularly useful in home-based interventions. Family members will typically talk to a therapist but not to each other. It is a very powerful intervention to ask two family members to talk to each other. For example, a family therapist might hold the following dialogue:

THERAPIST: Would you ask Johnny how he feels about school?

PARENT: Well, you heard him . . . how do you feel?

JOHNNY: I hate it.

PARENT: (to therapist) See, I told you so.

THERAPIST: (to parent) Can you ask Johnny to give us some examples of exactly what he hates about school?

PARENT: So exactly what do you hate?

JOHNNY: I hate the teachers. They pick on me.

PARENT: What do you mean?

JOHNNY: They accuse me of doing things I didn't do.

PARENT: Such as . . .

JOHNNY: Fighting, getting out of my seat in class. You know . . .

The family therapist thus becomes a facilitator, helping family members learn to communicate with each other.

Task Setting and Ending

In order to draw families into the treatment process, it is often helpful to assign a task at the end of each session that the family can work on before the next meeting (Boyd-Franklin & Bry, 2000; Haley, 1976; Minuchin, 1974). This is particularly important if there are long periods between sessions. A task should be straightforward and directed toward the family's empowerment. For example, the family therapist might ask a parent to visit the school once with the adolescent and speak to the guidance counselor about the adolescent's school performance. The parent should be encouraged to take the initiative in this area. If a parent is unable to do this independently (e.g., for work reasons or, in some cases, if they are too frightened), it may be helpful for the family therapist to contact the school or agency or offer to accompany the parent the first time.

Sometimes the task is a "family task." The therapist might ask a Latino or Asian family, with members who do not speak English, to talk together and choose an extended family member or close friend to invite to translate for them in the next session (see Chapters 3 and 8).

Sometimes "family time" can be prescribed. This often works well at the dinner table or before bedtime when a parent might be asked to call together all of his or her children and just ask them in turn to share how their day has been. Such tasks can help to facilitate family bonding and togetherness.

It is important that the family therapist follow up on these tasks early in the next session. At the end of a session, it is often helpful to summarize for the family members what has occurred and to help move them toward their positive goals, as in this example: "All of you have worked very hard today so that I could understand the things you have tried to change Johnny's behavior. We will work together to develop new ways in which the family can help him."

THE GENOGRAM

Genograms provide the family therapist with the opportunity to organize information about the family structure, including nuclear and extended family members (McGoldrick, 2011; McGoldrick et al. 2008) (see Chapter 8 for an example of a genogram). Some family therapists are trained to construct genograms early in the process of assessment with the family. However, when working with African American and other ethnic minority families, such as immigrant families who may have undocumented members, and who may have a healthy cultural suspicion of the process of therapy, as discussed in Chapter 3, clinicians are cautioned to join and establish a therapeutic alliance with all family members and to build trust before creating a genogram (Boyd-Franklin, 2003). This is important because exploration of the family's personal business may often be perceived as intrusive if it is done before trust has been established. In addition, family members may withhold important information and, in the worst case scenario, drop out of treatment if a therapist embarks on this process prematurely (Boyd-Franklin, 2003). Thus, it is often advisable to postpone constructing the genogram with the family until the second or even the third session when both therapist and supervisor are confident that the therapist has successfully joined. Families often do not reveal their full family genograms until they trust the therapist. Therapists should not be surprised if more family members are mentioned and the true picture emerges over time. For example, African American families may not reveal very significant "nonblood relatives," such as boyfriends or girlfriends, initially because of healthy cultural suspicion and a belief that family business should be kept in the family (see Chapter 3).

Genograms can be particularly helpful in situations where the family appears isolated from support systems. In some instances, particularly when a parent presents with a history of drug or alcohol abuse or serious mental illness, a family cutoff may have occurred from extended family members. The construction of a genogram can help identify potential family supports that might be reengaged when emotional cutoffs are addressed and healed.

IDENTIFYING AND PRIORITIZING PROBLEMS AND GOALS

In most cases, adolescents are referred with presenting problems. Therapists should review these problems with the family and add or incorporate any additional issues that are of significant concern to the parents or caregivers. It is important to look at all systems levels to identify factors that may contribute to or be involved in these problems, including the individual, family, extended family, peers, school, community, and outside systems (e.g., child protection services, the police, the courts, probation (Boyd-Franklin & Bry, 2000; Henggeler et al., 2009).

Once the problems have been identified and organized into a list, the therapist can work with the family to prioritize them. When this task is completed, therapists should then work with the family to identify clear goals. Therapists should review their progress in addressing the identified problems and assessing whether goals have been achieved regularly with their supervisor (and the supervisory group or team if available). (See the discussion of supervision in Chapter 9.) As family therapy continues, additional problems may be identified. They can be added to the list, accompanied by the factors contributing to the problems.

There are times when therapists feel pressure from the referral source, such as a school, to address a particular problem first. However, the therapist and the supervisor must remain vigilant about ordering priorities so that the problems potentially causing the most serious consequences are given the appropriate emphasis, and they should reprioritize when necessary. For example, as is described in Chapter 8, the therapist recognizes the seriousness of the academic problems of the adolescent who is failing two of his classes. He understands that the youth's association with delinquent, gang-involved peers is contributing to the problem, but he chooses to maintain his focus solely on the academic issues. In the interim, the adolescent becomes involved in a gang-related fight in the community, faces criminal charges, and comes under the jurisdiction of the juvenile justice system (i.e., the police, the courts, and a probation officer). A valuable lesson can be learned here. The therapist should clearly have prioritized intervening in the adolescent's involvement with delinquent peers earlier in the process of therapy (Dishion et al., 2003; Dodge et al., 2006). Both the academic and the peer-related issues urgently needed to be addressed. The failure to reprioritize intervening with delinquent peers contributed to other, more serious problems (Boyd-Franklin & Bry, 2000; Henggeler et al., 2009).

Do Not Overlook Concrete Problems

Many therapists are trained only to address psychological problems, which puts them at a disadvantage when working with the families of at-risk adolescents, particularly those who are poor. The advantage of the Multisystems Model is that it widens the lens of the therapist to incorporate into treatment other levels or systems impacting the family and interfering with the parents' or caregivers' ability to parent their children successfully. For example, the family that becomes homeless faces a crisis with many ramifications: (1) each child or adolescent is impacted individually; (2) the family as a whole is impacted; (3) all of the children or adolescents may need to be placed in different schools if the family is forced to move outside the area; and (4) once a family is homeless, a range of social service agencies might become involved with them.

In Chapter 4, we discussed the reality that many informal kinship care families may live in poverty. Often these families cannot pass the stringent guidelines required to become formal kinship caregivers and receive financial compensation commensurate with that received by licensed foster parents. In some cases, therapists might help the caregiver to problem-solve options and to empower them to apply for TANF funds (see Chapter 4).

Therapists may be aware of programs and resources, but it is important for therapists to remember that their task is to empower the parents or the caregivers to follow through on these referrals.

TARGETED FAMILY INTERVENTION

Targeted Family Intervention (TFI) is a home-based family therapy model developed by Bry, Greene, Schutte, and Fishman (1991). This intervention was intended to be used with the Achievement Mentoring Program (see Chapters 11–14) in the schools. At-risk adolescents who were provided both TFI and Achievement Mentoring improved their academic performance and reduced their at-risk behaviors more than adolescents who were provided with the school-based Achievement Mentoring Program alone (Boyd-Franklin & Bry, 2000; Krinsley, 1991).

TFI consists of communication training and problem solving (Boyd-Franklin & Bry, 2000; Robin & Foster, 2002). A major emphasis of this approach is on "catching the youth doing something good today" (Boyd-Franklin & Bry, 2000). Parental monitoring of adolescents behaviors is also an important part of this approach (Dishion et al., 2003; Veronneau et al., 2016). Home-based family therapy sessions are conducted in the home with adolescents and families referred by the school (i.e., teachers, counselors, principals, and other administrators (Boyd-Franklin & Bry, 2000; Krinsley, 1991). Once the TFI sessions have been completed, booster sessions have been shown to be useful 1 month afterward. The next booster session occurs 2 months after that, and the final booster session is 3 months later (Bry & Krinsley, 1992).

PROBLEM-SOLVING INTERVENTIONS

A challenge faced by many families of at-risk adolescents is that they often find themselves so overwhelmed by their problems that they become paralyzed. One task of the therapist is to help them prioritize the problem they want to address first. In addition, many families of at-risk youth may not be able to problem-solve successfully. Thus, many approaches to family therapy with these adolescents include an element of therapists helping families to learn problem-solving skills (Alexander, Waldron, Robbins, & Neeb, 2013; Boyd-Franklin & Bry, 2000; Henggeler et al., 2009; Robin & Foster, 2002; Sexton, 2011). Robin and Foster (2002) have delineated five steps in their problem-solving model: (1) define the problem to be addressed, (2) brainstorm possible solutions, (3) decide which solution to use, (4) develop plans for the implementation of the solution, and (5) renegotiate if the family is not able to resolve the conflict through the initial solution.

In the first step, the therapist asks each family member to define the problem as they see it (Robin & Foster, 2002). Robin and Foster encourage family members to reflect back each problem definition in a way that is "nonaccusatory and concise, and addresses behaviors, feelings, and situations, not personality characteristics of individuals" (p. 118). Therefore, throughout the problem-solving process, it is important that family members be encouraged to use "I" rather than "you" statements. If multiple problems are proposed, it is important for the family members to reach agreement as to the most important problem to be addressed. (Other problems should be recorded and addressed at a later point.)

In the second step, brainstorming possible solutions, the therapist encourages the family members to list a number of different ideas, avoid making judgments about these ideas until later in the process, and use their imagination because the therapist should give them unlimited leeway in suggesting ideas (Robin & Foster, 2002). The therapist might say something like, "I want you to think of the most creative, crazy ideas you can. Anything goes" (p. 122). These messages, by accentuating the positive aspects of problem solving, encourage the family members to explore novel, unusual solutions they may not have tried in the past. The therapist should write down the list of solutions.

The third step involves evaluating each suggested solution and deciding on the one to use. The therapist helps family members to discuss the positive and negative outcomes that might result from each proposed solution. The therapist can ask each family member to assign a plus or minus rating for the suggested solutions and then review the list of ratings with the family to determine their ranking from highest number of plus ratings from family members, followed by the one that received the next highest number of plus ratings, and so on. The goals are to help family members to reach a consensus around one idea or a combination of ideas that seem the most likely to resolve the conflict or problem, and to learn to negotiate with each other.

The fourth step involves helping the family to plan how to implement the solution they have decided to pursue. The plan needs to be detailed, including (1) behaviors in compliance with the plan, (2) positive outcomes for compliance, (3) behaviors not in compliance with the plan, and (4) negative consequences for noncompliance. Yet it is important that these plans be clear, straightforward, and as simple as possible (Robin & Foster, 2002). This plan should be recorded by the therapist. A further component of the plan involves helping the family to explore the problems that might occur during its implementation. Once this last element has been completed, a final plan can then be written, which includes methods the family has arrived at to address the possible problems they may encounter (Robin & Foster, 2002).

The therapist then reviews the plan with the family members. Some therapists have found it helpful to have all family members and the therapist actually sign the written plan. It is important to review the results of the plan implementation early in the next session. If the solution that was agreed upon and implemented was effective, it is important for the therapist to praise all of the family members and encourage them to continue to implement their plan. If it has not worked well, the therapist should reframe this experience as a normal part of the problem-solving process and predict that it sometimes takes a few times to find the best solution (Robin & Foster, 2002). The therapist should help the family to explore what may have gone wrong and then proceed to the fifth step: go through steps one to four again and renegotiate a new solution.

CONCLUSION

This chapter discusses our Multisystems Model. We have shared our conceptualization that the family, particularly the parents or caregivers, are the main vehicle for change and that we work to empower them to intervene effectively with their adolescents and with the other systems that may be impacting the youth's life (Boyd-Franklin, 2003; Boyd-Franklin & Bry, 2000). Because families of at-risk adolescents are often referred by outside agencies and systems, and because key members of the family may not attend office-based sessions, we have found home-based family therapy to be more successful at effecting needed change for these families. The next chapter explores multisystemic therapy (Henggeler et al., 2009), an evidence-based family therapy model that also incorporates home-based family therapy and intervenes at multiple systemic levels.

CHAPTER 7

Multisystemic Therapy

The last 30 years have witnessed a significant increase in the number of evidence-based family treatment interventions that have addressed the needs of families with at-risk youth, particularly those adolescents with antisocial behaviors such as conduct disorders, juvenile delinquency, violence, and substance abuse. These interventions have included (1) multisystemic therapy (MST) (Henggeler et al., 2009; Henggeler & Schaeffer, 2016; Schoenwald, Henggeler, & Rowland, 2016; (2) functional family therapy (Alexander et al., 2013; Sexton, 2011); (3) brief strategic family therapy (Szapocznik, Duff, Schwartz, Muir, & Brown, 2016); and (4) multidimensional family therapy (Liddle, 2005, 2016). Sexton and Lebow (2016) provide excellent chapters on each of these approaches.

This chapter focuses on MST (Henggeler et al., 2009; Schoenwald et al., 2016). Of all of the evidence-based family treatments listed above, the strategies and methods of MST are more similar to our own work than the other approaches. Although MST and our approach were developed independently, they have many features in common.

MULTISYSTEMIC THERAPY

MST was developed to address the clinical problems of at-risk youth and their families. Adolescents are considered at risk for the purposes of this program when they present with (1) antisocial behaviors such as violence, (2) involvement with the juvenile justice system, (3) status as a juvenile sexual offender, and/or (4) substance abuse issues (Henggeler & Sheidow, 2012). For almost 40 years, the program developers have published a number of clinical books on their interventions (e.g., Henggeler et al., 2009; Henggeler, Schoenwald, Rowland, & Cunningham, 2002), as well as a more specific approach for substance-abusing adolescents that combines MST with contingency management (Henggeler et al., 2012). In addition, this clinical and research team has published extensive outcome studies (see Henggeler & Sheidow [2012] for a summary of these studies).

The MST model builds on Bronfenbrenner's (1977) theory of social ecology. The theory of change underlying MST is based on the assumption that the interplay of risk factors at the family, individual, peer, school, and community or neighborhood levels contributes to the development of antisocial behavior in adolescents (Henggeler et al., 2002, 2009; Henggeler & Schaeffer, 2016). Thus, for interventions to be effective and change the behavior of at-risk adolescents, they must address the different levels of risk factors and incorporate protective factors for each level.

Inherent in the MST approach to working with this population is the assumption that caregivers are central in the process of change for adolescents. Therefore, a focus of treatment is to empower caregivers to become more effective with these youth. The therapist works collaboratively with the caregivers to identify family strengths (e.g., love, extended family members, strong cultural values) in order to overcome antisocial behaviors and improve functioning in all areas of the adolescent's life (e.g., family, school, prosocial peer group, and community). Consistent with many of the cultural strengths discussed in Chapter 3, this approach helps to mobilize supports for caregivers, including extended family members, friends, and neighbors.

MST Team Approach

Each MST team is composed of two to four master's level clinicians (psychologists, social workers, counselors, or marriage and family therapists), who each treat four to six families. This small number is in response to the demands of this intervention (Henggeler et al., 2002, 2009; Henggeler & Schaeffer, 2016). Each team has an experienced supervisor (doctoral level or advanced master's level), who meets with the team weekly for group supervision (Henggeler et al., 2009). In addition, a weekly team consultation session is held with an MST expert consultant who has had extensive experience with the model (Henggeler et al., 2002, 2009; Henggeler & Schaeffer, 2016).

Each therapist provides intensive home- and community-based services for approximately 3 to 5 months. Although, at first glance, this may appear to be a relatively short time period, given the serious presenting problems of many of the adolescents and their families, Henggeler et al. (2009) have emphasized that families often receive at least 60 hours of direct contact during this period and the team collectively provides coverage 24 hours per day, 7 days per week. Each team member, in addition to his or her flexible work schedule, is available on a rotating on-call basis and is provided with a dedicated cell phone for this purpose (Henggeler et al., 2009; Henggeler & Sheidow, 2012).

Nine Principles of MST

MST incorporates nine principles that are central to this treatment approach:

1. *Finding the fit.* The primary purpose of assessment is to understand the "fit" between the identified problems and their broader systemic context.
2. *Positive and strength focused.* Therapeutic contacts should emphasize the positive and should use systemic strengths as levers for change.
3. *Increasing responsibility.* Interventions should be designed to promote responsible behavior and decrease irresponsible behavior among family members.
4. *Present focused, action oriented, and targeting specific, well-defined problems.*
5. *Targeting sequences.* Interventions should target sequences of behavior within and between multiple systems that maintain identified problems.
6. *Developmentally appropriate and fit the developmental needs of the youth.*
7. *Continuous effort.* Interventions should be designed to require daily or weekly effort by family members.
8. *Evaluation and accountability.* Intervention efficacy is evaluated continuously from multiple perspectives, with providers assuming accountability for overcoming barriers to successful outcomes.
9. *Generalization.* Interventions should be designed to promote treatment generalization and long-term maintenance of therapeutic change by empowering caregivers to address family members' needs across multiple systemic contexts. (Henggeler et al., 2009, pp. 15–16)

In order to accomplish these principles, therapist engagement and connection with the family is necessary. The following discussion illustrates this process.

Client and Family Engagement, Developing and Maintaining Empathy

From the beginning of the assessment and treatment process in MST, it is essential that the therapist work on connecting and building a relationship with the client and the family. It is particularly important that the connection extends to the parents or caregivers as well as the adolescent. Similar to many other family therapy models (Alexander et al., 2013; Boyd-Franklin & Bry, 2000; Lebow, 2005; Sexton, 2011; Sexton & Lebow, 2016), MST emphasizes the importance of building the therapeutic alliance through client engagement. Developing empathy for the client and the family is essential to achieve this goal.

Empathy requires that the therapist be able to experience the internal world of each family member. Henggeler et al. (2009) have observed that it is much easier for therapists to maintain empathy and compassion for a client or family when they perceive the client as deserving or as a victim. It is much more challenging to maintain empathy with clients who seem to be unwilling to commit to changing negative behavioral patterns—for example, an adolescent who continually engages in antisocial behavior or a parent who resumes drug use.

With these challenges in mind, Henggeler et al. (2009) recommended that family therapists continually monitor and refresh their feelings of empathy for their clients. One intervention that these authors recommend for therapists who find themselves frustrated with a client is the "cup of coffee" intervention (p. 44). The therapist is encouraged by the supervisor to suspend efforts briefly to intervene, make change, or convince the client to change, and to have an informal meeting with the client in order to try to join with, and try to take the perspective of, the client. This strategy often results in the beginning of a therapeutic alliance and the rekindling of empathy in the therapist. Another important part of fostering client engagement and empathy is the use of warmth, expressed in different ways. It may include leaning in toward the client or even responding to a caregiver's hug at the end of an important session (Henggeler et al., 2009).

Reflective Listening

Based on the work of Miller and Rollnick (2009, 2012), reflective listening is a very important component of Motivational Interviewing and has now been incorporated into many family treatment interventions, including MST (Henggeler et al., 2009). Reflective listening requires the therapist to summarize the content and, even more important in some cases, the underlying meaning of the client's statements. It conveys that the therapist is listening and understands what the client is communicating.

Sometimes the therapist might focus on one word or concept ("Tell me more about feeling desperate."). In other cases, the therapist may focus on the underlying message ("You're feeling really frustrated right now and don't know what else to try.") (p. 46).

Reframing

Reframing is another important technique utilized in many family therapy interventions, including MST (Boyd-Franklin, 2003; Henggeler et al., 2009; Lebow, 2005; Minuchin, 1974; Nichols, 2011; Sexton & Lebow, 2016). The purpose of the reframe is to provide the family with an alternative way of viewing, describing, or labeling a situation or a person. For example, when treating the family of an at-risk adolescent, the therapist can reframe angry statements by parents as an indication of the worry or intense fear they feel for their child. When treating an enmeshed extended family in which everyone speaks for the adolescent, the therapist might tell family members that they "love her too much" (Minuchin, 1974).

Therapist Flexibility

The ability of the therapist to respond to an upsetting situation without judgment and with an ability to step in and problem-solve a solution is central to this approach. Sometimes this approach involves the ability to remain calm in a crisis situation or to not take it personally when clients are critical or dismissive of the therapist or the therapy. For example, it is not unusual for therapists to work hard over a number of weeks to put a plan in place for the adolescent. When the plan does not have the intended result, the family and the therapist may feel discouraged and frustrated. Despite the therapist's deep investment in the plan, his or her ability to recognize that something is not working and to try something different is an extremely important skill that can increase family engagement.

Other Strategies to Increase Engagement

Henggeler et al. (2002, 2009) have described a number of nonclini-cal strategies to increase engagement with clients. They recommended that therapists invite families to share photos when they discuss their genograms or that therapists ask about photos displayed in the home on a home visit. Bringing food to the family session may be a way to "get in the door" or to engage family members who normally stay in a back room for most of a home-based session (Henggeler et al., 2009, p. 48). Providing help with practical needs may be a way for therapists to join with a family. Offering concrete information about after-school or sports programs can be very helpful to families. This information can serve an additional purpose if the therapist uses this as a method to empower caregivers by suggesting that they follow up on a plan to investigate these services.

Assessment of Problems and Strengths, and Setting Goals

At intake, the MST therapist works with the family to develop a genogram to clarify the family structure and identify possible family supports (Henggeler et al., 2009; McGoldrick, 2011; McGoldrick et al., 2008). A list of presenting problem behaviors, including their frequency and duration, is developed. At each level (individual, family, school, peer, and community), both systemic strengths and weaknesses are listed. Once this comprehensive data is completed, the therapist clarifies the explicit overarching goals for treatment with the family. This genogram is later shared with the MST team (Henggeler et al., 2009). It is very important that these goals (1) are directly connected to the adolescent's presenting problems, (2) are written clearly, (3) target specific problem behaviors and focus on reducing them, and (4) provide standards for measuring whether the goals have been achieved.

Henggeler et al. (2009) described the overall analytic process of MST as follows:

1. The therapist aligns with the family and works with family members and key stakeholders to develop a clear consensus of the overarching goals.
2. The therapist works with the family and other sources of information, taking care to look within and between systems and to understand the "fit" of the referral behaviors (i.e., how they make sense) within the context in which the youth and family are embedded.
3. The team and family members prioritize hypothesized drivers of the identified problems and develop interventions to address the drivers.
4. These interventions are implemented, and any barriers to effective implementation are identified.
5. Finally, therapists assess the outcomes of their interventions from multiple perspectives to determine if they are having the intended effects. If not, the information gained during this process is fed back into the loop, and therapists work to develop new hypotheses and modified interventions based on these revised hypotheses. (p. 18)

One unique aspect of the MST model is the construction of *fit circles* (Henggeler et al., 2009, pp. 22–24), which are a part of the systemic assessment and the development of hypotheses about the possible causes of referral problems and other behavioral concerns. These fit circles evolve from the brainstorming sessions that therapists engage in with the family and conduct with the MST team members. During these sessions, broad issues at all systemic levels are considered as possible contributors to the problems. As new hypotheses are developed concerning the problems, new fit circles are developed.

Supervision, Team Meetings, and Weekly Review Process

Each week, in preparation for supervision with the MST team, the therapist completes a weekly review form (Henggeler et al., 2009). This form includes (1) the overall MST goals for treatment written in a clear behavioral format, including a clear statement of how completion of each goal will be measured; (2) the prior week's intermediary goals and an assessment of whether or not they were met; (3) the problems or barriers encountered that prevented achievement of those goals; and (4) any advances or successes in the treatment process. During the supervision session with the MST, two additional elements are integrated into the review form. First, the therapist and the MST team reexamine the referral problems and goals, and incorporate any new knowledge that they have learned during that week. If necessary, they develop new hypotheses about what might be driving or contributing to the problems and create new *fit circles*. Second, the therapist works with the MST team to develop new intermediary goals for the coming week (Henggeler et al., 2009).

This process of ongoing assessment, essential to evidence-based MST, maintains the clear focus of the therapist and the MST team on the goals and outcomes at each stage of the intervention (Henggeler et al., 2009).

Family Interventions within MST

Assessing Family Relations

MST therapists assess a variety of family relations, including parent–child interactions; quality of interpersonal relationships in terms of warmth and affection; parental control strategies; monitoring; and assessing the marital relationship (Henggeler et al., 2009). Therapists also perform an additional assessment concerning the various parenting styles—authoritative, authoritarian, permissive, or neglectful. As

Baumrind (2005) explained, authoritative parents display warmth and affection toward their children and have clear rules and expectations. Authoritarian parents demonstrate low warmth toward their children and may have an overcontrolling style that may often include physical punishment. Permissive parents often show a great deal of warmth to their children but do not provide them with clear rules, consequences for their behavior, or discipline. Neglectful parents may show little warmth or caring for their children and often show no interest in parenting. MST therapists learn about family styles and interaction patterns by questioning caregivers and children, observing family interaction patterns, and requesting that family members pay attention to, and keep a record of, particular behaviors (Henggeler et al., 2009).

Motivating Parents to Change and Sustaining Parental "Buy In"

Throughout their work, Henggeler et al. (2009) have emphasized the importance of therapists focusing on family strengths and keeping caregivers engaged in the process. This is crucial because many caregivers often feel burnt out and frustrated, and feel they have failed. Their sense of failure may often stem from the messages conveyed by schools, the police, juvenile courts, child protective services, and other agencies that they are to blame for their children's problems. It is important to engage caregivers in a discussion of the things they have tried to help their child. The therapist who implies that caregivers are to blame for the adolescent's problems will have difficulty establishing and maintaining a relationship with them and other family members.

One challenge that therapists face is trying to help parents to change their parenting strategies, particularly concerning discipline. Establishing discipline involves setting clear rules for the youth and developing consequences, including positive rewards and punishments. In tackling this challenge, the therapist works to brainstorm with the caregivers the types of rules that will address the problems that have been identified and the goals that have been set. In some cases, the therapist may engage in problem solving with the family, including both the caregivers and the adolescent. One challenge for many caregivers is that they may be unprepared for the responsibility of monitoring the adolescent closely. They often may not know the at-risk adolescent's friends and may have no sense of their activities outside of the home. Many parents learn that they have inadvertently rewarded their child for negative behaviors by allowing them to have privileges they have not earned. Privileges might include using a cell phone; playing video games; downloading and watching movies; being allowed to go outside; and getting special treats, such as ice cream, snacks, a trip to an amusement park, or shopping at the mall. Henggeler et al. (2009) recommended that MST therapists develop a behavioral chart with columns for rules, privileges, consequences, days, and whether the rule was followed (yes or no).

Many at-risk adolescents are very invested in their behaviors and their friends. Therefore, it may be helpful to prepare the caregivers for the possible resistance they may confront initially from adolescents as they attempt to provide more monitoring and structure. In this situation, parents or other caregivers will need the support of the family therapist and others in their support network to continue being consistent with the consequences they have developed (Henggeler et al., 2009).

The therapist may implement numerous family systems interventions that are standard in many family therapy models. For example, family members might be encouraged to engage in a problem-solving session around a particular problem (Robin & Foster, 2002). MST also incorporates structural family therapy techniques such as asking the more disengaged parent to talk with the adolescent directly about a particular issue (Minuchin, 1974). A task might be used within a family session, or as a homework assignment, in order to focus the family's energy on addressing and changing specific behaviors. When designing homework tasks, therapists are encouraged to keep them simple and to fit them to the needs and demands that the family faces. It is particularly important to follow up in the next session and review the outcome of assigned tasks (Henggeler et al., 2009).

Increasing Social Supports for Families

Caregivers in families of at-risk adolescents may feel overwhelmed, frustrated, and isolated, particularly when caregivers are working and/or are raising multiple children. They may need outside support to facilitate the positive change in an at-risk youth's life. Help may come in the form of obtaining financial assistance, monitoring adolescents after school while a parent is at work, or driving the youth to a sport practice or a game. Help may also be in the form of emotional support for parents, who may find it very difficult to set limits with adolescents who continue to act out. Sometimes the social support may be provided by someone in the community who is aware of all the resources available for youth (e.g., after-school programs, basketball leagues, job training programs).

Some families of at-risk adolescents face additional challenges, such as poverty or a lack of stability in their living situation, such as eviction, foreclosure, homelessness, or frequent moves, that leave them feeling they have no social supports. Sometimes parents who have had serious problems, such as drug or alcohol abuse or serious mental illness, may have had ongoing conflicts with family and extended-family members, resulting in severely damaged relationships and/or their separation from those individuals.

If that is the case, parents or caregivers may be reluctant initially to ask for help from family or extended family members and even to access social supports in their communities (Henggeler et al., 2009). In these situations, the therapist works with the caregivers to reframe the need for help and to focus on the serious situation the adolescent is experiencing.

For many African American, Latino and other ethnic minority families, blood and nonblood family supports may often exist but are not being utilized by the caregiver. (See Chapter 3 for more information on the cultural strengths regarding extended family that can be mobilized to help in times of trouble.)

Peer Interventions

Deviant peers, a major risk factor for adolescents, often contribute to antisocial and other problematic behaviors (Dishion et al., 2012; Dodge et al., 2006). Howell (2003) has shown that many adolescents engage in juvenile delinquent activities with their peers. Although proactive caregivers often sign their children and adolescents up for a basketball or other sports team in the community, or another positive youth activity through a church, YWCA or YMCA, or Boys or Girls Club, or other activities, many caregivers of at-risk adolescents involved in antisocial activities often have little, if any, connection to their child's peer group. Nor do they have knowledge of their child's life outside of the home (Henggeler et al., 2009).

MST therapists are trained to do an assessment of the adolescent's peer group (Henggeler et al., 2009). This assessment might involve questioning the youth, caregivers, other family and extended family members, teachers, guidance counselors, and other school staff; observing adolescents in their peer group at the school or in the community; and in some cases, interacting directly with peers. As indicated earlier, fit circles are then constructed which clarify the ways in which the peer group and other systemic levels contribute to an identified problem.

Interventions often focus on decreasing contact with delinquent peers and involving the adolescent in prosocial activities with new peers (e.g., sports, youth groups at church, school extracurricular activities, a job). Therapists work to help caregivers increase their contact with the adolescent's peers and, if possible, with the peers' parents or caregivers. With the family therapist's support, caregivers are helped to implement serious unpleasant consequences for the youth's involvement with problematic peers and to reward association with positive peers (Henggeler et al., 2009).

It is also helpful for the therapist to spend time with the adolescent discussing his or her dreams, interests, skills, or areas in which they feel they have ability or special gifts. This discussion might also be held with family members. The therapist can then work with the youth, the caregivers, family members, school, and other resources in the community to identify positive activities that would be of interest to the adolescent.

Gangs

Among the most serious indications of an adolescent's association with a deviant peer group is affiliation with a gang. Howell (2003, 2012) and Howell and Griffiths (2016) have investigated the impact of gangs on adolescent antisocial behavior and juvenile delinquency. Henggeler et al. (2009) have pointed out that groups of adolescents may appear to be gang affiliated if they dress in a certain manner or use gang symbols, but this might be an affectation, rather than evidence of formal gang membership. Moreover, research findings lend a note of optimism to the process of changing the behavior of youth who are gang-involved or connected with deviant peers (Henggeler et al., 2009; Howell, 2003, 2012; Howell & Griffiths, 2016). Only one-third of gang members remain in gangs for more than a year despite the perception that theirs is a long-term involvement. Moreover, many adolescents who have been gang members have been able to find positive peer relationships once they leave the gang.

The therapist can problem-solve with the adolescent; the family; concerned members of the school staff, such as guidance counselors, teachers, and the principal; and other involved professionals, such as probation officers, to explore possible alternative prosocial activities in the community (see Chapter 8).

School

As is indicated in Chapter 10, many at-risk adolescents present with school-related problems, such as school disengagement, academic failure, truancy, suspension, and fighting or other acting-out behaviors (Henggeler et al., 2009). As school is such an important part of the life and job of adolescents, it is extremely important that these issues be addressed before it is too late and the adolescent has been expelled or has dropped out (see Chapter 10). School dropout has both short- and long-term consequences. In the short term, not attending school, whether because of dropout or common pre-dropout experiences of truancy and repeated out-of-school suspensions, can often lead to increased time with peers involved in antisocial or delinquent and possibly criminal activities (Howell, 2003). In the long term, school dropout can impede the ability to earn a viable income as an adult.

Assessing the Fit of School Problems

Henggeler et al. (2009) have identified a number of issues that contribute to the fit of school-related problems: (1) individual factors (e.g., ADHD, cognitive problems, learning disabilities); (2) family factors (e.g., support for education and homework at home, parental monitoring, parental warmth, positive clear behavioral consequences, consistency); (3) poor connection between the family and the school; (4) deviant peers (e.g., peers who make fun of the adolescent for doing well in school); (5) school factors (e.g., resources, appropriate classroom settings, structure, willingness to work with the adolescent, the family and the therapist); and (6) neighborhood or community factors (e.g., poverty, crime and other safety issues).

It is particularly helpful if therapists can arrange to meet with school personnel, such as teachers, counselors, and school administrators, to assess the nature of the school problems. School personnel may not be receptive to discussing such sensitive issues on the phone without prior contact, so it may be helpful to send an email initially and later arrange for phone conference calls. If it is at all possible, observing the adolescent in classes can be particularly helpful. It can also be useful to ask teachers to define the problem behaviors and to identify both the antecedents and consequences of the behavior.

In some cases, the therapist may discuss with the caregivers and the school the possibility of referring the adolescent for psychological testing, which might include intelligence and achievement testing. Instruments such as the Conners Comprehensive Behavior Rating Scales can also be given to teachers and caregivers to get an accurate picture of the youth's behavior in different settings and classes. Family therapists will sometimes work with families to advocate for the referral for psychological testing and to follow up on the process. In some cases, such as situations in which the school is ruling out ADHD, the school may also recommend referral to a pediatric neurologist or psychiatrist for an assessment to determine if medication would be useful in helping the adolescent become less distractible in his or her classes.

School Interventions

Throughout this book, we have indicated that among the most important interventions are those that help to connect parents or family caregivers with the school. Caregivers, who may have been actively involved with their child's teachers when the child was in elementary school, often face far greater challenges once their child is in middle and high school. Students do not remain in the same classroom with the same teacher for each subject as they did in elementary school. They now have complicated schedules and multiple teachers. Some working parents may not have access to email or be able to make or receive phone calls at work, leaving them unable to have any contact with the school during the school day. These difficulties with communication can begin a dance of disengagement in which the school becomes frustrated and begins to label parents as disinterested, and hard-working parents feel increasingly judged by school authorities who make little, if any, effort to accommodate the parents' schedules. In these types of circumstances, the family therapist can be instrumental in establishing a positive collaboration between the parents and the school. Empowering parents or caregivers to learn to create and sustain connections with the school is a crucial skill that can contribute to their ability to advocate for the identified adolescent and all of their other children (Henggeler et al., 2009).

Meetings between the School and the Family

Often families of at-risk youth and school personnel become involved in a process of mutual blaming. In order for this attitude to be replaced with one of mutual collaboration, an in-person meeting is often indicated. It would be ideal if this meeting could occur at least once early in the process. Meeting in person will allow a positive connection to form that will sustain a collaboration even if crises with the adolescent arise along the way. Although helping to facilitate meetings between the school teachers, counselors, administrators, the adolescent, and the family may be one of the most critical actions a family therapist can perform, ironically, this can often be one of the most challenging interventions to arrange, particularly given the demands of working parents.

Finding Resources within the School System

Many family therapists who are not based in schools may not be fully knowledgeable about school-based services or resources within the school district that may address the needs of the at-risk adolescents they treat. School personnel are aware of the process of applying for a child study team evaluation to assess learning disabilities and behavior specialists to help teachers address behavioral issues in their classrooms. Connecting with these resources may be helpful when treating at-risk adolescents with issues such as cognitive problems that interfere with their ability to learn certain subjects, or ADHD that contributes to distractibility or hyperactivity, often leaving the students unable to stay focused in class. Parents and other family caregivers may benefit from a collaborative, brainstorming discussion with the therapist and teachers, counselors, administrators, or other school personnel. This discussion may be especially valuable to caregivers who are poor, have had less education, may speak a different language, or may be unfamiliar with the programs within the youth's school district.

In addition, as indicated in Chapters 10–14, some school systems may have available Achievement Mentoring Programs or tutoring that can help students facing specific challenges. Many students who are struggling with traditional academic subjects may have strengths in other areas, such as cosmetology, computer graphics, coding, auto mechanics, or nurse's assistant that might be a good fit with the vocational programs offered by some school systems (Henggeler et al., 2009). In addition to their appropriateness for some students, vocational programs offer adolescents preparation for a job in the field. This background may also serve as an entrée to community college programs, which may be most valuable for future job opportunities. Many employment areas now require educational credentials beyond a high school diploma.

School sports and other school clubs may be important opportunities for youth to engage in prosocial behaviors, increase their involvement with positive peers, and help to decrease time spent with delinquent peers. Family therapists and caregivers are more likely to learn about the availability of these types of activities within the school or community when meeting with school personnel. Therapists can then incorporate them into intervention plans.

Individual Interventions with Adolescents and a Parent or Caregiver

Even though MST focuses primarily on the involvement of parents or caregivers in family interventions with at-risk youth to address issues in the family, the adolescent, school, peers, and the community that may be contributing to the youth's presenting problems, there may be occasions when the family therapist needs to meet individually with caregivers or adolescents to address specific issues that may be interfering with their ability to accomplish the agreed-upon goals (Henggeler et al., 2009). This meeting might take the form of one or more individual sessions or ongoing regular interventions.

In the case of a parent or caregiver, the goal of MST is to empower caregivers to collaborate with the therapist and the adolescent to create and implement interventions that will change the problematic at-risk behaviors. The therapist may identify individual issues, such as depression, extreme anxiety, a feeling of being overwhelmed, or substance abuse or mental health problems that are interfering with the caregiver's ability to monitor the youth's behavior in all of the systems in which the adolescent is involved. The MST therapist may decide that individual sessions held with the parent or caregiver may be indicated to address the issue, rather than offer a referral to another therapist for individual therapy and thus involve an additional clinic or agency.

Similarly, if a youth presents with problems with aggression, impulsive behavior, or ADHD, or if he or she continues to choose delinquent peers, the therapist may decide to do individual interventions with the adolescent, in addition to the family therapy sessions. Another impetus for individual interventions is the at-risk adolescent's experience of severe trauma, such as domestic violence; physical or sexual abuse; witnessing of a killing, shooting, or dangerous gang violence in the community; natural disasters; terrorist acts; death of a loved one; and other traumatic losses or experiences (Cohen et al., 2006; Henggeler et al., 2009). If the assessment indicates evidence of PTSD and if the construction of fit circles related to a particular problem signifies that trauma treatment is necessary, trauma-focused cognitive-behavioral therapy (Cohen et al., 2006) may be indicated in addition to the family treatment. If the decision is reached to conduct individual sessions with the adolescent, it is important that the parents or caregivers are part of the planning, clear about the specific goals that will be addressed, and supportive of the intervention.

CONCLUSION

MST is an evidence-based family intervention for antisocial behavior in at-risk adolescents. It is strength-based and explores the fit between the presenting problems and the multisystemic levels (individual, family, peer, school, and community) that may impact the youth's life. Interventions are designed to address the causes of the problems at each level. Its goal is to empower parents or caregivers to gain the skills necessary to intervene effectively at each of these levels in order to address the identified risk factors, decrease antisocial behavior, and promote improved functioning.

Many of these interventions can be utilized by family therapists and other clinicians working with at-risk adolescents. Scott Henggeler, the developer of the MST intervention, offered the following caution, however:

Organizations and individual clinicians are free to borrow from [the] manuals and to adopt and adapt the concepts and clinical procedures they view as most useful for their purposes. The only caveat is that clinicians or organizations are not free to conclude that they are, for example, implementing MST in the absence of validated verification of such. (Henggeler & Sheidow, 2012, p. 53)

Therefore, although it is often helpful for therapists to incorporate aspects of MST into their work, it is important for them to recognize that MST is a complex, evidence-based treatment approach that is intended to be performed by licensed sites with rigorous training, approved supervisors, and careful oversight for fidelity. These issues are discussed in greater detail in Chapter 15. Therapists and program directors are also referred to the MST website (*http://mstservices.com*) for more detailed information about this approach.

CHAPTER 8

Multisystems Model Case Example

Case examples provided throughout this book have illustrated particular aspects of our work. This chapter, presenting a comprehensive case example of an at-risk Latino immigrant adolescent and his family, highlights the Multisystems Model (Boyd-Franklin, 1989, 2003; Boyd-Franklin et al., 2013).

The ecological environment of at-risk adolescents comprises many different systems (Boyd-Franklin, 1989, 2003; Boyd-Franklin & Bry, 2000; Henggeler et al., 2009). The adolescent in this case example is impacted by a number of system levels: (1) the individual; (2) his family; (3) the school he attends; (4) the court system; (5) the police; (6) his probation officer; (7) his community; and (8) his peer group, particularly with regard to the disproportionate influence of his gang-involved peers. Without the influence of his peer group, it is debatable whether the police, court, or probation systems would have been present in his life.

Treatment approaches and interventions described in this chapter include (1) the value of home-based family treatment; (2) the value of the combination of home-based family therapy and a school-based Achievement Mentoring Program; (3) the process of joining and engaging the adolescent and his family; (4) the importance of community outreach to engage family support systems, such as the church; (5) the significance of culturally competent interventions; and (6) the emphasis on the empowerment of the parents to take charge of monitoring the son's behavior and to become involved directly with the school and other systems (e.g., courts, probation, his peers) that impact his life.

CASE EXAMPLE

Description of the Family

Miguel, a 13-year-old adolescent from Mexico, was referred for home-based family therapy by Ms. Rodriguez, his ESL (English as a Second Language) teacher and his guidance counselor. Miguel's family consisted of his mother, Ms. Elaina Garcia (32), his father, Mr. Jaime Garcia (35), and his younger brother, Carlos (10). They lived in a low-income housing project in an inner-city neighborhood. His mother and father had left Mexico for the United States eight years earlier to find work and started saving money so that they could bring Miguel, then 5, and Carlos, then 2, to live with them as soon as possible. During that time, the boys lived with Ms. Garcia's mother in Mexico and were extremely close to their grandmother and extended family members in their home country.

Upon their arrival, Mr. and Ms. Garcia found the Catholic Church in their neighborhood and attended services; however, the services were conducted in English, and the Garcias were struggling to learn the language. Shortly thereafter, a neighbor suggested that they attend her small Pentecostal storefront church. The minister was from Mexico, spoke fluent Spanish, and all the congregation members were Spanish speaking. This church made them feel comfortable and welcome, and became a major support system for them. Through church members, that is, their "church family," they had referrals for job opportunities: Ms. Garcia joined the cleaning staff at a local hotel, and Mr. Garcia worked in a local restaurant. With both working long hours and availing themselves of overtime shifts, they were able to save enough money to bring Miguel and Carlos to live with them within 5 years. Miguel was 10 at the time.

Because they were undocumented upon arrival, the family lived in constant fear of deportation; however, with the help of their minister, Mr. Garcia was now in the process of being sponsored for a green card by his boss at the restaurant, who was also a member of the church (see Chapter 3). As the process had not been completed at the time of their referral for treatment, the family was still in fear of deportation.

Presenting Problems

Behavioral problems were the first areas of concern presented by Ms. Rodriguez, his ESL teacher, and the other teachers in Miguel's middle school. When Miguel had arrived in the United States to join his parents, his behavior in elementary school had not been problematic; however, once in middle school he became involved with, in Ms. Rodriguez's term, "the wrong crowd." These boys were rumored to be gang-involved, and

Miguel engaged in a number of fights in school and in the community with these peers, and also was truant on a number of occasions.

In addition, Miguel presented with a number of academic problems. Because he knew no English when he started school in the United States, he had to repeat the fourth grade. He had been transferred to an ESL class where he remained throughout elementary school and was now much more fluent in English. At the time of his referral, he had just begun the seventh grade in middle school. Although his homeroom teacher, Ms. Rodriguez, was an ESL instructor, he was otherwise mainstreamed. All of his academic courses were taught in English. His ESL teacher and his guidance counselor were concerned about his academic performance as well as his behavior. Although this teacher felt that he was very bright, Miguel seemed disinterested in his school work and was in danger of failing two classes.

The guidance counselor tried to contact Ms. Garcia to discuss her concerns for Miguel through three means: she sent a letter home with Miguel, she mailed a letter to their home, and she called the phone number in the school records. None of these efforts received a response. This was not surprising, as both letters and the phone message had been in English. When Miguel was involved in a serious fight at school that led to his suspension, a letter was sent to his parents; however, this communication was translated into Spanish by Ms. Rodriguez, Miguel's ESL teacher. It detailed the circumstances of Miguel's suspension: one of his friends had gotten into a fight with a boy from a rival group in school; when a second boy attacked his friend, Miguel jumped into the fight; and all four of the boys involved were suspended. It stated that Miguel would not be allowed to return to school until a parent attended a conference with the principal. This meeting was held with the principal, the guidance counselor, Ms. Rodriguez, the ESL teacher who translated for Ms. Garcia, and Ms. Garcia. The principal indicated that as a condition of Miguel returning to school, he and his family would need to participate in two programs: home-based family therapy offered through a university-based program and the school-based Achievement Mentoring Program. (See Chapters 10–14.) Because Ms. Rodriguez had already been trained in this program and because she spoke fluent Spanish, the principal asked her to serve as Miguel's achievement mentor, and she agreed. Miguel's mother, Ms. Garcia, also agreed and signed the paperwork—a release of information form and a contract consenting to family treatment.

Joining and Engaging the Family

Once the principal and the guidance counselor made the referral to the home-based family therapy program, the Director assigned Jorge

Batista, a master's-level psychologist who was fluent in Spanish, to be the therapist. Jorge was originally from the Dominican Republic and was currently enrolled in a doctoral program in clinical psychology. Jorge contacted the family by sending home a letter in Spanish and leaving a message in Spanish on the family's home phone. Normally, the family therapist would meet first with the family before meeting with Miguel individually, but there was no response from the family to Jorge's attempts to contact them by mail and phone, even though these communications were in Spanish. At the Director's suggestion, the guidance counselor introduced Jorge to Miguel, and they began meeting in the school's guidance office.

Jorge spoke with Miguel in Spanish, and they spent the first session discussing Miguel's favorite music, his interest in basketball, and his friends at school. Miguel shared their names and their customary pastime: playing video games on one of the boy's phones during lunch and after school. As Jorge and Miguel began to connect, Jorge mentioned that he was having trouble reaching Miguel's mother. Miguel laughed and told his counselor that the best way to connect with his mom was to call her on an "emergency" cell phone she had recently purchased so that she could be reached in urgent situations. This number was only known to family members. The school had never been notified of this way of contacting Ms. Garcia. Jorge encouraged Miguel to tell his mom to expect his call.

Jorge called Ms. Garcia on her cell phone and left a message in Spanish, introducing himself as the counselor who would be working with the family and Miguel, and stating that he would like very much to talk with her. Ms. Garcia called two days later, apologizing for calling in the evening and not returning his call sooner. She explained (in Spanish) that she worked long hours and was unable to make phone calls while at work. Jorge helped her to relax by letting her know that he understood that she worked hard. He told her that he had already met with Miguel in school and that Miguel had impressed him as a bright young man. He also indicated that he would like to work with her and her husband to help Miguel with the problems he was facing. Ms. Garcia cried and said that she and her husband would risk losing their jobs if they took time off to go to meetings at the school. (This is a common concern of poor immigrant parents.) Jorge told her that he understood her situation of wanting to help her son but being unable to miss work. He offered to conduct the session at their apartment at a time that would be convenient for them. She suggested Friday evening at 7:30 P.M. Their first meeting was scheduled for that time.

When Jorge arrived, Mr. and Ms. Garcia and the two boys were all present. Their apartment was clean, and although sparsely furnished, care had been taken with the décor—the slipcovers on the living room couch matched the curtains. When Jorge complimented them on their home, Ms. Garcia proudly stated that she had made the covers and curtains herself. The family seemed to relax a bit, and Jorge thanked them for being willing to meet with him after the long days they worked. He told them that he understood how hard it was for them to go to meetings at Miguel's school during the day. Mr. Garcia was thankful for Jorge's understanding but felt that the school thought that they did not care about their son. Jorge told them he would help them to make the school aware of how concerned they were about Miguel.

Ms. Garcia explained that because Ms. Rodriguez, the ESL teacher, had attended the recent meeting with the principal and served as a translator, this was the first time that she had understood what was being said at a school meeting. She knew just enough English to "get by" on previous occasions. She would nod, and say "yes," even when she did not understand. Jorge told them that he would attend meetings with them to make sure they understood what was being said. He also shared that many of the Spanish-speaking families he worked with brought a friend or family member whom they could trust to translate for them at meetings. Jorge asked if there was anyone like that who could help them in the future if he was not available. Mr. and Ms. Garcia were not sure, so Jorge asked them to help him draw a genogram (Figure 8.1), as this might indicate whether there was someone who could help the family. He also did a family ecomap (Figure 8.2) with them, to illustrate all of their possible support systems. Although most of their family lived in Mexico, they identified Ms. Garcia's sister, Angela, who had a 10-year-old son and lived nearby. They also identified their pastor, church family, and two neighbors in the housing project. At the end of this discussion, the therapist again asked if there was anyone who was fluent in English and Spanish who could come to some of the school meetings to translate for them. Ms. Garcia identified a woman who was part of her church family. The therapist asked her if she would find out if this woman would be willing to attend a meeting with her at school if necessary.

During the family session, Ms. Garcia mentioned that she was almost finished with dinner preparations and invited Jorge to join them. As this would give him a further opportunity to join with the family, he agreed. Mr. and Ms. Garcia smiled at his eager response. Jorge complimented the food, telling Ms. Garcia that dinner was delicious and as good as his Mama's. Through his relaxed style, his use of Spanish, his willingness to praise their attempts, and his agreement to share a meal with them, Jorge had engaged the family in a culturally competent manner and had established the beginning of a therapeutic alliance with all of the family members.

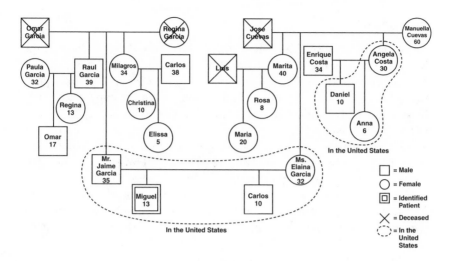

FIGURE 8.1. The Garcia family genogram.

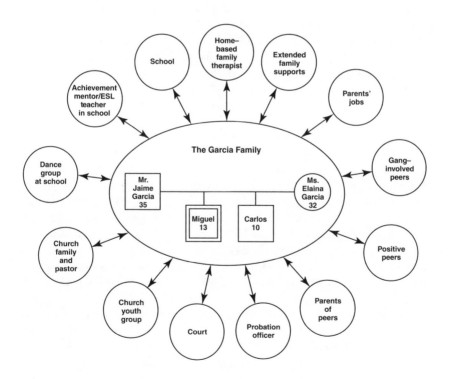

FIGURE 8.2. Ecomap for the Garcia family.

Assessment

In the next family session, they continued to discuss their concerns for Miguel and the problems that his parents felt needed to be addressed. Mr. Garcia said that Miguel would not listen to them and was irresponsible. They gave him the key to the apartment with the expectation that he would let his brother in after school, but sometimes Miguel stayed out with his friends. As a result, Carlos could not get into the apartment and had to wait at a neighbor's until Miguel showed up. Ms. Garcia often prepared nutritious food before her shift at work that only had to be heated up, but Miguel ate snacks instead. Mr. Garcia explained that when they returned from their long days at work, they would find Miguel watching TV with his brother with his homework not done and the house—which had been neat and clean when the Garcias left for work—in a mess.

Ms. Garcia said they were also very concerned about Miguel's behavior in school and in the neighborhood. She said that until the meeting with the school principal, she had no idea that Miguel was in so much trouble for fighting and truancy. She became even more concerned when the principal informed them of Miguel's friendships with boys who were suspected of gang involvement. Mr. Garcia echoed her concerns. He said they had sacrificed so much to come to this country so that their sons could get an education, and they did not want to see Miguel "throw it all away" because of friends who did "bad things."

Jorge asked Mr. Garcia if he would talk with Miguel about his concerns. Mr. Garcia told Miguel that they had brought them to this country to have a better life. He and his mother were working long hours to make this happen. He told Miguel he was concerned because instead of trying to help them, Miguel was getting in trouble in school and in the neighborhood, and not being responsible at home. The therapist encouraged Miguel to respond. He told his father he missed his family and friends back in Mexico. When he first came to the United States, he had no friends and it was very lonely. Now he finally had friends, and everyone was angry at him for having some fun. Mr. Garcia explained to Miguel that he understood, but that his friends were leading him into fights and being absent from school. Mr. Garcia revealed his fear that if Miguel continued getting into trouble before they had their green card, the whole family might be deported. The therapist summarized the parents' concerns as (1) Miguel's choice of friends who were getting him into trouble, (2) his truancy, (3) his behavior in school, and (4) his failing grades. In addition, the parents feared the possibility of deportation. Jorge reframed the idea that they obviously loved Miguel and were very worried about him. He also recognized Miguel's statement about how lonely he had been during his first few years in this country and understood his desire to have friends.

The family therapist talked with Miguel's parents about the need to establish clear communication with the school so that they could know how he was doing and be able to monitor his behavior. He encouraged Ms. Garcia to call Ms. Rodriguez, his ESL teacher and achievement mentor, as well as the guidance counselor and give them the emergency cell phone number so that the school could contact her if necessary. She agreed and did so the next day.

School

The family therapist continued his assessment by obtaining Mr. and Ms. Garcia's written permission to contact the school. He met with the principal, the guidance counselor, and Ms. Rodriguez. Miguel's ESL teacher was concerned that he was in danger of failing two of his classes. The principal shared this concern about Miguel's failing grades, but he was also troubled by Miguel's fights with other students in school, his truancy, and his increasing involvement with friends rumored to be gang-involved. The principal also mentioned his suspicions that on the days Miguel was truant, he was spending his time with the boys who were such negative influences on him. Ms. Rodriguez suggested a tutoring program in which college students at a nearby university volunteered at the middle school to tutor students to improve their academic performance. Jorge emphasized to the school authorities present that Ms. and Mr. Garcia shared the principal's concerns and that they were very worried about Miguel, but that they were hard-working people who could not get time off to come to school. The principal recommended that they try to attend the parent–teacher meetings as they were held in the evenings, one of which was scheduled for the following week. The family therapist arranged with Ms. Rodriguez; the teachers in the two classes he was in danger of failing, math and science; and his guidance counselor to have a meeting with Mr. and Ms. Garcia and Miguel in the last slot of the scheduled parent–teacher meeting, 7 P.M.

The parents agreed to attend the meeting with Miguel, and the family therapist also agreed to attend. When they arrived, Ms. Rodriguez welcomed the parents in Spanish. Mr. and Ms. Garcia thanked her and the teachers for being willing to stay so late as they were unable to get off from work to attend meetings during the school day. The guidance counselor acknowledged how helpful it was that they were willing to come in the evening.

The family therapist made a list of the school's concerns, and the parents and the professionals agreed on the following goals: Miguel would (1) improve his grades, particularly in the courses he was failing; (2) attend school every day; (3) curtail his friendships with the delinquent peers and become involved in activities with more positive students; and (4) stop fighting in school.

The goals regarding grades were addressed first. Both his math and science teachers explained that Miguel had failed all tests in both subjects, and unless he could raise his test scores on subsequent exams, he would not pass either course that semester. Miguel explained that math and science were always hard for him, but tests now included much longer questions and word problems. He had so much difficulty with English that the time he spent trying to understand the questions left him no time to answer them.

At that point, Ms. Rodriguez introduced a young university student named Maribel, a Spanish-speaking tutor who volunteered to work with middle school students in need of help and who would work with Miguel in school. Maribel asked Miguel if he would be willing to work with her while he ate his lunch in school three days a week to work on his homework and improve his grades, and he agreed. She told Miguel that she would give him a note to his parents in Spanish after each tutoring session. Ms. Rodriguez, in her role as his achievement mentor, explained to Miguel and his parents that she would be working with him once a week and would be checking in with his teachers to see how he was doing in his classes, his attendance, and his tutoring. She would also be giving his parents feedback on how he was doing in school. Because his truancy was such a big problem, she agreed to leave a message on his mother's cell phone once a week to confirm that he had attended school. It was clear that Ms. Rodriguez already had a good rapport with Miguel and his parents. At the family therapist's request, she also agreed to be in touch with Jorge on a regular basis to update him on Miguel's progress. At the end of the meeting, the therapist asked the family if they would be willing to work in the next family session on rewards and consequences for Miguel.

Rewards and Consequences for Miguel's Behavior

In the next home-based family therapy session, the therapist reviewed this meeting with Miguel and his parents. The therapist raised the question of rewards for Miguel for attending school and doing his school work, and what consequences there would be if he did not. Initially, the father objected to providing rewards to Miguel for doing what was expected of a boy his age. In response, the therapist talked with the father about the power of positive reinforcement to encourage Miguel to stick to his commitments. The therapist helped the parents, Miguel, and Carlos to engage in a problem-solving session to discuss a possible behavior plan, and to point out the rewards and consequences. The therapist explored with Miguel and his parents what Miguel considered his favorite activities. His parents mentioned how much he loved playing video games on his mother's cell phone. The family agreed that for each day that Miguel attended school; went to all of his classes; did all of his in-school assignments; and brought home a positive note signed by his tutor and as soon as he showed his parents that his homework was completed, he would be allowed to play with his mother's cell phone for a half hour. If he forgot the note or did not complete his homework, he would not be allowed to play video games that evening. If he missed a day of school, he would be grounded for the next week and would miss the opportunity to play with the cell phone for a week.

Things had begun to improve in school for Miguel. He was attending school every day and was working with his tutor and his achievement mentor. The therapist checked at the beginning of each session to see how things were going in school and whether Miguel's parents had received any calls from Ms. Rodriguez. The parents stated that Miguel had regularly shown them his homework and the notes from his tutor. Most of the notes were positive, and so Ms. Garcia had allowed him to play video games on her cell phone for a half hour. One day, however, Miguel did not bring his report from his tutor home, and Mr. Garcia enforced the consequence. Miguel was not given his mother's cell phone and could not play video games that evening. The therapist praised the parents and Miguel for their willingness to follow through on the behavior plan.

Individual Therapy with Miguel

The Multisystems Model often involves interventions at the individual level (Boyd-Franklin & Bry, 2000; see Chapter 6). Because of the seriousness of Miguel's involvement with gang-involved peers, the therapist met Miguel once a week for an individual therapy session at the school in addition to the family therapy session in the home. The individual sessions initially focused on discussions with Miguel about his dreams for himself. He talked about his love of music and dance, particularly hip hop. His dream was to be a performer or to be a DJ playing music for parties and clubs. The therapist explored this goal with him in great detail. As Miguel began to show improvement in school, his dream changed slightly to incorporate education, and he began to add a desire to graduate from high school and go to a community college.

The therapist utilized Motivational Interviewing (Miller & Rollnick, 2009, 2012) in his individual sessions with Miguel and worked hard to establish a therapeutic relationship with him. He used reflective listening (Miller & Rollnick, 2009, 2012) to demonstrate his understanding of Miguel's experience and convey a great deal of empathy for him. In describing how lonely he felt during his first year in the United States, Miguel noted the long hours his parents worked and his lack of friends. Then he started to make friends and he wasn't lonely any more, but he now realized that these friends were leading him into trouble and, as hard as it was for him, he knew he had to give them up. Jorge reflected how hard it was for him and how upsetting it must be to finally have friends and to be told to give them up because they caused trouble.

In the coming weeks, the therapist and Miguel talked about the tough decisions he often had to make with regard to his friends. The therapist used decisional balancing, a motivational interviewing technique (Miller & Rollnick, 2009), to help Miguel to look at the pros and cons of his actions. They talked about the pros and cons of staying in school versus being truant all day or part of a day. During this session, Miguel revealed that he was very scared that if he kept getting into trouble, he would end up "doing time" in a juvenile correctional facility or in prison like some of his friends. In the individual sessions, his therapist helped him to weigh the excitement of "playing hooky" from school against the fear of incarceration.

One day Jorge joined Miguel in the cafeteria for lunch and sat at the table with Miguel and his friends. It was obvious to the therapist that Miguel was a "follower" and this confirmed the information that Miguel's teachers had given the therapist. The group of boys Miguel seemed to be very involved with were older, half of them were in the eighth grade. The original leader of this group was serving a sentence in a state juvenile correctional facility; the current leader of the group, taller and stronger than the other boys, was 15 years old and in the eighth grade, having been held back twice since he had migrated from Honduras.

In his meetings with Miguel, the therapist learned more about the fights Miguel got into at school. They were all related to his peer group. He told the therapist that it was expected that they would watch out for each other and that they would back each other up if threatened. Thus, Miguel felt he had no option other than fighting if someone from another group threatened him or one of his "boys." During this process, Miguel's ambivalence became clear to Jorge—he was truly frightened by the prospect of incarceration and wanted to avoid what he called "trouble," but he felt obligated to be loyal to his friends. The therapist began to work with Miguel on delineating the problems that resulted from his association with these peers.

The Crisis

Six weeks after the family therapy began, it became clear that Miguel's association with a negative, gang-involved peer group needed to be addressed when a crisis occurred. The therapist learned from this experience that, given the danger posed to Miguel, the influence of negative peers should have taken a primary focus earlier in the treatment.

After weeks of excellent school attendance and a positive attitude toward his school work, some of Miguel's friends persuaded him to leave school before the last period on a Friday afternoon. They were "hanging out" near a neighborhood McDonald's when a gang fight broke out among another group of boys. As the situation escalated, Miguel and his friends were pulled into the fight. The police were called, and all of the boys were arrested. Ms. Garcia was contacted by the police and had to leave work to go to the police station. Miguel was released into her custody and given a pending court date in the next week.

Ms. Garcia, in a panic, called the family therapist. An emergency session in the home was arranged for that evening in which the whole family discussed this serious situation. Mr. and Ms. Garcia were obviously very upset, and Miguel was visibly shaken. In response to the therapist's question about what had occurred, Miguel admitted that on Friday afternoon his friends had convinced him to leave school an hour early. He shared that a number of the older adolescents were members of a gang. A group of boys from a rival gang had showed up and a fight developed. Initially, Miguel and some of his friends were bystanders, but then they were attacked and were pulled into the fight.

Mr. Garcia was very angry and told Miguel that this was why he had been telling him to stay away from these boys who kept getting him into trouble. As this was a serious situation, the therapist reframed Mr. Garcia's anger as fear for his son. Ms. Garcia told the therapist the court date, and he agreed to accompany the parents to court.

Only Ms. Garcia and Miguel attended the court appearance, as Mr. Garcia had been threatened with loss of his job if he took time off to go to court. Ms. Garcia shared the same concern for her job with the therapist. While at court, the therapist and Ms. Garcia had the opportunity to talk with Miguel's court-appointed legal aid lawyer, who indicated that if he told the judge that Miguel was already involved in therapy and had no prior arrests, it would help Miguel's case. At disposition, the judge gave Miguel probation because he had not had a history of prior arrests, but his other friends, all of whom had prior arrests, were sentenced to a juvenile correctional facility. The judge mandated that Miguel continue in family therapy and that he meet with his therapist individually. At the same time, however, he warned Miguel that he would be assigned to a probation officer and that if he was arrested again, the consequences would be more severe.

Once the probation officer was assigned, the therapist contacted him and asked him to attend a family therapy session at the Garcia home. The probation officer agreed. In the next family therapy session, the therapist emphasized that Miguel's peer group had become a major problem. Miguel, still shaken from the court appearance, agreed. The probation officer made it clear that if Miguel was arrested again, he could be sentenced to a juvenile correctional facility. The threat of jail was very powerful for both Miguel and his parents. The probation officer also addressed the issue of his truancy since this was the circumstance that had led to the fight and the subsequent arrest. The therapist told the probation officer that he would be arranging a case conference at the school to address these serious concerns, and the probation officer agreed to attend.

Multisystems Case Conference

To address the issue of his truancy and his involvement with gang-involved peers, Jorge called an urgent multisystems case conference at the school. Because both parents expressed concerns about losing their jobs and because the therapist emphasized the importance of both parents being present for the meeting, the therapist asked Ms. Garcia to contact Ms. Rodriguez and Miguel's guidance counselor to see if they would be willing to attend this important meeting in the evening. Given the seriousness of Miguel's crisis, both agreed to meet the parents at 6:00 P.M. the following day for the multisystems case conference at the school; the tutor was also asked to attend, and she readily agreed. The therapist next asked Mr. Garcia to contact the probation officer, who agreed to come as well. The case conference therefore included the family therapist, the probation officer, Ms. Rodriguez, Miguel's guidance counselor, the tutor, Miguel, and both of his parents. During this multisystems case conference, the family therapist and Ms. Rodriguez translated the meeting into Spanish for the parents.

In their discussion of the truancy, the therapist helped Miguel, his parents, Ms. Rodriguez, the guidance counselor, and the probation officer to list the factors that were contributing to his truancy. They listed the following factors:

1. Friends encourage him to miss school.
2. Parents are working for long hours, and no one is monitoring his behavior.
3. Sometimes he misses a whole day of school.

4. More often, he signs in at his homeroom in the morning and then leaves school with his friends during the course of the day.
5. There is poor communication between the school and the parents.
6. He has contact with negative peers.
7. He needs to be connected with prosocial friends.

Miguel agreed to attend school every day, and Ms. Rodriguez, in her role as his achievement mentor, agreed to check in with his teachers regularly to see how he was doing in his classes. The guidance counselor agreed to take responsibility for checking the school records for Miguel's attendance every day.

The therapist also raised the issue of Miguel's involvement with gang-involved peers and how it contributed to his behavioral problems and arrest. The probation officer agreed that this was a big problem and that if Miguel continued to associate with these negative peers, it might result in a violation of his probation and a consequent sentencing to the juvenile correctional facility. It was clear that Miguel took this threat very seriously. He agreed to sign a contract not to be involved with the negative peers either in school or in the community.

The therapist raised the concern about Miguel beginning to connect with more positive peers. Ms. Rodriguez shared that there were two boys in her ESL homeroom class who had been Miguel's friends in elementary school, were "good kids," and were involved in positive activities, such as a dance group run by the gym teacher. In this group, students learned and rehearsed hip hop dance routines after school, culminating in a dance performance at the end of the school year. The dance performance was the highlight of the year for the students who participated and was well attended by teachers and other school staff, students, parents and other relatives, and members of the community. When the therapist asked Miguel about these boys and about the dance group, Miguel seemed more alert and involved than he had been at any other point in the session. He agreed to meet with the therapist during their next individual session to discuss this and to follow up on the dance group.

The probation officer agreed to be in touch with Ms. Rodriguez, the parents, and the family therapist to monitor Miguel's progress. He made it clear to Miguel that the information he obtained from those sources would be part of the report he had to submit to the judge. The family therapist thanked everyone for coming and underscored the importance of maintaining contact between the parents and the school. Mr. and Ms. Garcia were concerned about maintaining contact with the school if it meant having to take time off from work. The therapist, sympathetic to the Garcias' fears about losing their jobs, asked Ms. Rodriguez for a suggestion. They decided to hold a conference call twice a month that would be scheduled to coincide with Mr. and Ms. Garcia's lunch breaks. Ms. Rodriguez and the guidance counselor told them they would give them the conference call line and that they would speak to them from the guidance counselor's office every other week to update them on Miguel's progress. Ms. Rodriguez agreed to translate the guidance counselor's comments into Spanish for the parents.

Peer Interventions

As they began to discuss alternatives in his next individual session with his therapist, Miguel's fears that he would end up "doing time" in a juvenile correctional facility or eventually a prison like his friends had increased greatly as a result of his arrest and the court appearance. As the therapist once again helped him to balance the "fun of cutting school" to hang out with his friends against his fear of incarceration, it became clear to Jorge that Miguel at last was ready to understand the consequences of his actions and their impact not only on himself, but on his entire family, given his father's fear that they might be deported if Miguel's behavior continued to bring them to the attention of the police, the judge, the probation department, and other authorities.

In the next individual session, Jorge followed up with Miguel on the two positive boys in Miguel's ESL homeroom class that Ms. Rodriguez had mentioned. When the family therapist, who wanted to increase Miguel's contact with them, broached the subject of the dance group run by the gym teacher, Miguel looked very down. He wanted to be part of this prestigious group; however, only students with good grades were eligible for participation. and his current grades were too low. Moreover, practices took place after school when he was expected to take care of his brother.

The therapist thought if he and Miguel could meet with the gym teacher, there might be a way to make it possible for Miguel to qualify. The gym teacher was willing to listen to Jorge and Miguel and came up with a reward for Miguel that would allow him to join the group—it was conditioned on him getting an A in all of his classes! The therapist discussed the challenge of going from an F to an A so quickly. The gym teacher conceded that this was an unrealistic expectation and offered a compromise: if Miguel went to all of his classes, attended school every day, worked with his tutor, and received at least a C in each of his classes, he would be allowed to rehearse with the group. He also stated that in order for him to appear in the final performance, however, he would have to obtain at least a B average.

This gave Miguel the motivation not only to improve his grades but also to increase his contact with positive peers—the two students in his ESL class homeroom who were good students and participants in the dance program. The therapist used many of his individual sessions with Miguel to discuss his progress toward this goal and to problem-solve issues as they arose in school. They discussed his two friends in the ESL class, and Miguel began to "hang out" with them more often, eating with them in the lunch room and playing video games.

The therapist also began to explore with Miguel how he would respond if his former peers wanted to hang out together after school or on weekends, engage in truant behavior, or tried to pull him into fights. He did role plays with Miguel in which the therapist played a former peer who was trying to lure him into "playing hooky" from school. They arrived at a response that would give Miguel a face-saving way to handle the requests of his peers that might result in negative behavior: "No man, I can't. This probation officer is breathing down my neck, and I don't want to end up in jail." When this role-played situation actually took place with one of his gang-involved peers, Miguel included an addition to the statement he and his therapist had devised to handle this troublesome issue: his probation officer had already come to school to check on him. This is an important intervention for at-risk adolescents who are attempting to change their association with negative peers and who are still in the same school or community (Boyd-Franklin & Bry, 2000; Henggeler et al., 2009).

Family Interventions Regarding Prosocial Peers and Activities

In the next family therapy session, the therapist raised the issue of positive peer involvement with Miguel and the family. Miguel reported his eagerness to be involved in the dance program and his agreement to work to bring his grades up to a C in order to take part in the rehearsals and a B to achieve the goal of participating in the end-of-the-year program. The therapist asked Mr. and Ms. Garcia for their thoughts on the matter, and they expressed their excitement for him. The therapist asked Mr. Garcia to talk to Miguel in the session about what he would need to do to pull up his grades and to participate in the after-school rehearsals. This presented a roadblock, as Mr. Garcia was insistent that Miguel had the responsibility to take care of his brother after school. Miguel was upset and asked if there was anyone else who could take care of Carlos after school. The therapist helped the family to do a problem-solving exercise and to construct a list of possible alternatives. He emphasized that the opportunity for Miguel to earn the right to be part of this after-school program was a strong, positive reward for his hard work with his tutor and in his classes. In addition, it was an opportunity to help to connect him with friends who would be a positive influence. Mr. and Mrs. Garcia agreed that this was crucial for Miguel and that they would try to find someone in their social network who could help with Carlos after school. (The resolution of this problem is presented in the following section.)

In a family session a few weeks later, the family therapist spoke with Mr. and Ms. Garcia about the importance of knowing their sons' friends and their parents. When he asked them whether they knew any of these friends, they spoke honestly that their long work hours did not give them the opportunity. The therapist helped all four family members to problem-solve this issue and try to find a possible time when Miguel and Carlos could invite some of their friends to their home. Miguel suggested that Saturday afternoon might be a good time when he could invite his two friends from school to play video games. Carlos talked about a friend he would like to invite. Ms. Garcia considered this possibility with the condition that both boys would have to complete their chores in the house first.

The therapist asked Mr. Garcia if there was a way they could tie this special opportunity as a reward for a great deal of effort at school. The parents agreed that (1) if Miguel was able to get positive daily reports from all of his teachers for attendance and for completing his work; (2) if he was able to raise his grades to Bs in all of his classes for 2 weeks; and (3) if both boys completed all of their chores on Saturday for 2 weeks, they would allow them to invite their friends for a few hours on a Saturday afternoon. The therapist turned to Mr. and Ms. Garcia and asked if they might use this opportunity to connect with the parents of these boys. He explained that as adolescents become older teenagers, it is increasingly more difficult to know their friends and their parents. Ms. Garcia asked Miguel if he could get the phone numbers of his friends' parents. They all agreed that Ms. Garcia would call their parents to get permission for them to visit once Miguel had demonstrated that he could meet his behavioral goals of school attendance, completing his homework and class work, and raising his grades to a B in all of his classes. She also spoke with Carlos about contacting the parents of his friend. It took a month before Miguel was able to raise his grades to a B in all of his classes. Jorge checked in each week and validated Miguel for his efforts and helped empower the parents to stick to the agreement. Both boys had been dedicated to cleaning the house and attending to their chores on Saturdays during that month. When Miguel was able to achieve his goals, the entire family celebrated. Ms. Garcia contacted his friends' mothers and the mother of Carlos's friend and arranged for a visit on the following Saturday. The therapist praised the whole family for solving this problem together and for sticking to their plans.

SOCIAL SUPPORTS

In the next family session, the therapist asked Mr. and Mrs. Garcia to talk about possible supports for the family. Who did they turn to for help? Who were their extended family members and close friends? Who might help out with Carlos after school in order for Miguel to attend the dance program? The therapist pulled out the piece of paper on which they had drawn an ecomap and genogram in an earlier session. With a magic marker, he began highlighting those individuals on the genogram (Figure 8.1) and the ecomap (Figure 8.2) who had been supportive of the family in the past and who might help with Carlos after school. Ms. Garcia again volunteered that her sister, Angela, lived nearby and that her son, Daniel, was Carlos's friend. She and Mr. Garcia agreed that they could trust Angela to bring Carlos to her house after school and to help him start his homework. The therapist also followed up with the parents to see if they had contacted their friend from church to interpret for them, if needed, during important meetings at the school or the court. Ms. Garcia reported that this friend was retired and had agreed to help.

This led to a broader discussion of their social supports. Both became very animated when they spoke about their experiences at their Pentecostal church; they were enthusiastic about their minister and the members of the congregation. Since the church was so small, everyone was "like family." Mr. Garcia also proudly reported that the minister's wife was starting an English class after church on Sunday and that he and Ms. Garcia were planning to attend. The therapist expressed his appreciation of the help offered by the church, and praised the parents for finding such an important support system for their family.

The therapist asked the boys how they felt about the church and whether they had friends there. Carlos quickly listed a group of friends. Miguel said that he used to have friends there but not so much now. When the therapist explored this issue, it became clear that Miguel had pulled away from his friends at church as he had gotten more involved with his at-risk friends while at school and on the weekends. Ms. Garcia described the youth group at the church and the pastor's efforts to help adolescents gain some work experience by matching them with people and small businesses in the community that needed odd jobs done (raking leaves, cutting grass, washing cars, shoveling snow, and carting away trash) and would compensate the adolescents for these efforts. The therapist asked Ms. Garcia to discuss this possibility with Miguel. She spoke with her son about his desire to earn money and how this youth group might give him an opportunity to do so. She also indicated that it would give him something positive to do on the weekends. The therapist asked if the minister might be willing to attend a family therapy session. The father suggested that they might be able to have their next family session at the church on Wednesday night following the prayer meeting. The therapist, eager to involve and empower the father, asked him to contact the minister. The father called the next day to report that a meeting was scheduled for 7:30 P.M. the following Wednesday at the church.

When the therapist and the family arrived, the minister, Reverend Avila, introduced them to Mateo Arrandando, a member of the congregation who was studying to become a minister. He confided to Miguel and his parents that he had been in a gang and in trouble with the law when he was a teenager and had ended up in a juvenile correctional facility. He shared with them that he had been paying for this mistake ever since. Many of his friends had spent years in prison, having been charged as adults.

In the last year, Mateo had become involved in the church and was helping the minister to work with the youth group. Mateo and the minister discussed the weekend work program that they had developed to help adolescents in the church become involved in positive projects on the weekends and to earn some money for themselves. Miguel talked with them about wanting to save up money for his own cell phone. Mateo offered to work with him in the youth group, to help him get jobs, and to mentor him as he worked toward his goal. The therapist asked Mr. Garcia if he would be willing to keep Miguel's earnings for him until he had saved enough to purchase the cell phone. His father agreed, and Miguel considered this arrangement to be a good idea as well. The therapist thanked the minister and Mateo for their help.

Achieving Goals

As the last marking period in school was approaching, Miguel was doing well and had attended school and each class every day. The therapist went with Ms. Garcia for a meeting at the school to discuss Miguel's progress. At the therapist's suggestion, they were accompanied by Ms. Bolana, the friend from church whom Ms. Garcia had contacted to help translate for her in the session. (This was an important intervention because the therapist was preparing the family for completion of their work together and they needed to identify someone who could serve as a translator for the family once therapy ended.) The meeting was held during Mr. and Ms. Garcia's lunch break and Mr. Garcia called into a speaker phone in the guidance counselor's office during the meeting.

In the meeting, they learned from Ms. Rodriguez that Miguel had pulled up his grades to Bs in all of his classes and had been rehearsing with the gym teacher and the dance group in preparation for the performance. These after-school rehearsals and the visit to the Garcia home had led to a closer relationship between Miguel and his two positive friends. He was continuing to work hard with his tutor to maintain a B average so that he could achieve his goal of participating in the performance at the end of the school year.

In the next family session, the therapist praised Mr. and Ms. Garcia and Miguel for their hard work and for their follow-through on their agreements. He also praised Miguel's parents for their ability to work closely with the school to monitor Miguel's behavior and to give him rewards and consequences despite their demanding work schedules. Miguel's time was now occupied with more positive peers during and after school, and he was working with other members of the church youth group on the weekends. Now that he was working on the weekends, he was not available to "hang out" with delinquent peers as he had been accustomed to doing prior to the intervention with the minister. At the end of the school year, the therapist attended the dance performance, participation in which had so motivated Miguel that he brought his once-failing grades up to a B average.

A final home-based family therapy meeting was held at the end of June. To celebrate the successful completion of the school year, Ms. Garcia surprised the therapist with a delicious dinner. Mr. Garcia gave Miguel a wrapped box containing his new cell phone that he had worked so hard to earn through the church work experience program for adolescents. Mr. and Ms. Garcia indicated that Miguel and Carlos would both be involved in a camp program at the church that summer. Miguel, who had just turned 14, and a few of the older boys in the church would serve as counselors, earning a small salary each week. The therapist praised the parents for planning ahead to occupy both of the boys' time during the summer when the parents would be busy at work.

A follow-up meeting in October of the following school year indicated that Miguel was doing well in school and had continued to be involved with Ms. Rodriguez, his achievement mentor; Maribel, his tutor; the after-school dance program conducted by the gym teacher; and the weekend youth program at the church. His probation officer continued his oversight and reported that Miguel was doing well and had had no further incidents in the community.

Discussion

As indicated earlier, this case illustrates the Multisystems Model (Boyd-Franklin, 1989, 2003; Boyd-Franklin & Bry, 2000; Boyd-Franklin et al., 2013). At the time of his referral, Miguel was at risk for school failure and was beginning to show signs of involvement with gang-involved peers. The fight in his community that had brought about his subsequent arrest and court appearance raised his risk level significantly, but this crisis also presented him the opportunity to change the trajectory of his life.

The Combination of Home-Based Family Therapy and School-Based Achievement Mentoring

This case also illustrates the combined effectiveness of home-based family therapy and the school-based Achievement Mentoring Program (see Chapters 10–15). The home-based family therapist was able to reach out to the family at times that were convenient for them in a home setting where they were most comfortable. His ability to communicate in Spanish and his knowledge of their culture were both assets in the treatment process. As Chapters 10 through 14 illustrate, the school-based Achievement Mentoring Program helped to engage Miguel in his school, which led to his improved academic performance. In addition, Ms. Rodriguez, his achievement mentor, was also his ESL teacher. She knew the school and his other teachers well. She was also aware of the hip hop dance program offered by the gym teacher, Miguel's positive peers in her class, and the tutoring program, composed of students from a nearby university, and she was able to suggest these additional supports for Miguel in the school. Her ability to speak Spanish made it possible for her to communicate effectively not only with Miguel, but with his parents as well. She became an additional link between these Spanish-speaking parents and the school. Therapists and schools are encouraged to search for staff in their schools and clinics who are fluent in Spanish and who may be willing to reach out to immigrant parents like Miguel's.

The Impact of the Crisis

The crisis that occurred in this case reveals an important lesson for clinicians who work with at-risk adolescents. Even though there was evidence of contact with gang-involved peers, the therapist chose to focus first on the adolescent's academic problems, concluding that his failing two subjects posed a serious issue for Miguel and could have resulted in his having to repeat a grade in school. This was absolutely correct and understandable; however, the issue of his gang-involved peer group also needed to be addressed. Postponing the attention to the at-risk peers by as little as a month put Miguel in more imminent danger and at increased risk in his community. Given how quickly activities with at-risk or delinquent peers can escalate and result in very serious consequences, clinicians are encouraged to begin to address strategies for decreasing contact with these peers and increasing involvement with prosocial peers and activities early in treatment (Boyd-Franklin & Bry, 2000; Dodge et al., 2006; Henggeler et al., 2009).

The multisystems interventions allowed the therapist to empower the parents first by accommodating their work schedule so that they could take a more proactive role in their son's life and school and second, by monitoring his behavior. Research has shown that parental monitoring is one of the most important protective factors for at-risk adolescents (Dishion et al., 2003). By helping the parents to develop a positive relationship and clear communication with the school, the door opened for his parents to play a more direct role in their son's academic life. The family therapist was also able to support the parents by reframing their relationship with the school from "unavailable and disinterested" to "hardworking and concerned for their son." The mother's initial meeting with the school allowed for more flexibility. With the reframe in place, his achievement mentor/ESL teacher, the teachers whose classes he was failing, and the guidance counselor were all willing to meet with the parents at the end of a parent–teacher night. Technology was also utilized in a later meeting to allow both parents to participate in a meeting at the school through a conference call during their lunch hours. These connections modeled for the parents the creative ways in which they could maintain a cooperative partnership with their son's school despite their inability to attend in-person meetings during the day. This alliance was crucial to sustaining positive changes over time.

Reaching Out, Focus on Strengths, and Cultural Sensitivity

This case illustrates the many ways in which home-based, school, and community interventions utilized outreach to engage a family that would not have been able to participate in traditional office-based therapy. As indicated earlier, the therapist's flexibility; his willingness to reach out to the parents; his ongoing acknowledgment of their strengths, including their willingness to meet with him late in the evening and their obvious caring for their son; and his cultural sensitivity in the process of engagement were all important to building a therapeutic alliance with them. The therapist's cultural sensitivity was exemplified first by his ability and willingness to speak to them in Spanish. His recognition of their work demands and his enjoyment of the food they shared with him were all a very natural part of the engagement process. He was also very understanding of the parents' fears that Miguel's problems with the school, police, courts, and probation departments would bring them to the attention of the immigration authorities and lead to family members being deported. These fears are very common among immigrant families in the current political climate.

Another aspect of the therapist's cultural awareness and sensitivity was his willingness to explore their religious and spiritual support system provided by their church family and their minister. As indicated in Chapter 3, such support systems can be a tremendous asset and strength in the lives of many ethnic minority families with at-risk adolescents. Churches such as the one the Garcias attended often provide positive activities and programs that can engage children and adolescents after school, on weekends, and especially during the long summer vacation when they are more likely to spend large amounts of unsupervised time in their communities while their parents are working. For example, the summer would have been a crucial period in which Miguel might have been recruited to become more actively involved in his friends' gang lifestyle. His parents had also begun to generalize the things that they had learned in family therapy and had involved Miguel and his younger brother in a positive camp activity for the summer. In many ways, this involvement with positive peers and activities also served as a protective factor not only for Miguel, but for his younger brother as well.

This case also illustrates the critical importance of training Spanish-speaking therapists who can work with clients such as the Garcia family and the need for clinics, schools, achievement mentoring programs, agencies, and master's and doctoral programs to recruit such individuals. Many therapists and teachers who do not speak Spanish have resorted to using the troubled youth as a translator. This is definitely a mistake since it reverses the role of the parents vis-à-vis their adolescent. Since the at-risk youth is presenting with problems, it is also less likely that he or she will give an accurate translation. In cases where no Spanish-speaking therapists are available, we have sometimes recruited a bilingual undergraduate from a local university to accompany the therapist to the home and translate for the family. We reached out to all student organizations on campus, including Latino, African American, and Asian groups, to recruit volunteers who were fluent in Spanish. Many of these undergraduates were also very willing to volunteer at the school as tutors and translators when necessary. One of the undergraduate professors even arranged for these students to receive credit for their work. Schools and clinics are encouraged to be creative and to reach out and develop multisystems partnerships with nearby universities. These experiences as tutors and translators have also proved helpful in recruiting young people who are fluent in Spanish and members of other ethnic minority groups to enter the fields of teaching, social work, psychology, counseling, and family therapy.

It is also helpful to have a Spanish-speaking coworker encourage the family to identify a member of their support system whom they can trust to translate for the family if the family therapist does not speak Spanish and other supports are not available. The family was also fortunate in that Ms. Rodriguez also spoke Spanish. This might not be the case throughout the at-risk youth's future years in school. Therefore, prior to completion of the therapy, the therapist also utilized the strategy of identifying someone in their support system who could function as a translator, so that the parents could continue to be informed of their son's involvement with the various systems in his life. It was also important to put this support in place so that the parents could participate in school activities for his younger brother, Carlos, over time.

Empowerment of the Parents

One of the most important aspects of the Multisystems Model is its emphasis on empowering the parents to take increasing responsibility for the interventions for their son throughout the process of home-based family therapy (Boyd-Franklin & Bry, 2000). MST also emphasizes the need for this empowerment (Henggeler et al., 2009). For example, to increase the connection between the parents and the school, the therapist asked the mother to call Ms. Rodriguez, the achievement mentor and ESL teacher, and the guidance counselor and give them her new cell phone number. In this way, the mother was empowered to create the connection with the school staff herself, rather than the therapist doing this for her. Similarly, he asked the father to contact the probation officer to ask him to attend the multisystems case conference. Later he encouraged the father to contact his pastor to arrange a meeting at the church to discuss youth activities for Miguel. These interventions were important means to directly reengage the parents with the school and the other systems involved in their son's life.

Two of the challenges presented by these parents are common for immigrant families: (1) working long hours in jobs that do not allow time off for school and court appearances, and (2) the challenge of needing someone to translate for them in important meetings with the school and other systems. Both of these issues presented opportunities for the therapist to engage and build relationships with the parents. He held evening meetings at the parents' home, conducted family sessions in Spanish, and initially translated for the parents at the school and court meetings. Gradually, however, he began to empower the parents to take charge of these issues. For example, he asked the mother to contact the achievement mentor and the guidance counselor to arrange the time for a meeting at school. He also helped the family to identify a friend from the church who was retired and therefore available to attend meetings at school to translate for the parents. These interventions were important ways to empower the parents to advocate for their sons and for these experiences to generalize into the parents' monitoring of their sons' behavior in the future. The therapist also praised the parents for using the supports provided by the church to allow monitoring and productive activities for both boys during their summer vacation while the parents were working.

Another important aspect of the empowerment of the parents involved the therapist's efforts to encourage them to invite the friends of both boys to their home and to connect with their parents. This is a challenge that many parents face, particularly those living in inner-city areas. As Jorge discussed with them, as adolescents age, enter middle and high school, and connect with new groups of friends, it becomes increasingly difficult for parents to monitor their youth's peer networks. As parental monitoring and contact with their peers is one of the most important aspects of parental empowerment (Boyd-Franklin & Bry, 2000; Dishion et al., 2003; Dodge et al., 2006; Henggeler et al., 2009), the therapist was able to impress on the parents the importance of connecting with both boys' friends and their parents or caregivers so that this pattern could become established before their sons grew older, when it might be too late. It also illustrates another value of family therapy in general and home-based treatment in particular. Rather than just meeting with Miguel alone or just with his parents, the entire family was seen together, including his brother Carlos. Therefore, the home-based family therapy had a direct positive impact on his life as well.

CHAPTER 9

Supervision and Training of Home-Based Family Therapists

For family therapists, overburdened with the demands of large caseloads, the pressures of managed care insurance companies, and the challenge of families who present with many life stressors (Boyd-Franklin, 2003; Boyd-Franklin & Bry, 2000; Boyd-Franklin et al., 2013), a supervisory process that focuses on the positive can serve as a life preserver. Just as our therapeutic methods emphasize the empowerment of clients, our supervisory philosophy is based on the empowerment of family therapists and supervisors.

Parents who feel accused, blamed, and judged by family therapists or other systems (e.g., schools, child protective services, the police, the courts) tend to blame and scapegoat their children and adolescents. In like fashion, therapists who feel blamed and unsupported by their supervisors or agencies tend to be harsh in judging or diagnosing the clients and families they treat. In order for family therapists to be able to see strengths in the families they work with, supervisors must model that approach. In this respect, our model of supportive supervision is not only an investment in the personal and professional development of therapists, it also has a direct link to clinical outcome (Boyd-Franklin, 2003; Boyd-Franklin & Bry, 2000; Boyd-Franklin et al., 2013). This chapter presents an in-depth exploration of supervisory and training techniques that will enable therapists to help the families they treat to achieve goals without suffering the burnout that all too often accompanies the treatment of families burdened with multiple problems.

THE NEED FOR AN ORIENTATION PROCESS AND TRAINING

Programs and agencies, under pressure to handle large caseloads, may view a comprehensive orientation process for new staff members as a luxury they cannot afford, especially when there is a rapid turnover of clinicians. It is certainly not in the best interests of the families we treat when new therapists are expected to function without the benefit of a thorough orientation. While a manual can explain agency policies and provide a careful overview of information new workers will need, a well-developed orientation process may be helpful in assessing the new therapist's strengths and weaknesses and, in the latter case, to provide additional training when indicated. In the absence of this orientation, in the best-case scenario clinicians seek out more senior therapists in their program or agency; in the worst-case scenario they are forced to begin immediately with a large caseload and little preparation.

Training Model

Since many master's and doctoral students as well as beginning therapists (e.g., psychologists, social workers, marriage and family therapists, and counselors) may have had limited exposure to families with at-risk adolescents, it was our intention in writing this book that it can serve as a training textbook, preparing therapists to work with these families. It will also augment the knowledge of clinicians who have received training, whether it consists of ongoing training for practitioners already in the field through their clinics, programs or agencies, or graduate school programs. Students in master's and doctoral programs can be trained to do this work in a semester-long course or in an intensive short-term (one- or two-week) course.

Prior to implementing the Multisystems Model and reaching out through home-based family therapy, it is essential that therapists first familiarize themselves with the issues often facing the families of at-risk adolescents. The chapters in Part I provide a helpful cultural and contextual introduction for therapists working with at-risk youth and their families. The presenting problems of these at-risk adolescents and their families, and the risk and protective factors at the individual, family, peer, school, and community levels are explored in Chapter 2. As many families of at-risk youth are from African American, Latino, and other ethnic minority groups and/or are from poor families, we have found it helpful to include intensive training on cultural competency (see Chapter 3). Other patterns common among families of at-risk adolescents include kinship caregiving (see Chapter 4) and multigenerational experiences of issues such as child abuse, teenage pregnancy, domestic violence, drug and alcohol abuse, and incarcerated or gang-involved family members (see Chapter 5).

The second part of the book introduces our Multisystems Model, the importance of reaching out to families whose cultures may include a suspicion of therapy, and the challenges for many poor families when multiple systems, such as child welfare, schools, the police, and the courts, have a great deal of power in their lives. Chapter 6 instructs clinicians in the basic concepts of the Multisystems Model and the process of home-based family therapy (Boyd-Franklin 1989, 2003; Boyd-Franklin & Bry, 2000; Boyd-Franklin et al., 2013). Many aspects of the MST model, an evidence-based treatment developed by Henggeler et al. (2009) (see Chapter 7), are consistent with ours, and training in this model is helpful to therapists who will be working with clients at many systemic levels. The Multisystems Model case example in Chapter 8 illustrates the process of intervening at different systems levels and will be very instructive for new trainees as well as experienced staff. As indicated earlier, because of the difficulties of this work, clinicians need supervisors who take a very hands-on, frontline approach to supervision, and who are available and can be reached when crises develop.

FRONTLINE SUPERVISION

The Multisystems Model and home-based family therapy require a very active treatment approach in which outreach plays a vital part. This can occur on many levels. As discussed in Chapter 3, because of the "resistance," hesitation, and suspicion of many communities toward mental health treatment, credibility must be established on a community level, as well as with each family. Therefore, it is very important for agency directors and clinical supervisors to have a frontline presence in the community or communities they serve. Many agencies often omit this first level of frontline supervision; others engage in community outreach only in the initial stages of the establishment of a new service or research program but fail to follow through by maintaining *ongoing* contact with the community.

One method of frontline supervision and administration that addresses the need for ongoing contact is "networking," whereby someone in a position of authority in an agency is well connected to key leaders and resources within the community. Networking serves many purposes. First, it can help to establish the positive "word of mouth" in the community that is crucial to a program, research project, or an agency's credibility. Second, designating one person to maintain ongoing contacts in the community will ensure that the clinic or agency is acting with up-to-date information, since it is not possible for individual family therapists to have key contacts in each school and multisystems agency, let alone to be cognizant of each agency's personnel changes. As shown in Chapter 8, knowledge of churches in the community can be invaluable to a family therapist who must negotiate one of these complex systems in partnership with a client or family.

Another component of frontline supervision is that supervisors and agency administrators know the families as well as the communities they serve. We have found it useful as supervisors to make occasional home visits with our supervisees, to initiate and attend meetings with community agencies, and to work in partnership with other community programs on shared grant proposals or collaborative community initiatives.

For clinicians to feel competent and supported in the "hands-on" work this treatment approach requires, it is essential that supervisors and agency administrators model this philosophy. For example, in Boyd-Franklin and Bry (2000), when a support group was being organized in a local community, supervisors co-led the first few group sessions; this helped them to understand the issues that supervisees encountered and to join with the community and establish a visible presence there.

As therapists change over time, supervisors and administrators can act as a bridge and "introduce" new workers into the community. For these new staff members and students, it is also often helpful for a supervisor or a senior, more experienced family therapist to accompany them on their first few home visits and/or multisystems case conferences, in order to support and observe. Later, the supervisor or senior therapist can give direct, nonjudgmental, and supportive supervisory input about the new clinician's home-based family intervention skills.

Another opportunity to engage in hands-on supervision occurs when a family is in crisis. We often utilize these occasions to do a consultation session with a supervisee in which the supervisor sits in on a session with a client or family, especially since a family crisis presents an opportunity for change. A supervisor or consulting clinician should be careful not to undermine the credibility or power of either the family therapist or the parental figures in the family. The manner in which the supervisor's involvement in the session is broached to the family or client should stress the collaborative efforts of all parties to find a solution. It might be expressed in this way: "With your permission, I would like to invite Dr. _____, my supervisor, to come out and meet with us for our next home-based session. We can brainstorm together about how to solve this problem."

It is also often helpful to invite a family to come in for a "live interview" at the program, agency, or clinic, in which the supervisor or consultant can meet with the family therapist and the family to explore solutions to a particular issue. Once again, it is essential that this be proposed within a collegial, collaborative framework. It is particularly important that new staff members or student trainees not undermine their credibility with their clients by presenting themselves as needing the intercession of supervisors and consultants, or by communicating that they occupy a low position in the agency hierarchy. Observing this type of interview can also be instructive for students and trainees, so holding it in a room with a one-way mirror, or videotaping with the family's consent, might be pursued. Readers are cautioned, however, that despite the training benefits of this approach, many families, particularly those from ethnic minority groups, may have negative associations with one-way mirrors or videotaping (i.e., police stations) (Boyd-Franklin, 2003). Therefore, therapists should not initiate this process unless they have a strong therapeutic alliance with all members of the family, particularly the parents or caregivers, and *all* family members are in agreement.

Frontline supervision also requires enhanced availability on the part of supervisors as well as a process for emergency consultations. Many of the clients discussed in this book have difficult life circumstances, and crises do not occur on a convenient 9-to-5 schedule. It is important that a mechanism be developed for handling such occurrences on evenings and weekends. Some programs contract with a local emergency room or crisis intervention unit. Others establish a system in which different staff members or supervisors are "on call" on a rotating basis. It is important that supervisors and key administrators also be available for consultation in these circumstances.

It is crucial, however, to be mindful that therapists and supervisors also need protection within this model of frontline supervision. Endless "on-call" days can lead to burnout and undermine the effectiveness of both staff and supervisors. Some agencies have established "comp time," so that therapists who become involved in a family's crisis regardless of their work schedule may be reimbursed by coming in later or leaving earlier when the crisis abates. In order for a "comp time" program to be successful, a record-keeping system must be developed and maintained.

Group Supervision and Team Building

Although many programs provide individual supervision for clinicians, we have found group supervision, involving a supervisor and two to four supervisees, helpful on a number of levels (Boyd-Franklin, 2003; Boyd-Franklin et al., 2013; Henggeler et al., 2009).

1. It is a powerful learning opportunity, particularly for those therapists who are just beginning to do this work, such as new clinicians,

externs, interns, and postdoctoral students. As participants in group supervision offer ideas and suggestions in each other's cases, the knowledge gained increases their ability to intervene creatively with their clients and families.

2. Group supervision provides an excellent opportunity for staff members or trainees to begin to bond with each other and learn the process of intervening on different systems levels (Boyd-Franklin et al., 2013). Effective multisystems work requires an on-call process that may involve coverage by different team members at different times. Hearing each other's cases and becoming familiar with them makes this process more feasible (Henggeler et al., 2009) in addition to facilitating team building. The team-building process is one possible antidote to burnout for clinicians, as a close-knit team provides ongoing support for all members. We have often found that it is particularly helpful to have team members who are at different levels of expertise (e.g., staff and trainees, or advanced trainees with beginners) (Boyd-Franklin et al., 2013). As the more experienced members share their knowledge with newer staff, it validates the achievement of these more experienced members and provides support for newer staff.

3. This process inevitably creates opportunities for peer supervision. As we indicated in Chapter 5, many families of at-risk adolescents present with frequent crises. It is helpful for therapists to have the support of more experienced staff when such crises occur, in addition to on-call supervisors.

4. Group supervision is a more effective use of a supervisor's time than one-on-one meetings.

THE MANAGEMENT OF CRISES

Throughout this book, we have shown how crises can often serve a purpose for clients and families (see Chapter 5). It is also important to understand the function that repetitive crises often serve for family therapists. Some family therapists, particularly early in their careers, find that solving crises puts them in a position of power vis-à-vis their clients. They begin to feel competent in the work and validated for offering a much-needed service. Often new therapists feel the need to be seen as change agents by family members and are very empowered by this process. This can also occur with experienced family therapists. Well-meaning clinicians can inadvertently fall into the trap of always responding in "crisis mode," as indicated in Chapter 5.

An important supervisory issue in many of these cases is the process of helping family therapists to explore their own role in repetitive crises. The need to feel empowered by "solving" a family crisis may occur at the expense of the empowerment of the parents or caregivers (Boyd-Franklin, 2003; Henggeler et al., 2009; Kagan & Schlossberg, 1989). It is also crucial for staff members to be aware of what constitutes an actual crisis. An anxious student, trainee, or therapist may respond to a family's definition of a "crisis" without an independent determination that it is a true emergency.

OTHER SUPERVISORY DILEMMAS

Helping Therapists to Raise Difficult Issues with Clients When Necessary

Another supervisory dilemma that can occur often is when new or inexperienced family therapists feel a need to be loved and appreciated by their clients. Although this may result in positive consequences in the beginning stages of treatment, that is, it can facilitate joining and lead to the development of a good initial therapeutic alliance in which clients show up regularly for sessions, an "excellent" relationship may often come at a price: Despite the family's regular attendance at meetings with the therapist, no change is occurring, or a major therapeutic impasse develops around a treatment issue. The challenge for the supervisee, the supervision group, and the supervisor is to identify the impasse and explore the issues that are getting in the way of the process of producing change for both the family and the clinician.

Even an experienced clinician often finds himself or herself in a dilemma when the therapist has worked hard to establish a therapeutic bond with a client and family, but begins to suspect that a family member "in recovery" may be experiencing a relapse in drug or alcohol addiction. There is often a fear that raising this issue will disrupt this therapeutic alliance. Once again, timing, sensitivity, and the framing of such an intervention are crucial in both the clinical and the supervisory process. The following case illustrates these issues.

Case Example

Barbara McMann (age 40) and her family were referred for treatment by child protective services because workers at that agency were concerned that Barbara's substance abuse might be interfering with her parenting and leading to neglect of her children. This Irish American family included Mark (age 15), Beverly (age 10), and Carl (age 5). The family was supported by public assistance and was living in a trailer park. The child protective services workers informed Barbara that if she was not able to overcome her addiction to cocaine and maintain her recovery, her children would be removed from her home.

The family therapist joined with Barbara and learned of her strong desire to keep her family together. After 2 months of sessions, the family therapist was able to convince her to go into a drug detox program, and subsequently to attend an inpatient rehab program for 28 days. The family therapist also empowered Barbara in a session to negotiate with her mother to keep her children for the length of these programs. Barbara also role-played with her therapist the process of discussing this with her children, which also empowered her. Before her entry into the detox program, a family session was held in which Barbara explained to her children what she would be doing, and she told them that they would be in their grandmother's care while she was on the inpatient detox and rehab units. With the family therapist's support, she frankly answered their questions about her addiction.

After her discharge, Barbara appeared to be a new person. She took her recovery very seriously and attended an outpatient rehab program and a number of Twelve-Step (Narcotics Anonymous) meetings per week. She also became more actively involved in parenting her children and in the home-based family therapy sessions.

Barbara had been in recovery for about 5 months when a crisis occurred: Her mother, who had been a major support to her, died suddenly of a heart attack. The family therapist, who had grown close to Barbara and her children, felt very sorry about Barbara's loss and admired her recovery struggle. There were no overt signs of Barbara's relapse. Unfortunately, the therapist missed the more subtle indications, such as the cancellation of several sessions, which would have alerted a more experienced clinician that the death of Barbara's mother might have precipitated a resumption of drug use.

After three successive weeks of Barbara's canceled sessions, the family therapist met with her supervisor and her supervisory group, who worked with the therapist to recognize the signs of Barbara's relapse. The family therapist was able to talk honestly about her fears that addressing this issue with Barbara might endanger the therapeutic alliance with her. The supervisor and the group helped the family therapist to role-play some ways to raise the issue with Barbara about her return to substance use. The emphasis was placed on Barbara's wish as a mother for a drug-free, positive life for her children. They also discussed the importance of the family therapist's emphasizing her caring for Barbara and her children.

With this direct supervisory help, the family therapist was able to raise this issue with Barbara in a positive manner, get past her denials of her current substance use, and convince her to enter a drug program that would provide housing and support groups for her and her children. This was very important to Barbara, as she did not want to lose custody of her children while she sought help.

Cultural and Racial Issues in Supervision

Prior to the last 10 years, many training programs in family therapy, social work, psychology, and psychiatry were structured around what Hardy (1989) described as the "theoretical myth of sameness . . . or the belief that all families [or clients] are virtually the same" (p. 18). Hardy successfully challenged this mindset, and subsequent scholars (Helms & Cook, 1999) extended Hardy's view to encompass the other figures in the treatment process, in addition to clients: "The cultural orientation or predisposition of each of the participants in the [therapy] process—supervisor, supervisee, and client(s)—may . . . be invisible, but is a meaningful dynamic in supervision" (p. 291).

As more ethnic minority therapists and supervisors enter the field, there is an increased likelihood of cross-cultural or cross-racial supervision (Boyd-Franklin, 2003; Falender et al., 2014; Helms & Cook, 1999). In addition, the ever-increasing diversity in the United States (McGoldrick et al., 2005) has also increased the likelihood of cross-cultural and/or cross-racial treatment. Accordingly, in recent years, the process of cross-cultural and cross-racial treatment has received more attention in the literature (Falender, Shafranske, & Falicov, 2014; Helms & Cook, 1999), as have the issues related to cross-cultural supervision as well as multiculturalism and diversity in supervision (Boyd-Franklin, 2003; Falender et al., 2014).

A number of scholars have offered guidelines for cross-cultural and cross-racial supervision (Boyd-Franklin, 2003; Falender et al., 2014; Helms & Cook, 1999). Boyd-Franklin (2003) explored this issue from the perspective of supervisors and therapists of different ethnic and racial backgrounds and has presented guidelines for supervisors of therapists from Black, White, and other ethnic backgrounds working with Black families. Supervisors must feel comfortable themselves when discussing these issues with supervisees, if the supervisees are to feel comfortable in exploring these issues with their clients and families. Falender et al. (2014) have explored the issues of multicultural supervision and issues of diversity in supervision in a much broader context involving gender and sexual orientation issues, as well as ethnic and racial differences.

Supervision as a Process of Negotiation

When a supervisor is introduced to a new staff member or family therapist, it often takes time to establish a positive working relationship and to develop an open, honest context in which the family therapist's skills can be evaluated. This process is complicated when, as in many clinics and agencies, the supervisor is responsible for evaluating the supervisee's progress prematurely, before the supervisor has had the opportunity to make an informed judgment.

Another potential pitfall is a supervisor's inadvertent overestimation or underestimation of a supervisee's experience and competence. A common example of underestimation occurs when clinicians with several years of experience in office-based family therapy are doing home-based family treatment for the first time. If they are approached by supervisors as beginning therapists, they might be resentful. However, if the supervisor conveys respect for their past experience, the therapist will be more likely to welcome ongoing consultation to assist them in the transition to home-based interventions.

In many forms of clinical work, supervision is viewed as a hierarchical, power-based relationship with the supervisee in the inferior position. Particularly in the home-based or outreach modality, such structure is contrary to effective treatment progress and to the development of counselors' competence. It is helpful to approach supervision as a process of negotiation—to frame it as consultation, which implies a partnership and not a hierarchy.

Family therapists should be encouraged in their first supervisory meetings to talk about their past experiences in the field. They should also be encouraged to discuss what they perceive to be their strengths and the areas where they feel competent. They can then be encouraged to identify areas in which they need help to grow or learn more. During the subsequent evaluation process, supervisors and supervisees can explore and discuss the progress achieved in meeting these goals. If care is taken by the supervisor in a group situation to empower more experienced staff by asking and validating their opinions, benefits will accrue to both experienced and newer clinicians.

It is also helpful for supervisors to let clinicians know that their supervisory style is open to input and negotiation. For example, as we currently supervise graduate students who are relatively inexperienced, we have found it useful to be directive in the early stages of supervision. Although this approach is also indicated when supervising therapists who are new to both family therapy and home-based approaches, it can be perceived as condescending or infantilizing by more experienced clinicians. Therefore, we have found it helpful to acknowledge our supervisory style in the initial sessions and to let our supervisees know that we see supervision as an ongoing negotiation process geared to facilitate their learning. As they become more confident, supervisees can then take more risks and begin to negotiate the type of supervision that is most helpful and empowering for them at progressive stages of their development. Often the shifts in feelings of competence are subtle, and it is helpful for supervisors to discuss this openly with their supervisees. A flexible supervision style that accommodates and is responsive to the needs of the supervisee is particularly important for staff members or trainees who have had the same supervisors for many years, although it is recommended that experiencing a number of different supervisors can enrich the experience for supervisees.

Mechanisms for Building Skills, Providing Support, and Developing Teamwork

One of the many parallels between supervision and clinical work, as emphasized throughout this book, is that often "helping" is not "empowering." Supervisors should be vigilant about empowering clinicians to take more and more responsibility for developing treatment plans and strategies. Four mechanisms are particularly helpful for empowering clinicians through skill building, support provision, and the development of teamwork: (1) use of an outside consultant, (2) clinical case conferences, (3) multidisciplinary teams, and (4) peer supervision.

The Use of an Outside Consultant

The practice of home-based, school, and community interventions is clearly demanding. Many agencies and programs have handled this dilemma by hiring an outside consultant, as needed, to advise on specific issues. Outside consultants may be utilized in helping to address organizational issues or staff burnout; to train staff members and supervisors in a specific content area that is new to them; to explore an area of cultural competency with a particular ethnic or racial group; or to offer assistance with cases demanding specific expertise, such as those involving alcoholism and drug abuse, chronic abuse or neglect, child custody, violence, and juvenile delinquency (Boyd-Franklin & Bry, 2000; Boyd-Franklin et al., 2013; Henggeler et al., 2009).

We have found it very useful to invite a colleague from outside our program to join us, our staff, and our students to explore particular issues, such as community entry, interface with other multisystemic agencies, and partnership with other programs. Both of us have had extensive experience in serving as consultants to other programs and agencies and are grateful to our colleagues who have been willing to consult with us in our own clinical and research efforts.

Case Conferences

Some agencies have adopted regular case conferences (or, in some instances, "difficult case conferences") in which all staff members, supervisors, and administrators work together, sometimes with the help of an outside consultant, to brainstorm the treatment of especially challenging cases (Boyd-Franklin et al., 2013). Despite the difficulty of the case, such sessions may be refreshing and refueling. They can also contribute to an atmosphere of ongoing learning and professional development and serve as an antidote to burnout for all staff, supervisors, administrators, and trainees.

It is helpful to agree on a format for presenting cases at these conferences. Typically, cases are written up or presented orally, or some combination of these methods is used—for example, a PowerPoint presentation accompanied by handouts. In addition, visual aids can be offered: a family tree or genogram (McGoldrick et al., 2008) can be drawn to illustrate multigenerational family patterns; or an ecomap (Boyd-Franklin, 2003; Boyd-Franklin et al., 2013; Hartman & Laird, 1983) can be included to show the involvement of the client or family with different multisystems agencies (see Chapter 8).

Case conference presentations often include the following key areas:

- Presenting problems
- Description of client and family history
- Case diagnoses
- Formulation
- Treatment plan
- Treatment summary
- Questions for discussion

In addition to the knowledge gained in such sessions, important implicit messages are conveyed: We are all in this work together; no one person has all the answers; all of us can learn from each other; asking for help is a positive thing; ongoing learning and training are important for all of us, no matter what our level of experience; and training is an antidote to burnout (Boyd-Franklin, 2003; Boyd-Franklin & Bry, 2000; Boyd-Franklin et al., 2013).

Multidisciplinary Teams

One advantage of working in the fields of mental health, home-based family intervention, medical and health services, social services, and education is that they often bring together individuals from very diverse professional backgrounds and experiences (e.g., teachers, school administrators, family therapists, psychologists, social workers, counselors, psychiatrists, other physicians, nurses, child welfare workers, outreach workers, police, probation officers, judges). These individuals often approach a problem from very different perspectives. Although such diversity may sometimes lead to misunderstandings and difficulties in communication, it can also be an enriching experience.

Unlike agencies or programs in which clinicians see clients for treatment in their office, home- or community-based therapists are often out in the field and can sometimes feel isolated and disconnected from colleagues. These frontline family therapists often need a sense of a "home base" of their own. Staff meetings and multidisciplinary team meetings can serve the purpose of countering isolation and can reinforce the sense of connectedness to the project or program. Multidisciplinary team meetings offer different professional perspectives on a problem. If these meetings are held regularly (possibly in combination with regular case conferences), they can contribute greatly to the process of team building.

These team meetings are also an excellent time to share resources, including contacts with individuals in other agencies and schools. Staff members can interact with colleagues trained in different family therapy models, or more individually focused behavioral, cognitive-behavioral, or psychodynamic approaches. Team meetings also present an excellent opportunity to identify the "agency experts" on different multisystems institutions. For example, a social worker with considerable child welfare experience may be able to help staff members interact more effectively with child protective services. A psychiatrist with years of hospital-based experience may be able to help nonpsychiatric mental health workers to recognize the reasons for prescribing current medications and to understand the medical terminology of other physicians. If this sort of interaction takes place within a collaborative, supportive framework, multidisciplinary team meetings can be enriching for all involved.

For administrators, these meetings can serve both a team-building and an organizational purpose. They provide an opportunity to discuss intake cases with staff members and to discuss treatment plans. They serve the purpose of helping to orient new staff members and trainees to the "culture of the program." Finally, they provide an opportunity to strategize about issues affecting the entire agency, such as funding, managed care, census of clients, and new programs and directions for the agency.

Peer Supervision

In the current atmosphere of budget cuts and managed care demands, family therapists should be prepared for the possibility that they may not be provided with adequate supervision. What is considered "supervision" at some clinics or social service agencies can constitute little more than administrative monitoring of required paperwork at its worst or case management at its best, rather than a process of receiving regular clinical or case supervision. Other clinics or agencies may provide excellent case supervision for students, interns, and trainees but may abruptly discontinue supervision once a family therapist, psychologist, social worker, or psychiatrist has completed training and obtained licensure. This is unfortunate because limitations on the process of supervision decrease the clinical effectiveness of family therapists and may increase the likelihood of staff burnout. In home-based family treatment as well as all multisystems work, even experienced workers need ongoing clinical case supervision and consultation.

One way to counter this deficit is for family therapists to form peer supervision groups with other workers from their own agency, or possibly from other agencies. This can be planned around lunchtime: Everyone can bring a brown-bag lunch and spend an hour once a week discussing cases. The case conference format can also be utilized, or a more informal structure can be tried. It is essential, however, that meetings be regularly scheduled. It is helpful for meetings to be arranged for an entire year in advance, so that participants reserve those dates on their calendars. If lunchtime meetings do not work out because of competing schedules, some therapists have found it beneficial to arrange early morning or after-work meetings once a week. Even if they are scheduled for once or twice a month, sessions can be extremely helpful if they meet the two necessary conditions of regularity and predictability.

Family therapists often underestimate the value of peer supervision: One does not need an "expert" in order to learn; regular case discussions sharpen the clinical skills of all therapists (Boyd-Franklin et al., 2013). It is helpful if a clear ground rule is established early on that only clinical case material or multisystemic case issues will be discussed during this time, as problems can arise when discussions meander off-topic (e.g., if clinicians use this meeting to "vent" or complain about organizational problems). It is also helpful to rotate presentations so that all members of the group may benefit from the peer supervisory process.

Supervision and Training as Antidotes to Burnout

Boyd-Franklin (2003) and Boyd-Franklin et al. (2013) discuss regular staff training as an "antidote to burnout." Supervision often provides a direct "lifeline" for family therapists. Ongoing training offers an opportunity for all therapists to keep their skills current and developed. Recent developments in the field, such as the impact of managed care and the funding priorities of state and national agencies, are appropriate topics for training. Special topics and current developments in various areas (e.g., cultural competency, cross-racial treatment, drug and alcohol dependency, physical abuse and neglect, sexual abuse, domestic violence, gang violence) can be offered. It is not always necessary to go outside an agency to find speakers. Senior staff members with expertise in a particular area can feel empowered if they are invited to give presentations to the rest of their colleagues. Also, since few agencies have budgets extensive enough to send all staff members to professional conferences, one staff person can attend the conference with the understanding that he or she will then do in-service training for other staff members. It is helpful if this responsibility is rotated so that everyone benefits (Boyd-Franklin et al., 2013).

Professional Growth and Development

Another casualty of cost cutting has been a decrease in attention to the ongoing professional growth and development of therapists. This is a major loss because these discussions can also serve as an antidote to burnout. Successful supervisors and administrators often make the time to discuss professional development plans with each staff member at least once a year. This support, though minimal in time, has many benefits in terms of staff morale and energy. Regular discussion of continuing education programs being offered by professional organizations can provide an incentive for further growth and training. Although few agencies can afford to pay for this training, this is a situation where a "comp time" arrangement is appropriate: Staff members can arrange with their senior administrator to work additional hours in order to be allowed to attend a training activity.

Career plans and further education can also be discussed with supervisees. Sometimes these goals must be conceived of as "long term" since they might constitute "overload" in a trainee's current situation. It is important that future plans be discussed individually in a supportive atmosphere and that all staff members, and not just the "chosen few," have the benefit of this encouragement.

The Need for Clinician Self-Care

In a recent book, *Therapy in the Real World,* Boyd-Franklin et al. (2013) devoted a chapter to the need for clinician self-care. As we have indicated throughout this book, working within a Multisystems Model with families of at-risk adolescents is rewarding and fulfilling, but it is also very challenging and demanding. Henggeler et al. (2009) recommended that caseloads for full-time clinicians encompass only four to six families at a time because of the intense nature of this work. Many of the families that we treat have members who have experienced multiple traumas (e.g., physical or sexual abuse, homicides or deaths of close family members, community violence). In addition, many experience the traumas related to poverty, homelessness, racism, discrimination, and other societal issues. Hearing repeated experiences with these issues can be exhausting for clinicians, and they can begin to feel overwhelmed. In some cases, particularly in hearing repeated descriptions of violence, shootings, killings, physical or sexual abuse, and other traumas, clinicians can experience vicarious traumatization (Dass-Brailsford, 2007) in which they begin to feel the effects of these traumatic experiences. Thus, in addition to the organizational supports of reasonable caseloads, it is important for clinicians themselves to recognize the signs of compassion fatigue or burnout that may result from the demands of their work (Dass-Brailsford, 2007). Boyd-Franklin et al. (2013) have given extensive examples of self-care that individual therapists can practice as well as organizational interventions that clinics and agencies can include that can serve as "antidotes to burnout" (Boyd-Franklin, 2003; Boyd-Franklin et al., 2013).

EMPOWERMENT OF FAMILY THERAPISTS AND SUPERVISORS

In summary, as we have stated throughout this book, our primary goal is *to empower families, family therapists, and their supervisors*. Isolation is a major problem for families and for family therapists. Therefore, we encourage all supervisors and family therapists to use training conferences and agency outreach, as well as in-house case conferences, as an opportunity to build support networks for themselves. It is crucial that family therapists find peer networks and supervision that can sustain them in this exciting and challenging, yet difficult and demanding, work. It is our hope that this book will provide a knowledge base that will empower family therapists and supervisors to do their jobs even more effectively.

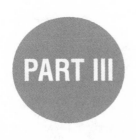

ACHIEVEMENT MENTORING

AN EVIDENCE-BASED,
SCHOOL-BASED INTERVENTION

CHAPTER 10

School Engagement, Disengagement, Dropout, and a Learning Theory Approach

with Patricia Simon

Public education offers cognitively and developmentally appropriate training, in a gradually less sheltered setting, until adolescents are at least 18 years old. Yet some youth tragically disengage from this protective factor while they are still eligible to receive it. When adolescents fail to take full advantage of public education or drop out of it altogether, the human potential of the approximately 20% of youth who do not graduate from high school often remains untapped. If students do not learn the necessary skills of attending school regularly, paying attention to what authority figures teach, following instructions for assignments in class, regulating themselves to complete assignments at home, and using initiative to find extracurricular activities that suit them, they probably will not have those skills as adults when they are necessary to earn a living and advance in careers, thus limiting their ability to access and maintain responsible, financially sustaining employment. What can

Patricia Simon, PhD, is Associate Research Scientist in the Division of Prevention and Community Research, Department of Psychiatry, Yale University School of Medicine.

schools do so that adolescents do stay engaged, learn, and develop skills for adulthood?

Although there have been recent improvements in national high school completion rates (U.S. Department of Education, 2014), many low-income, urban, and/or minority group members disproportionately fail to earn diplomas. While 85% of White students complete high school, the completion rate is 76% for Hispanics and 68% for African Americans. When graduation rates were analyzed with more specificity, it was found that since 1980 Mexican American students have been the most likely to repeat grades and drop out of school (Jensen & Sawyer, 2013). More than ethnicity and race, low socioeconomic status, particularly among urban adolescents, is the strongest predictor of failure to graduate from high school (U.S. Department of Education, 2014). In some urban areas, only 50 to 55% of high school students graduate. Failure to graduate often results in other negative outcomes, such as increasing the likelihood of (1) delinquent behaviors (Henry et al., 2012), (2) substance abuse (Bachman et al., 2008), (3) alcohol abuse and dependence (Roebroek & Koning, 2016), (4) welfare dependence (Belfield & Levin, 2007), (5) incarceration (Lochner & Moretti, 2004), (6) unemployment (Symonds et al., 2016), and (7) low wages when employed (Symonds et al., 2016).

What interferes with adolescents staying in school and taking advantage of this opportunity to learn information and, even more importantly, learn personal habits that will lead to advantages for the rest of their lives? Are there malleable factors that might increase the percentage of all youth—regardless of race, ethnicity, family income, and neighborhood—who graduate from high school? If there are modifiable predictors, can they be changed, and will such change lead to more school completion? Research has indicated that school engagement is the primary conceptual model for explaining differential high school completion rates and subsequent adult outcomes (Fall & Roberts, 2012).

SCHOOL ENGAGEMENT

The concept of school engagement has been explained by various researchers as: (1) encompassing what students "*feel* and *do* to be academically successful" (Finn & Zimmer, 2012, p. 98); (2) "the attention, . . . investment, and effort students" put into work related to school (Marks, 2000, p. 155); and (3) manifested in students who "concentrate on their work, are enthusiastic about it, and are deeply interested in academic content" (Pressley & McCormick, 1995, p. 328).

The concepts of school engagement and disengagement were first discussed as part of Finn's participation-identification theory in 1989 (Finn, 1989). Subsequent decades of observational, correlational, predictive, and mediation research have further refined Finn's concept, so that school engagement now is understood to be multidimensional and to include four, continuously distributed (low to high) interdependent components, each with its own indicators (Reschly & Christenson, 2012): (1) an *academic* component involving observable behaviors such as homework and class work completion that result in report card grades; (2) a *behavioral* component that encompasses abiding by written and unwritten classroom rules and is indicated by the number of disciplinary problems; (3) a *cognitive* component that comprises internal processes, such as deliberate decision making and problem solving; and (4) an *affective* component that involves a sense of belonging at one's school and acceptance by teachers and peers (Finn & Zimmer, 2012).

Development of School Disengagement

Finn (1989) has always seen school engagement as a dynamic process, either expanding over the duration of schooling as a child increasingly participates in routine classroom activities, succeeds academically, identifies with school, and exerts more and more initiative; or, conversely, decreasing as a student loses interest in what school offers, participates less in the classroom, complies with fewer behavioral expectations, and feels more passive and alienated. Thus, the signs of developing student disengagement are increasingly poorer grades; more discipline referrals; heightened negative feelings about teachers and peers; and fewer beliefs in self-improvement.

Both academic and nonacademic factors can impact student engagement. Research has shown that disengagement can be influenced by a number of variables. Lower socioeconomic status, for example, has been identified as a factor in greater and increasing disengagement (Li & Lerner, 2011). A longitudinal study showed that stressful family events, parenting practices and attitudes, student factors, and negative experiences over time beginning during the first year in school interact to influence school engagement trajectories (Alexander, Entwisle, & Hoorsey, 1997). Students may be consistently disengaged over time or fluctuate from disengaged to engaged status (Tuominen-Soini & Salmela-Aro, 2014). Thus, school disengagement does not decline in a straight line. Eccles et al. (1993) has attributed the variability of school engagement over time to the "person-environment fit" (Eccles et al., 1993, p. 22).

Disengagement is particularly concerning once students start high school because, as Reschly and Christenson (2012) pointed out, they are approaching a time when they will no longer be legally mandated to attend school. They can drop out, or they can also stay in school and fail to earn a diploma. In fact, a surprisingly large number of students remain in high school for 4 years but do not earn diplomas due to failure to pass graduation tests and insufficient credits (Christenson et al., 2008).

Three scenarios have been suggested as frameworks to explain the school dropout process: adolescents may be pushed, pulled, or fall out of school (Jordan, Lara, & McPartland, 1994). Students may be *pushed out* of school, particularly in low-income, urban communities, as a result of harsh school discipline policies. For example, students who frequently receive out-of-school suspensions primarily because of behavioral issues may often fall far behind in their academic work and report lower levels of school bonding, thus contributing to greater likelihood of school dropout (Catalano, Oesterle, Fleming, & Hawkins, 2004). Those who leave high school in less than 4 years often leave because of discipline problems (Rumberger & Rotermund, 2012). Students may be *pulled out* of school by factors unrelated to school, such as illness; teen pregnancy; or their families' financial circumstances, which might necessitate the need for a student to obtain full-time employment. Students may *fall out* of school when they receive insufficient personal and educational support for academic problems and thus experience lower academic engagement (Whitaker, Graham, Severtson, Furr-Holden, & Latimer, 2012).

Protective and Risk Factors and Disengagement Trajectories

According to Johnson, McGue, and Iacono (2006), once students reach the age of 11, school engagement is the most decisive factor influencing academic achievement, surpassing others such as family characteristics. Eccles, O'Neill, and Wigfield (2015), in their examination of the research, identified student protective factors that lead to positive educational trajectories as (1) high aspirations (life dreams), (2) confidence in one's ability to achieve those aspirations, (3) good academic record, and (4) few behavior problems.

Although the configurations of risk factors are different for different children (Bry, McKeon, & Pandina, 1982; Rumberger, 2004), signs of school disengagement can often be identified in students well before the age at which dropout is an option. Predictions of school dropout have been made with accuracy as early as kindergarten (Pagani et al., 2008), sixth grade (Balfanz, Herzog, & MacIver, 2007), seventh grade, and ninth grade (Janosz, LeBlanc, Boulerice, & Tremblay, 2000). In addition, the pathways to dropout vary among students. In a Montreal longitudinal study, Janosz et al. (2000) identified four patterns which they characterized, in order of prevalence, as "quiet dropouts," "maladjusted dropouts," "disengaged dropouts," and "low achievers." Forty percent of the students who did not complete high school by the time they were 22 years old were classified as "quiet dropouts" because they did not show obvious risk factors and, in fact, had been considered motivated students at prior points in their schooling. Another 40% exhibited extensive issues with both academic performance and behavior (the "maladjusted dropouts"). Ten percent of the dropouts consistently had earned at least average grades and displayed no behavior problems but had shown little motivation in school (the "disengaged dropout"). In contrast with the disengaged dropout, the 10% characterized as "low achievers" received failing grades as a result of their low motivation but, in common with the disengaged dropout, demonstrated no behavior issues. Delineating dropout patterns in this manner revealed three potentially modifiable influences—low motivation, behavior problems, and failing grades—which, if addressed at a sufficiently early stage of schooling, may reverse negative trajectories.

COMPONENTS OF SCHOOL ENGAGEMENT

Academic Component

The observable behaviors of a student that are related to learning constitute the academic aspect of school engagement. This component also includes student attentiveness in class, time on-task in class, completion of in-class assignments and homework assignments, and participation in extracurricular school activities. Students need to attend school regularly and be on time for this essential learning to occur, National data show that absences increase over time into high school for all students (Balfanz & Byrnes, 2012). Bry and George (1980), and Reyes, Gillock, Kobus, and Sanchez (2000) found that the attendance of at-risk students in the eighth and ninth grades had deteriorated to such an extent, when compared to other students and even their own prior record, that it was reasonable to conclude that they had already started the process, albeit gradually, of dropping out of school. Another indicator of this population's disengagement with academics was also present—failing courses and repeating a grade in school.

Bachman et al. (2008) found that one in four boys and one in six girls are held back before they start high school. According to their research, repeating a grade between the first and eighth grades negatively affects academic achievement thereafter. Other researchers have corroborated the end of eighth grade as a pivotal point in determining the trajectory of an adolescent's life. Whereas grades drop for *all* urban students as they enter high school (Rosenkranz, de la Torre, Stevens, & Allensworth, 2014), having a low grade-point average (GPA) by the end of eighth grade is associated with increased chances of being held back, being suspended or expelled, and eventually dropping out of school before graduation (Bachman et al., 2008). Examining the cumulative effect of several indicators of academic school disengagement, the Rochester Youth Development Study showed that it was related to high school dropout and problem behaviors in adolescence and early adulthood (Henry et al., 2012). Moreover, the effect of academic school disengagement on future problem behaviors appears to be mediated by high school dropout.

Behavioral Component

The behavioral component of school engagement involves abiding by school rules, both written and unwritten (Finn & Zimmer, 2012, p. 104). Inherent in this characteristic is valuing customs and standards appropriate in various social environments. Caring to please others, particularly adult authority figures such as teachers, motivates students to learn the rules and endeavor to obey them. Awareness of how one's behavior impacts others, and the self-control not to indulge the impulse to break a rule, are important. Also important are communication skills. Being able to listen to adults and answer their questions in polite, respectful, socially acceptable ways are necessary to stay out of trouble.

Academic performance and behavior should not be seen as isolated from one another. Finn and Zimmer (2012) pointed out that every model of school engagement emphasizes the interaction between the academic and behavioral components. As only 10% of dropouts in the Janosz et al. (2000) study were "low achiever dropouts," poor academic performance by itself does not account for elevated school dropout rates. Interestingly, Janosz et al. (2000) found that low academic achievement could be predicted by early oppositional behavior. This finding stands to reason as a youth's antisocial behavior disrupts learning opportunities (Finn & Zimmer, 2012) and as the adolescent is otherwise preoccupied and is not paying attention to the teacher's instruction. Such misbehavior also has the consequence of teachers being less inclined, however unconsciously, to give the adolescent individual help. In addition, when misbehavior merits classroom exclusion (e.g., in the case of being sent to the office of a school authority figure such as a guidance counselor or the principal, or in the case of in-school or out-of-school suspension), the youth misses crucial teaching time and in-class practice of essential information, such as math facts and methods. Subsequently, the adolescent may be unable to pass tests when they are given. As negative school experiences accumulate, it may be surprising that an adolescent comes to school at all and less surprising that he or she will drop out as soon as legally possible (Whitaker et al., 2012).

Researchers' findings suggest that students may engage in learning-disruptive behavior problems at school because they have not been taught effective social skills at home. Instructive research on understanding the trajectory from early behavior problems to low academic achievement to school dropout has been conducted by Patterson, DeBaryshe, and Ramsey (1989) and Dishion and Patterson (2016). In studying the connection between certain parenting styles and children's behavioral and academic problems in school, they observed that families can inadvertently train children to use coercive, antisocial methods to influence other people when they employ coercive parenting methods at home. Parents who use coercive methods (threatening, bribing, etc.) to influence their children to do what they want them to do (e.g., chores) inadvertently teach their children to use aggressive methods (irritability, temper tantrums, destruction of property, rage, etc.) to avoid doing what the parent wants them to do. At home, the adolescent avoids or escapes his or her parents' threats by doing something so aversive (e.g., deliberately waking up a sleeping baby) that the parents' attention is diverted to handling the negative situation their adolescent has created (soothing the crying baby). Thus, the adolescent avoids not only doing the chore, but also the punishment for not doing the chore. The youth then has learned the habit of using aversive behaviors as a method to stop interactions that are not desired. Such adolescents learn to influence other people not through polite, effective, respectful communication but through aggressive behavior.

When they get to school, students who prefer socially acceptable ways of influencing each other avoid the coercive student. The student can be a friend of only other coercive students. This behavior also impacts relationships with teachers. Having been taught by parents a coercive way of trying to force others to do what they want, such students will become irritable or audibly reject help from or insult a teacher who tries to help them learn in class. In order not to stimulate a "scene" or to be rejected or insulted in front of the other students, a teacher will unconsciously avoid interaction with the student who has not learned polite, respectful, and effective communication with others. Therefore, it is not surprising that researchers found that adults with higher levels of social competence were more likely to have graduated from high school than those adults with lower levels of social competence (Hamre & Pianta, 2006).

Affective Component

The affective aspect of school engagement refers to emotional feelings of belonging to and valuing the school social community and being wanted and accepted there (Finn & Zimmer, 2012; Reschley & Christensen, 2012). As is true of the other elements of school engagement, the affective component can exert influence on other components, such as academic and behavioral performance (Monahan, Oesterle, & Hawkins, 2010). For example, McNeely (2005) found that for both middle school students and high school students, school connectedness (feeling respected and "feeling cared for") was a stronger predictor of higher grades and lower behavior problems than any other predictor they tested. Finn and Zimmer (2012) reported that this affective component of school engagement was an *indirect* influence on students' academic performance in the classroom.

School belonging tends to decrease in middle school (Anderman, 2003). Over the course of high school, it remains stable for boys, but it continues to decline for girls (Gillen-O'Neel & Fuligni, 2013). One possible explanation for declines once students enter middle school is that at this stage they often have multiple teachers, which may make the sense of connectedness more attenuated. Research has demonstrated the importance of teachers to the affective component of school engagement. From as early as kindergarten, a child's perceptions of teacher–child relationships are associated with youth participation in positive academic behaviors (Papadopoulou, 2016). Positive relationships with school adults and peers enable learning to take place and give students reasons to please adults. Perceived teacher support buffers the effects of low-income and minority group status on academic achievement (Fall & Roberts, 2012). Recently, Stepney (2016) found supportive relationships with school faculty, staff, and peers to be related to higher GPAs in Hispanic adolescents.

In a systematic review, teacher–student relationships (affective school engagement) were found to predict other forms of school engagement, that is, psychological engagement, academic grades, school attendance, disruptive behaviors, suspension, and dropout (Quin, 2017). Fruiht and Wray-Lake (2013) found, for all ethnic groups and all ages from childhood through young adulthood, that having a teacher–mentor was more predictive of school achievement than being mentored by an individual other than a teacher, such as a family member, friend, or other individual from the community. Taking further the analogy of going to school as the job of an adolescent, relationships with other students, that is, peers, are comparable to relationships with coworkers—a crucial determinant as to whether school (or work) is a positive or negative environment. Urga (2003) looked specifically at peer relationships and found that a sense of acceptance by classmates who valued academics mediated a positive relationship between overall school belonging and academic achievement.

Conversely, researchers have documented that the lack of the affective aspect of school engagement, termed social distrust, can result in negative responses (Bushman et al., 2016). For example, Chung-Do, Goebert, Hamagani, Chang, and Hishinuma (2015) recently documented a relationship between a low sense of school connectedness and violent attitudes in Asian and Pacific Island youth. Williams and Guerra (2011) found that social trust in school between adolescents and adults leads to less peer violence (bullying). This research indicates that one predicate for safer schools would be for adults to reach out to at-risk adolescents and offer a positive, life-changing connection. Unfortunately, one-third of at-risk youth report that they have never had an adult who acted like a mentor while they were growing up (Bruce & Bridgeland, 2014). And a 2015 study by the Center for Promise, titled "Don't Quit on Me: What Young People Who Left School Say about the Power of Relationship," found that a substantial portion of the youth attributed leaving school to negative relationships with adults or peers. It is especially noteworthy that many of these adolescents were high school seniors close to graduation.

Cognitive Component

The cognitive component is described as positive attitudes about school, "perceived relevance and motivation to learn" (Reschly & Christensen, 2012, p. 9), and a self-concept of being competent in school. The latter aspect is called "self-efficacy" by Bandura (1997) and is defined as the belief that one can actually meet the challenges that one will face. Stepney (2016) found level of self-efficacy to be a protective factor for low-income Hispanic high school students whose GPAs reflected the presence of school engagement. An exploration of school dropouts by Fall and Roberts (2012) revealed the interdependent nature of the various components of school engagement. They found that students' emotional sense of social support from teachers and peers (affective component) predicted cognitive perception of competence (cognitive component), which, in turn, predicted academic achievement (academic component), low behavior problems (behavioral component), and less school dropout. Finn and Zimmer (2012) included employing active decision making and problem solving in the cognitive component. The National Research Council (2013) concluded in a "Reforming Juvenile Justice" report that there are three important ingredients for healthy youth development: having (1) a supportive adult authority figure mentor, (2) an association with prosocial peers, and (3) the capacity to engage in autonomous decision making.

Students with high cognitive school engagement see themselves

as being able to control their destiny. Their self-confidence and persistence increase self-reliance over time (Cleary, 2015). They become
more autonomous learners and independent, responsible citizens. These
qualities clearly indicate perceptions of agency in the student, forming a
strong contrast with Seligman's learned helplessness concept (Peterson,
Maier, & Seligman, 1993). Eccles et al. (2015) found that, although self-
perceptions of competence tend to decline gradually in all children as
they progress from grade 1 to grade 12, self-perception of competence
together with subjective valuing of school work nevertheless predict subsequent academic achievement and related behaviors.

POTENTIALLY MODIFIABLE ASPECTS OF SCHOOL ENGAGEMENT

School engagement is so strongly associated with adult success that all
professionals who work with adolescents—teachers, counselors, coaches,
principals, administrators, other school personnel, therapists, recreation
specialists, police, judges, probation officers, residential staff, camp
counselors, and all who train and supervise these professionals—are
committed to enhancing and supporting adolescents' involvement and
success in school, starting with kindergarten. As the research we have
cited in the preceding paragraphs makes clear, youth with low school
engagement can be identified by both school professionals' face-to-face
experiences and from school records. Some factors that predict school
engagement, such as income, parenting, neighborhood, race, ethnicity,
and previous educational experiences, cannot be modified by professionals working solely with adolescents. That should not, however, discour-
age caring adults from interceding in adolescents' lives in the areas in
which they can make a difference. The stakes are high. Whether or not a
youth earns a high school diploma makes a difference throughout adult
life in accessing job and relationship opportunities. Furthermore, the
habits and skills that students learn during this process will prove vital
to maintaining economic security, stable adult relationships, and social
supports.

In-depth examinations of research into the etiology and prevention of
life-altering substance abuse (Bachman et al., 2008) and life-determining
youth violence (Bushman et al., 2016) point to bolstering and maintaining school engagement to prevent negative outcomes. Bachman et al.
(2008) offered a powerful conclusion stressing that interventions are not
wasted on even previously low-achieving students:

> Overcoming . . . educational problems is particularly important
> . . . Educational research is showing that there are successful alter-
> natives to grade retention and ways to help children deal with

and overcome . . . educational failures. For example, teachers and curriculum developers can provide students with experiences in which they feel *competent* and lessons that highlight the *value* of their schoolwork [emphasis added]. . . . Even students who struggle in school can remain motivated to persist in the face of failure, provided they believe that additional effort can result in personal growth and success. . . . Educational programs and additional support for low-achieving students are among the best ways to decrease adolescent substance use and delinquency. (p. 279)

In a parallel fashion, Bushman et al. (2016) stated that

[a]cademic achievement during the school years, along with school engagement, predict *lower* rates of youth violence. . . . Such findings may reflect a variety of cognitive and emotional self-control skills associated with school readiness and success, as well as the effectiveness of schools in engaging children and preventing dropout. (pp. 21–22)

They go on to recommend that "general efforts in schools should focus on creating climates where students feel engaged and feel a sense of belonging. Of particular importance is the development of mechanisms that can build social trust between youth and adults" (p. 28).

Thus, intervention programs need a bidirectional focus—decrease school disengagement-related problem behaviors and increase students' sense of efficacy, belonging, and competence. In addition, interventions must be targeted and individually designed to meet each student's specific combination of needs related to school engagement and the dynamic roles they play over time in each student's development and school experiences. Given the heterogeneity in students' combinations of risk factors and protective factors, it is especially important that programs are not developed within a "one-size-fits-all" framework.

LEARNING THEORY AND SCHOOL ENGAGEMENT MODIFICATION

The concept of school engagement delineates empirically identified and extensively confirmed student-centered variables that correlate closely with academic achievement, behavior problems, high school completion, and adult success. School engagement's continuous variables reflect ranges of reactions and responses that children and adolescents have during their educational experiences. Examples of these variables, as discussed earlier, include class work completion, time on-task, homework completion, discipline referrals, expectations regarding teachers, and sense of acceptance by peers. Students' reactions and responses provide stakeholders (notably, researchers, parents, educators, and other professionals who work with adolescents) with current indicators and prospective predictors of the degree to which each is taking advantage of his or her education and the likelihood that the individual will complete high school and obtain a diploma. The variables also offer targets for programs designed to improve school engagement so that more at-risk students can derive benefit from education and graduate from high school. Measuring the variables in a randomized, controlled trial can demonstrate whether a program improves aspects of school engagement, and thus the probability of graduation, or whether it does not.

Although the concept of school engagement functions well to delineate *which* student responses and reactions need to be improved to increase the likelihood of graduation, it does not provide insight as to *how* student responses and reactions can be changed. For that, a dynamic, comprehensive theory of human development is needed to pinpoint exactly *what* determines change in people. With that information, mechanisms can be targeted and altered in programs designed to change students' school engagement-related responses. Learning theory fills the void by offering a comprehensive explanation of moment-to-moment determinants of individuals' responses and reactions. If the mechanisms identified by learning theory as determining student reactions and responses could be altered to change school engagement variables, positive outcomes for at-risk students might be achievable.

Features of Learning Theory

Learning theory attempts to explain everything people do (Ramnerö & Törneke, 2008). This includes what we see people do, when someone acts, and what we do inside, when we think, feel, and remember. Learning theory considers acting, thinking, feeling, and remembering together because it uses the same principles to explain whatever people do, think, feel, or remember. Learning theory's first assumption always is that any action, thought, feeling, or memory has been *learned* through universal learning processes.

The function of theories is to provide hypothesized explanations for why people do what they do. We can then make educated guesses as to how to change what they do. The results of interventions based on these guesses will reveal whether or not the theory is useful. That is, do the theory's hypothesized explanations about why people do what they do enlighten and assist our ability to change what they do or not? We have found learning theory to be useful in guiding effective interventions to change what at-risk youth do.

One feature of learning theory is its focus on the present. It explains moment-to-moment, discrete actions, feelings, thoughts, and memories, instead of longer-term patterns of what a person does, thinks, feels, or remembers, as would be the case with a personality characteristic. In common terminology, the discrete, learned things that we do moment to moment would be referred to as habits and skills. Since the assumption of learning theory is that whatever we do is learned, this suggests that every time we act, feel, think, or remember, we may learn something that will result in our doing the thing differently the next time. Skills and habits are in a continuing process of change. Because everything is the result of learning, everything can be changed through new learning.

Thus, learning theory offers an optimistic, instead of pessimistic, view of people. People are not seen as having entrenched, unchangeable, permanent characteristics. Correspondingly, what people do, think, feel, and remember are not seen as pathological but, rather, as learned responses and reactions, cultivated in the same manner as all other learning. Therefore, a student may exhibit a "skill" deficit or a maladaptive "habit," attributable to the same universal learning processes that account for all human functions. The skill deficit or maladaptive habit does not need to be pathologized because it is malleable and capable of constant change.

Another implication of learning theory is that thoughts (e.g., expectations), memories, and feelings are not permanent either. They are learned as the result of moment-to-moment learning experiences, so they are continually changing. This means that one's own beliefs (thoughts) about things may not be "true," just as is the case with feelings and memories. Our feelings may often change. Our memories may not be accurate. Instead, each is something that we learned under specific circumstances and is subject to continued change. This applies to the expectations, feelings, and memories of other people as well. Learning theory does not see them as permanent or accurate either. Thus, the things that teachers, students, and parents say, think, feel, and remember were learned under certain circumstances, and new learning experiences will change them. Learning does not require awareness of the determining consequences. Thus, professionals, teachers, students, and parents alike are probably unaware of 90% of the *actual* consequences (immediate payoffs) that determine our behavior moment to moment. This is one reason why we do not tend to ask adolescents, teachers, or parents *why* they do things. We fear they will give (and hear themselves stating) an inaccurate (learned) reason for their past actions, thinking, feelings, and memories based on what they have been taught through previous consequences, instead of being able to report the actual immediate consequences that determined their behavior. Rather than ask the why question, we would rather ask students to generate ideas on what they could do differently in the future. Monitoring actual student responses and consequences (Carbonaro, 1998) provides more accurate records of skill learning and maladaptive habits than asking students why they do things.

Learning Theory's Central Mechanism of Change

According to learning theory, we learn through the immediate consequences of what we do, think, feel, or remember. As immediate consequences or proximal "payoffs" are the most likely mechanisms of change or change agents, the most helpful question to ask when trying to understand why an at-risk adolescent did something is, "What events followed immediately?" or, depending on the context, "What immediate effects did the act, thought, feeling, or memory episode have?" What purpose or function might the act, thought, feeling, or memory have had at that moment?

When an occurrence of a consequence makes a discrete act, thought, feeling, or memory *more likely* to occur in the future, the consequence becomes, in technical terminology, a *reinforcer.* When applying this learning principle to work with at-risk youth, the common phrase is "catching a kid doing something good today."

The more often adolescents are noticed and "consequated" (praised) immediately for doing, or saying, or feeling, or thinking something that increases their school engagement, the more often they will do that in the future, which augurs well for their chance to graduate. Immediate acknowledgment (reinforcement) of positive behaviors needs multiple repetitions, as past behavior has momentum (tends to persist even when conditions change). Nevin (2000) described behavior change as analogous to changing the course of a large cargo ship or a large bus. Thus, most learning takes multiple repetitions over a long time. There is little "one-trial learning." For at-risk adolescents to unlearn maladaptive habits and to learn instead the skills necessary to take advantage of public education, repetition with a coach who consistently provides appropriate consequences is necessary, in much the same way one learns multiplication tables or spelling words.

When an occurrence of a consequence makes a discrete act, thought, feeling, or memory *less likely* to occur in the future, the consequence, in technical terminology, is a *punishment.* Another way that a discrete act can become less likely to occur in the future is if an incompatible, alternative act brings about more "payoff" than the habitual act (Daniels, 2016). For instance, a student may have the habit of skipping class to avoid expected embarrassment (punishment) if a teacher asks her to describe a homework assignment that she did not do. Her habit of skipping class could become less frequent if she began expecting, instead, an offer of help from the teacher (or someone else in the classroom) who would assist her to complete the homework during the class.

Positive results are a function of continuous reinforcement of responses that increase and maintain school engagement (Biglan, 2015). Eccles (2008) suggested that programs to enhance school engagement should be conceptualized as "nutrition models" rather than as "inoculation models." A short-term "inoculation" program will not suffice because the immediate consequences for actions, thoughts, feelings, and memories need to persist for an entire lifetime. As adolescents continue with their education past the initial intervention, the frequency of reinforcement can be reduced, but actions, thoughts, feelings, and memories consistent with school engagement must continue to be recognized and acknowledged in order for the new learning to continue.

Generalization of learning across people, environments, and time must also be considered when planning and implementing programs, as research has indicated that new skills and habits learned in one environment do not automatically transfer to another (Forehand, Breiner, McMahon, & Davies, 1981). Therefore, positive consequences for exhibiting school engagement must be provided by multiple people in multiple settings across time. For instance, parents should be told about signs of a youth's engagement in school and be asked to praise them at home (Jurbergs, Palcic, & Kelley, 2010). School engagement support programs should continue beyond one school year so that students find the same reinforcement contingencies to be in place when they return to school after summer vacation. All personnel in the school should look for and acknowledge school engagement in students even when they are not directly involved in teaching or interventions with at-risk adolescents. Mayer, Sulzer-Azaroff, and Wallace (2013) spell out multiple additional ways that skill and habit learning can occur and be maintained in the school setting.

Learning can also occur through observing someone else being reinforced for a new action, thought, feeling, or memory, and imitating the reinforced behavior. Bandura (1977) established that direct experience with immediate reinforcement is not necessary for every new action, thought, feeling, and memory to be learned. This insight is valuable because, without the ability to learn through observation—what Bandura called observational learning or modeling—learning would be painstakingly slow. Because learning can occur through observation or modeling, students can learn school engagement (and disengagement) from each other and adults in the school. Thus, school personnel should model school engagement-related skills and habits themselves if they wish students to conform to school rules. For instance, after taking a student out of class for a meeting, a guidance counselor or teacher should not say, "I will not give you a hall pass today. We will just hope that no hall monitor sees you going back to class." Through modeling, a student learns a negative behavior by observing school personnel disregarding school rules. Understanding learning theory will help school personnel to appreciate their vital role in enhancing school engagement training for at-risk youth (Biglan, 2015).

Practical Implications of School Engagement: Affective and Cognitive Components

All individuals, no matter where they are, want to make a difference—to have the power to affect the world versus being invisible and helpless. This also is true of children and adolescents when they enter a new classroom—an experience relevant to the affective component of school engagement. Does the student feel wanted, recognized as a unique individual, and able to generate positive responses from people in this new school environment? When the answer is "yes," the student becomes progressively more motivated to attend school and gets more of that personal recognition, acceptance, and opportunities to create daily, pleasant events with teachers and peers. Engaged students will be making decisions, doing problem solving, taking initiative, and eventually becoming autonomous learners who see themselves as agents of their own destiny (Cleary, 2015). On the contrary, when the student's experiences in a new school environment are not empowering and positive, the student becomes progressively less motivated to attend school, less inclined to look for personal recognition and social support from teachers and other students, and less able to generate positive daily experiences. Their school engagement decreases over time while their academic performance deteriorates to the extent that they eventually may have to repeat a grade, and their discipline referrals mount, initially for absenteeism and then additionally for rule infractions during school.

Two processes that parallel these scenarios representing engaged students are (1) motivation to please school authority figures and (2) valuing education. When students see that their efforts can cause positive responses (reinforcers) from teachers, they will be motivated to please those teachers and other school personnel more often, in order to generate more positive responses. Correspondingly, if students find that they have frequent rewarding experiences in school, they will value education more and seek increased educational experiences. Eventually, if such experiences are repeated in different classrooms year after year, the processes of pleasing adults and learning may become intrinsically motivating, instead of extrinsically motivating.

The positive experiences must continue, however, if students are to maintain their expectations of academic competence and personal recognition in school. It only takes approximately a year of negative experiences before students' expectations of good relationships with teachers are lowered, along with their decreased valuing of school (Cleary, 2015). Recall that students in the "Don't Quit on Me" study reported dropping out of school their senior year because of negative relationships with teachers and/or other students (Center for Promise, 2015). If positive expectations regarding school continue into adolescence, students will choose not only to attend school regularly, but also voluntarily to stay in school more hours a week in order to participate in extracurricular activities, a decision that, in turn, leads to a greater sense of belonging to a school and greater preparation for adulthood success. Interestingly, the processes described earlier (increased motivation to please teachers and valuing school when students feel they have the ability to generate their own pleasant social experiences) work in reverse too. Teachers (and parents) feel more positive about a student when the adults see they are having a positive impact on that adolescent. For instance, teachers will feel more kindly toward students who show in class, in a paper, or a test that they learned what the teacher taught them or did what the teacher asked them to do. Likewise, parents feel more loving toward their children when they see evidence that their child has paid attention to something the parent taught or requested.

Another result of a positive sense of efficacy at school is that these students develop a positive future orientation and are more likely to have an active "life dream." Conversely, one of the saddest situations one can witness is the student who is unable to visualize a "life dream." Some of these students do not expect successful adulthoods; others, most distressingly, do not even expect to live long enough to become an adult. In *Hillbilly Elegy*, a memoir about growing up in Appalachia, Vance (2016) concluded: "What separates the successful from the unsuccessful are the expectations they had for their own lives" (p. 194).

Practical Implications of School Engagement: Academic and Behavioral Components

To take advantage of the education that schools provide, students must already possess, or must acquire, myriad essential life skills and habits, or what is called "school readiness." Schools tend to assume that all students already have these skills and habits. Many at-risk students, however, do not start school with these necessary skills and habits. Teachers may interpret students' failures to exhibit the skills, not as a lack of knowing them (which can be learned) but as willful refusals, resulting in negative characterizations of students, such as intentionally "resisting" teachers' requests, "rebelling" against school rules, being "unmotivated" to learn, being "lazy," being "uncooperative," being "irresponsible," or having "uninterested" parents.

Furthermore, although many students arrive at school with learned habits that will help them to succeed academically and behaviorally, thus giving rise to the mistaken belief that this is true for all students, at-risk students often arrive at school with habits learned at home or in their community that will interfere with their learning. For example, some students do not have the habit of asking for help. They may have learned that asking for help results in refusals, or even more negative consequences, such as being punished. Another habit that may have been learned, but ill serves students in school, is to avoid a situation when you have not met an adult's request. When not completing a task assigned by a parent may have resulted in harsh punishment, a student may be absent from school or "skip" a specific class because homework has not been completed. Another self-defeating habit may be the failure to ever make a decision or to take initiative. This habit may be learned when a parent or older sibling has made all decisions for the child and the child expects to fail or be punished for taking initiative. A final example is that of a student who may have learned a habit, ingrained through interaction between siblings and parents at home, of loud and insulting personal interchanges.

All of these habits, which are adaptive for students in another setting, must be unlearned and replaced with more school-appropriate habits in order for students to benefit from their education. Unlearning established habits and learning new ones does not happen easily. It may take a long time and require specifically designed habit-development strategies. Methods based on learning principles can be applied over time with ample guided practice, in the same way that gradual methods and guided practice are applied over time to teach good driving habits.

To succeed academically, students must not only attend school but possess a multitude of demanding skills. Students must have the skill of *attending to adult authority figures,* that is, listening to and following adults' instructions and requests. Students also must be able to *complete challenging individual assignments in school* (on-task time). Additional skills are involved in *completing and turning in homework assignments.* *Communication skills* are important—particularly communication with adults. *Help-seeking and help-accepting skills* are beneficial. As students grow into adolescence, the *skill of empathy* makes relationships go smoother. Being able to analyze another's point of view and to become aware of one's own impact on others turns puzzling social interactions into understandable ones. Abiding by school rules—the behavioral component of school engagement—requires some of the same attending, self-control, self-regulation, communication, and empathy skills as does succeeding academically.

The practical implications of school engagement are daunting. It is a tall order for schools to provide knowledge to all adolescents, given that a significant portion of students—those who are considered at risk—require modifiable aspects of their school engagement to be targeted and then individually addressed in order that they too can acquire knowledge and graduate. To optimize the success of efforts to improve the outcomes of at-risk youth both in school and as adults, programs to modify aspects of individuals' school engagement should be theoretically guided and evidence-based (Mihalic & Elliot, 2015).

CONCLUSION

Approximately 20% of American adolescents do not graduate from high school, which not only deprives society of their full human potential but also increases their individual chances of poverty, incarceration, and substance abuse as adults. Conceptualizations that best explain differential high school completion rates are school engagement and disengagement. Most children begin school curious, eager to learn, and engaged. Some young people, however, gradually become disengaged over time, shown by their decreased effort on classwork, more discipline problems, feelings of rejection by teachers and peers, and reduced beliefs in their academic competence. Implications of this understanding are that several serious adult problems, such as unemployment and crime, might be prevented if more adolescents' sense of competence and success in school could be maintained or restored until graduation. Learning theory suggests that this may be accomplished through individual coaching, practice, and ample acknowledgment from school personnel who view school engagement as discrete skills that adolescents at risk can learn and who perceive disengagement as maladaptive habits that adolescents at risk can replace.

CHAPTER 11

The Achievement Mentoring Program

The Achievement Mentoring Program (hereafter the Program) is an adult-delivered, evidence-based, school-based program for at-risk preadolescents and adolescents who show signs of school disengagement, such as low grades, behavior problems, poor relationships with teachers, and/or a lack of confidence, or interest, in doing schoolwork. This preventive intervention is based on learning theory and has been judged by several organizations to be promising or strongly evidence-based for preventing behavioral and academic problems. Some of those organizations are: Blueprints at *www.blueprintsprograms.com/factsheet/achievement-mentoring,* the National Institute of Justice at *www.crimesolutions. gov/ProgramDetails.aspx?ID=402,* and the National Dropout Prevention Center at *http://dropoutprevention.org/mpdb/web/program/134.* In accordance with practical considerations, achievement mentors are caring adults who reach out to at-risk individuals in school without the youth having to ask for help. Over time, a mentor coaches a mentee in communications skills, rule abiding, goal setting, and self-efficacy. The achievement mentor also monitors and encourages school attendance and work completion through weekly problem solving, recognizing small gains and keeping parents informed of progress. In the simplest terms, the Program is designed to increase the skills necessary for school engagement and to change the habits that interfere with acquiring knowledge. Because learning requires repetition and practice over time, at-risk students participate in Achievement Mentoring during at least two consecutive school years (Bry, 1982).

The demonstrated outcomes of this intervention include (1) improving academic performance (Bry, 1982; Clarke, 2009); (2) reducing behavior problems (Bry, 1982; Clarke, 2009; Holt et al., 2008; Taylor, 2010); (3) increasing students' sense of acceptance in their school and perceptions of their teachers (Clarke, 2009; Holt et al., 2008); and (4) enhancing their decision-making abilities (Holt et al., 2008). By targeting these four components of school engagement, students in the Program become more likely to stay in school and graduate than at-risk students who have not received this intervention (Bry, 2001a). Prior to implementation, teachers and other professional staff who will deliver the Program receive intensive training, and, once implemented, providers receive ongoing support. Individual professionals working in the schools (e.g., teachers and counselors) can also decide to implement Achievement Mentoring on their own.

OVERVIEW OF THE SCHOOL-BASED ACHIEVEMENT MENTORING PROCESS

Teachers nominate students in the fifth through eleventh grades whose academic and/or behavioral records indicate they may be at risk for not graduating from high school. The students are then assigned a trained adult achievement mentor. Achievement mentors fall into two categories: (1) a staff member, that is, a teacher or a counselor, employed by the school; or (2) a professional employed at a community agency that provides services to schools. Full-time teachers or guidance counselors will mentor two at-risk students, and professionals employed by outside agencies will mentor 15–20 at-risk students, since this is their full-time job.

Achievement mentors can meet with youth individually once a week during the school day for 15–20 minutes, or with small groups of between two and six students for longer sessions up to an entire class period. The small-group process involves completing all of the steps of Achievement Mentoring with each student individually while the others wait in a circle for their turn, with the option of offering constructive comments if they wish. Most achievement mentors, however, find it easier and more efficient to take mentees out of classes one at a time for individual mentoring.

Before meeting with a student, the achievement mentor completes a Weekly Report Form (WRF), while having a brief (3- to 5-minute) consultation with one of the student's teachers concerning the student's academic performance and behavior during the prior week (see Figure 11.1) The WRF, which is reviewed by the achievement mentor with each student, serves several purposes. First, it is an opportunity for mentees to receive face-to-face acknowledgment and praise for specific examples of positive school engagement. As achievement mentors reinforce their praiseworthy academic work and classroom behavior, mentees are encouraged to take credit for this which, in turn, should foster self-efficacy beliefs. A blank copy of the WRF (Form 11.1) is available for readers to duplicate for their use at the end of this chapter; an enlarged version that can be downloaded and printed is provided online (see the box at the end of the table of contents).

Second, after reviewing the WRF with the achievement mentor, each student chooses a new, small step as a goal for the next week to increase their school engagement. The achievement mentor helps them to refine the step so that success is probable; that is, it is both small enough and feasible within the context of the student's life circumstances. It is very important that the achievement mentor be knowledgeable about the realities of each mentee's life, as empathy—putting yourself in the shoes of your mentee—is necessary to the success of this intervention. Details of the implementation are planned carefully with the mentees, including identifying problems that might prevent goal attainment and deciding how such problems might be overcome. New school engagement skills are practiced. Before the session ends, students write their goal for the upcoming week at the bottom of the WRF (see Figure 11.1). Each weekly Achievement Mentoring session conforms to this structure for the 2-year period.

After the mentoring session, achievement mentors inform teachers about the positive step that the student has chosen to take. Teachers are encouraged to look for positive behaviors in the classroom that are related to that step. Achievement mentors also involve parents in this process and give them a monthly report on their adolescent's progress, highlighting something positive that the youth has done in school. Incorporating teachers and parents into the Program multiplies the positive messages the youth receives from the achievement mentor, as teachers and parents will be alert to signs of increased school engagement and praise them when they see them.

Achievement Mentoring as a School-Based Intervention

For a mentoring program to be effective, mentors need to know (1) with whom to intervene, (2) where to contact adolescents who need intervention, (3) what goals to target, (4) specific intervention strategies, and (5) a means for assessing whether or not goals are attained. We have found that working with the schools is useful because schools can

Weekly Report Form (WRF)

WRF	Teacher: *Brown*	Subject: *Lang. Arts*	Date: *4/10*	

Details about the YES's/NO's refer to behaviors—actions the teacher sees the child doing

	Monday	Tuesday	Wednesday	Thursday	Friday
In School	(YES) NO	(YES) NO	(YES) NO	(YES) NO	(YES) NO
On Time	(YES) NO	YES (NO)	YES (NO)	YES (NO)	YES (NO)
Materials for Class *Pen, text*		(YES) NO	**Did Classwork** *no participation*		YES (NO)
Satisfactory Behavior *Polite, cell phone*		YES (NO)	**Did Homework** *zeros*		YES (NO)
			Marks/Grades *0, 0, 66, 0, 68*		

Details about the YES's:	Details about the NO's:
Good attendance.	*Doesn't pay attention.*
Polite	*Cell phone. Never*
On time Monday!	*raises hand.*
Passes some quizzes	*Starts, but doesn't finish classwork.*
	No homework done, so gets zeros.

Goal for this week generated by pupil	Tell Mrs. Brown no cell phone.

FIGURE 11.1. Weekly Report Form (WRF) completed by an achievement mentor during a brief teacher interview.

identify the adolescents who need help; schools are where adolescents are located; school officials can help to present the mentoring to parents; school records contain the information that is required, and schools can provide the feedback necessary to evaluate the effectiveness of the intervention.

Development of the Achievement Mentoring Program

One author of this book (the Program developer, Bry) was engaged by her county government to develop and implement a prevention program for county secondary schools to help at-risk students avoid juvenile delinquency, substance abuse, and criminal involvement. Given this mandate, the Program had to fit into the existing school structure and had to be practical for schools to execute.

The Program developer started with the premise that the major "job" of adolescents is to succeed in school. She knew that if they do not experience the pleasure that comes from succeeding at the tasks put in front of them (payoffs) and from knowing that the successes resulted from their own actions (self-efficacy), students would look for payoffs and self-efficacy elsewhere. For example, they would look for ways they could feel successful outside of school through activities such as gambling, stealing, bullying, and/or fighting; they might find that they could gain pleasure through drugs or alcohol; they might identify adults who seem successful in crime or gang involvement as their role-models, and so on. Therefore, the best way to prevent students from finding alternative sources of payoff and self-efficacy would be to help them succeed in school. This is consistent with learning theory, which holds that payoffs motivate everyone's behavior—those of both adolescents and adults (Ramnerö & Törneke, 2008). Because the original goal was to make the Program a long-term, established offering in all secondary county schools—urban and suburban—the Program developer realized that learning theory concepts would need to be applied to the schools as well as to the students. The Program needed to make life easier, rather than harder, for personnel to have in their schools; or the Program would not be continued. In other words, the Program would have to offer a "payoff" for them.

In addition to learning theory, program development was guided by research and the Program developer's prior 8 years of experience practicing individual and group psychotherapy with at-risk youth. This background made the Program developer aware of how difficult change is and what strategies could be applied to make change more likely.

As a clinical psychologist, the Program developer's previous association with schools was limited. She had been a successful student herself and, as a clinician, had treated children and adolescents who often complained bitterly about difficulties with teachers and schools. During development of the Program—a process that entailed spending 4 days a week in schools for 3 years—her admiration for educators and other personnel who work in the schools grew exponentially. She understood what a challenging job and difficult circumstances they managed to overcome with skill, persistence, and dedication every day.

As the Achievement Mentoring Program developed, the Program developer took note of how students, teachers, other school personnel, and parents reacted to each component of the intervention. They taught her, through their responses, what worked ("paid off") for them and what did not. This allowed the Achievement Mentoring Program to be shaped and later refined by the input of the stakeholders, a trial-and-error process designed to result in a payoff for all parties.

ASPECTS OF THE ACHIEVEMENT MENTORING PROGRAM

Selection of At-Risk Students for Achievement Mentoring

Although school staff, such as principals, vice principals, guidance counselors, school psychologists, social workers, and child study team members, should have input as to student selection, both authors of this book have found that teachers are best equipped to identify students who are in danger of dropping out before high school graduation, and thus in need of interventions such as Achievement Mentoring. This was confirmed by the Program developer's experience in her initial effort to find Program candidates. She examined the school records of every student to find those with some failing grades; teacher comments such as "Student is capable of doing better work," or "I do not know how to motivate this student"; a higher than average number of absences; and/or referrals for discipline problems. After that painstaking review, she compiled a list. Next she interviewed teachers to develop a list of students needing intervention—a far less cumbersome process. This second list was identical to the first, thereby corroborating the idea that asking teachers for nominations was the most efficient selection method. Conducting such interviews also presents Program administrators with an opportunity to inform teachers about the Achievement Mentoring Program. An additional advantage of involving teachers in the nominating process is that they become invested in the success of Achievement Mentoring, having chosen the student participants themselves.

Teachers can choose at-risk students by identifying them either in June for the following school year or at the end of September after observing them for a month in their classrooms. Teachers who have taught in a school for more than a year may also be able to identify candidates based on their knowledge about family members' experiences in the school and other relevant factors indicating that the youth may be appropriate for this intervention. For example, they may have taught older siblings or even parents who had dropped out of school; they may know of the student's problematic relationship with parents; or they may be aware that the youth is in foster care. Because Achievement Mentoring is a relatively low-intensity program, it is not appropriate for students with serious mental health or substance abuse disorders. Although truancy is an indication of school disengagement, students would need to attend school an average of at least 3 days a week to benefit from Achievement Mentoring. To alleviate concerns that being chosen for Achievement Mentoring might add to stigmatization of at-risk students, the Program is described as one for "students who could do better in school." Schools typically assign students to Achievement Mentoring in the same way that they assign some students to remedial reading or to nonacademic subjects, such as advisory or a career explorations class. When schools do this, parental permission is not required; however, as parental involvement in Achievement Mentoring is important to positive outcomes, some schools will not enroll a student in the Program without obtaining parental consent.

In this case, school personnel with whom the parent is familiar, such as the guidance counselor or the principal, contacts the parents. The Program is described, and the parents' permission for their children to participate in the prevention program is requested. A guidance counselor follows up with a phone call. This method of recruitment increases the acceptance rate, as the achievement mentor may be unknown to the parents. The language used to describe the Program also affects the acceptance rate. It should be presented in a positive manner, again stressing that it is aimed at "students who can do better in school." Because most of the parents of at-risk adolescents are used to getting critical messages from the school, the positive tone is often a welcome surprise and encourages an affirmative response.

The acceptance rate for Achievement Mentoring is very high: at least 88% of the caregivers agree to enroll the at-risk adolescent in the Program. The retention rate for adolescents is even more noteworthy: a full 100% stay in the Program (Krinsley, 1991). When the selection of students is finalized, the school holds a luncheon for the mentees and the mentors so that the students can be introduced to the Program and their individual mentors in a positive, stress-free manner.

Achievement Mentors

Experience has shown that achievement mentors should be educators or other helping professionals in a related field, such as guidance counselors, community youth workers, social workers, nurses, psychologists, professional counselors, school administrators, substance abuse counselors, and other human service workers. Employees of a school have certain advantages over employees of community agencies in helping at-risk students become engaged in school, in that (1) school employees are known to, and have the respect of, other school employees; and (2) they are familiar with the school's rules and customs, as well as the habits and patterns of their colleagues. (See the case example in Chapter 8, in which the achievement mentor was a teacher in the school.)

Professionals who do not work in the school, however, can earn the respect of the school staff and, with effort, can gain the knowledge needed to function effectively in this new environment. (See the case example in Chapter 13, in which the achievement mentor was an employee of a community agency providing services to students in the school.) In addition, achievement mentors who are employed by outside agencies are not restricted to the present school and are free to follow mentees who may change schools during the Program. For example, mentees may be sent to an alternative school for a specified period of time, or a mentee may change schools if his or her family has moved.

All achievement mentors, whether employed within or outside of the school, must feel comfortable with, respect, and care about at-risk youth. School personnel and human service workers who specialize in working with high-achieving students, or those with specific academic interests, would probably not be best suited to serve as achievement mentors. It is not in the students' best interests to have personnel assigned as achievement mentors who do not welcome the opportunity to help at-risk youth. Therefore, this function should not be added to any staff member's job responsibilities without his or her consent.

Mentoring Sessions

Achievement Mentoring is a school-based program because school is a natural environment of at-risk students. The Program does not require that the students do anything beyond what they usually do in a school day—they are not expected to arrive early or stay late to meet with a mentor, for example. The mentoring sessions are integrated into the regular school day because disengaged students usually will not spend any more time in school than is required. We do not expect enthusiasm or initiative on their part. After all, the notion that an intervention could be useful is our idea—not theirs. We characterize our approach to recruiting at-risk adolescents as "respectfully persistent and patient." Achievement mentors find and reach out to students wherever they are in school.

It is also important for achievement mentors to realize that when the Program is introduced, school personnel may not be initially optimistic about its success. For this reason, during recruitment, we ask teachers for the names of students they are concerned about—not students whom they think will benefit from the intervention. Their confidence in the Program will come with time. Therefore, it is particularly important for achievement mentors' supervisors and trainers to be clear and verbalize their optimism about the Program for both the mentors and the school personnel, until they begin to witness the positive results themselves.

It is to the school's advantage that Achievement Mentoring occurs during the school day as budgets are not strained with overtime costs to implement the Program. Logistical concerns involving conflicts with mentoring teachers' noninstructional responsibilities, such as cafeteria or hall monitoring; attending meetings; and bus duty, can be addressed by replacing achievement mentors with other staff members. Conducting mentoring sessions during the school day does have some drawbacks, however. For example, as Achievement Mentoring sessions are conducted when the students would otherwise be receiving classroom instruction, teachers may express some hesitation at first about a student missing important schoolwork. As classroom teachers learn more about the Program from the mentor and are able to see for themselves the improvement in school engagement the at-risk students' exhibit as a result of being in the Program, they realize that the benefits of Achievement Mentoring accrue to them as well. For example, it is common for mentors to be told, "You can take her out of my class for 20 minutes a week because she is more likely to pay attention to the lesson or do the seat assignment after she returns." There are some teachers, however, who remain adamant in refusing to allow students to attend mentoring during instructional time. As teacher agreement is necessary, mentors will have to find another time during the week to see the student, even though a student's or mentor's lunch break may be the only option remaining.

Weekly mentoring sessions take only 15 to 20 minutes for several reasons. First, there are time constraints for achievement mentors who are full-time teachers. When meetings last only 15 to 20 minutes, teachers can see both mentees during one prep period, even allowing for the time it takes to go to the mentees' classrooms and escort them to the mentoring sessions. The brief meeting time also encourages the mentor to stick to the meeting agenda.

Short meetings also are important for mentee buy-in. Based on past experiences with adult authority figures in the school, students often are wary and even fearful about meeting with their mentor. They may be anxious that they will not know what to say or that they may say something that would elicit the adult's disapproval. They also may have concerns that their statements in sessions could be misconstrued and communicated to others in the school in a distorted way. In addition, the longer a meeting lasts, the more students may anticipate that their failures or behavior problems will be brought up. Mentors' first challenge is to demonstrate that Achievement Mentoring will not bring negative consequences to their mentees. The mentor ideally will show that mentoring can bring immediate desirable benefits. Once at-risk students learn that the meetings are predictably short and focused on pleasant topics, they will be less likely to dread mentoring. In this manner, it is beneficial for mentoring meetings to end *before* students want them to end, with the result that students want more mentoring rather than less. The proof that mentoring is a pleasant activity rather than one that is feared occurs when a mentee is accompanied to the session by a friend who expresses the desire for mentoring as well.

Life Dream

Life dreams are an important aspect of Achievement Mentoring. During the first mentoring meeting, as mentors and mentees are learning about each other, the mentor will ask the student, "If your life goes well, what do you see yourself doing at 25 years old?" As projecting his or her life a decade or more in the future may not be the way an adolescent or preadolescent is accustomed to thinking, the mentor often spends some time asking more questions and repeating back what the student says until the student's actual image of adulthood is elicited. This answer is called the mentee's "Life Dream."

The mentor accepts this life dream without condition. For instance, if a student dreams of being "a pediatrician," the mentor does not say, "You could be a nurse by the time you are 25, but you could not have finished medical training by then," "That training costs a lot of money," or "You have to take a lot of science courses for that." Likewise, if the student says, "I want to be a rap star or an NBA basketball player," the mentor, irrespective of any misgivings he or she may have about the student's choice, accepts this life dream at face value as well. Mentors accept and remember their mentees' life dreams so that they can function as incentives to gain knowledge and learn adaptive skills in school. For instance, when mentees say they are not interested in math and will never need to do math outside of school, the mentor can connect the necessity of knowing math to the student's life dream and ask, "How will you know your patients, customers, and/or agents are giving you the right amount of money?"

When students reveal a life dream, they are not only entrusting the mentor with precious information about themselves, but they are also confiding something that may make them vulnerable to the criticism or ridicule of others. Mentors want mentees to trust that they will make their lives easier instead of harder. Thus, mentors should not share the mentees' life dreams with anyone else, including teachers, parents, and best friends, as it might leave mentees vulnerable to being laughed at or criticized for lofty ambitions, for thinking they are better than others, or for thinking they have talents that others consider nonexistent.

Program Duration

As we described in Chapter 10, school disengagement is a process that occurs over many years. Therefore, it also takes a long time to unlearn established habits of disengagement and to learn the complex attitudes, expectations, and skills necessary for school engagement. Furthermore, if new school engagement habits, skills, thoughts, and relationships are going to help mentees in their adult life, they must persist across time, places, people, and things. Abrupt changes can disrupt new learning. It follows, then, that if positive changes have started to occur for students who have participated in Achievement Mentoring for one school year, continuity is required to help them generalize and increase school engagement in the following school year when they are faced with unfamiliar circumstances.

Thus, it is not surprising that data from repeated, controlled studies of long-term Achievement Mentoring outcomes show that at-risk students have to be in the Program during 2 school years for positive effects to endure (Bry, 1982, 2001a; Clarke, 2009; Taylor, 2010). In addition, by the time they reach secondary school, disengaged students may have already participated in one or more intervention programs designed to increase school engagement. Even if these programs had been pleasant experiences, and the student formed close relationships with the teacher or other adult conducting the intervention, once a new school year began or the program was otherwise completed, this adult typically vanished from the student's life. After that happens a few times, students have an expectation of abandonment and develop social distrust (Bushman et al., 2016), maintaining a psychological distance between themselves and the adults who promise to help them.

Achievement mentors repeatedly report that they do not feel really appreciated by mentees until the second year of the program. The Program developer experienced this phenomenon herself. During the first year, mentees showed little enthusiasm for the Program, but they dutifully attended mentoring sessions and accepted the routine of the mentor taking them out of class, conducting a mentoring session, and returning them to class 20 minutes afterward. They communicated an unspoken feeling of having had little choice, which was their attitude about school in general, although they seemed to appreciate being taken out of class.

Their affective connections to the program and to the achievement mentor changed, however, when the mentor showed up in the school Guidance Office the following school year, asking for copies of her mentees' schedules. After one of the mentees saw her there and learned that she would be working with her mentees again that year, almost all of them "happened" to visit the Guidance Office that day with cheery greetings for her. The students, many of whom had become used to abandonment, seemed very pleasantly surprised that the mentor kept her promise to continue working with them for a second year.

Weekly Teacher Interviews

One unique method of Achievement Mentoring is that mentors arrive at every weekly mentoring session, except the first one, with the standardized WRF, which includes the results of the brief interview mentors have had with one of the student's teachers. The teacher is asked what the student's attendance, promptness, and behavior were like during the past week. The teacher is also asked whether or not the student did classwork, had school materials (pen, texts), and handed in homework. The WRF is filled out in the mentors' own handwriting (see Figure 11.1).

The information obtained from teachers' reports serves to structure the meeting with the student, as mentors have expressed concerns about the difficulty they often have conducting give-and-take conversations with the at-risk youth. It is customary for adolescents and preadolescents, particularly with adult authority figures, to offer little in the way of communication. For example, when an adult asks, "How are things going?" the most common answer given is, "Fine." This response impedes information gathering and often may lead to a mentor mistakenly making assumptions when accepting the student's words at face value. For example, on one hand, the mentor may naively say something like, "I am glad things are going well," and then lose credibility with the youth because, in fact, the student was just in a fight, was suspended from school, or failed Science for the marking period. On the other hand, the mentor might also learn of a positive event as a result of the teacher interview. Perhaps the student recently arrived to a class on time for the first time in 2 weeks, which would give the mentor an opportunity he or she would not want to miss—catching a kid doing something good today. Another advantage of interviewing a teacher before each mentoring session is to save time. Even if a mentee is cooperative and forthcoming, reviewing with the youth what has happened in a course the previous week would not be the most effective use of a short 15- to 20-minute session. Finally, if the youth is to change, progress will take longer if only the youth's perception is considered. Mentoring can be far more helpful once others' observations of the youth are incorporated into the discussion. Disengaged youth often do not see themselves and their school persona in the same way as others do. For instance, disengaged students often are surprised to learn that teachers want them to succeed and will notice small signs of growth in them. When their mentor reads these positive observations from teachers on the WRFs, students receive reinforcement for their efforts.

Students also learn from the WRFs exactly what teachers and schools are looking for from them. Disengaged students typically believe they cannot win in school because to them the standards of the school are capricious—they fail for different reasons on different days—and they become convinced that they cannot do anything right. They are often unaware of what skills will help them feel effective in school and which of their habits interfere with their gaining self-efficacy. At-risk students can learn from WRF content that there indeed are consistent, basic, minimum expectations and standards of conduct in schools, which students are capable of meeting once they know what to focus on. Those minimum expectations are listed on the WRF (see Figure 11.1). The content in their WRFs also reflect what teachers care about the most in their students. Because individuals learn in different ways, students are both shown in the form and told verbally of their teacher's observations.

Only one of each mentee's teachers is interviewed each week, so that at-risk youth are not overwhelmed with so much feedback that they shut down. In schools where students have multiple teachers, achievement mentors will have the students' schedules listing teachers. It is ideal for mentors to interview teachers in sequence; for example, if there are six teachers, each teacher will be interviewed once every 6 weeks. In reality, however, such precision may be impractical. Mentors may encounter a teacher they interviewed 4 weeks previously, or a teacher whose turn it is to be interviewed may not be available. As it is necessary to have new feedback from one teacher per mentee each week, if a recently interviewed teacher is the only one available to be interviewed, it is sufficient for the purposes of the Program that the mentor interview this teacher again. Mentors should make every effort to see each teacher at some point, as the teacher who is hardest for a mentor to find might have the most important feedback. This is true even when the teacher is not an academic instructor. For example, a mentor may learn from the physical education teacher that a student may not be promoted because he or she has not been changing into gym clothes for the class.

Trial and error have shown that there is no good substitute for face-to-face interviews with teachers. If blank WRFs are given to teachers to fill out themselves, the feedback will not necessarily be as constructive for the mentees. On another hand, if mentees are given the WRFs to ask their teachers to fill out, the personal encounter with teachers can often be so overwhelming and unpleasant for students that they will stop asking teachers to fill them out. That is, teachers may be so happy that disengaged students are asking for feedback that they list every area for improvement they can think of, rather than focus on priorities. An additional problem might arise from feedback expressed in personality characteristic terms, such as "You were rude and disruptive," or "You must be more mature and responsible," instead of behavioral observations.

Given the time constraints teachers are under, mentors' interviews with them are necessarily brief. Even under these circumstances, however, the interviews can be a two-way street. In addition to the rich, up-to-date, monitoring data mentors receive from teachers, the interviews inform the teachers about the Program methods and invest teachers in their students' reaching Achievement Mentoring goals. Teachers also can be made aware of positive actions, behavior, thoughts, and feelings of mentees and their parents. For example, when teachers do not hear from parents, particularly when teachers have made previous attempts to contact and/or meet with the parents, they frequently conclude that the parents do not care about their child's schooling. A sentence or two from the mentor explaining the parents' challenges and deep interest in their children's education can change that preconception (see Chapter 8). Relatedly, teachers can assume that a youth with behavior problems deliberately provokes the teacher. Assurance from a mentor that the adolescent has expressed the goal to stay out of trouble in the classroom each day can offer a new perspective. Furthermore, when the mentor repeatedly asks teachers to relate something positive the youth did during the past week, teachers will start looking for those instances themselves and acknowledge them to the at-risk youth. The more coordinated the positive responses are to at-risk students' improvements in school engagement in various environments, the faster the student will learn new skills or unlearn interfering habits (Mayer et al., 2013). This is consistent with the learning theory assumption that behavior is a function of the environment's response to similar behavior in the past.

WEEKLY MENTORING SESSION STEPS

Although Achievement Mentoring activities may seem simple and routine, challenges need to be acknowledged. One such challenge is logistical: finding a convenient time and place to meet for 15–20 minutes. Consistency is preferable, so that the student need not experience uncertainty or anxiety about whether or not they will meet and, additionally, the student can learn to count on the mentor. The achievement mentor reaches out 99% of the way to the student. If the arrangement is for mentees to arrive at the meeting place unaccompanied by the mentor, and the student is not at the meeting place on time, mentors consult the student's schedule and locate the mentee. If the student cannot be found, the mentor acknowledges the missed meeting to the student. Because mentors do not want mentees to feel criticized or blamed for not being available and thus avoid seeing their mentor in the future, the message simply will state, "I missed seeing you today," instead of, "Where were you? I could not find you." Achievement Mentoring is a "no dropout" program (unless parents, who originally consented to their youth's participation, revoke permission). Although no parent has ever withdrawn their adolescent from the Program, it is important for achievement mentors to remember that, in the end, parents have the power to determine their child's treatment.

Along with a strong personal belief in the value of the Achievement Mentoring, and ample, enduring Program and institutional support for their work (see Chapter 14 for an in-depth discussion of institutional supports), mentors must have "thick skins." Even though achievement mentors play a much larger role and have greater importance in their mentees' lives than the mentees typically acknowledge and the mentors may realize (Holt et al., 2008), mentors may not feel appreciation, respect, or gratitude from students or parents. This should not be unexpected, as neither the student nor the parents asked for the mentees to be in the Program.

For mentors, one way to earn that appreciation and respect is to show appreciation and respect to mentees and parents. Mentors should make the mentoring process as transparent as possible to students and allow for student decision making consistent with the original premises of the Program. For example, the mentor tells the student that teachers will be interviewed, and relates the questions the mentor asks teachers; the mentor tells the student before contacting a parent and informs the student of what the mentor intends to tell the parent; and the mentor can ask if the student would like the mentor to tell something specific to a teacher, parent, or school administrator. Mentors can also ask mentees to predict what their teachers will say in mentor interviews with teachers. This inquiry can encourage students to monitor the impressions they make, and teacher feedback may provide opportunities for students to modify inaccurate views of how they are perceived.

Achievement mentors should continually ask directly about their mentees' lives, multiple identities, cultural traditions, and concerns rather than assume understanding. This is true even when the mentor has the same or similar racial, ethnic, and cultural background as the mentee. Given that, at a minimum, the mentor's education, power, and income will often diverge greatly from those of their students and the students' families, mentors will be seen as being different from their mentees and many of their parents. Mentors should also be aware that many parents often do not feel comfortable visiting schools or talking to school personnel because of their own negative and/or embarrassing experiences as students. In addition, parents often feel criticized by schools when their children's performance and/or behavior is deemed inadequate, even though parents are doing the best they can (Alexander, 2001). The recommendation that mentors praise their mentees and the parents whenever speaking to the parents may help to compensate for preexisting negative impressions conveyed by school staff and encourage parents' willingness to talk to mentors in the future.

Step 1: Check-In

Even though the Achievement Mentoring Program's primary purpose is to enable students to feel successful in school, mentors should not launch each session with a discussion of schoolwork. Students may have recently experienced a decisive nonschool-related event that has caused them to be preoccupied, such as a family member's illness, an eviction notice, a new pregnancy, an injury, or the disappearance or return of a special person. Thus, each session should start with a check-in question. If the student relates an important event in response, the mentor should apply Active Listening Skills (see Chapter 12 for an extensive discussion of these skills) when engaged in follow-up. The mentor's questions should not concern anyone other than the mentee and how this event impacted him or her. Achievement Mentoring is narrowly focused on changing the mentee. This is different from a family therapy model, which would be designed to change parents as well as students, or teacher training; however, the changes mentees may undergo as a result of effective Achievement Monitoring can change families and teachers too, as has happened in another school-based mentoring intervention, the Lunch Buddies Program, in which mentors work with at-risk students in the lunchroom (Gregus, Craig, Rodriguez, Pastrana, & Cavell, 2015).

Step 2: Show the WRF to the Mentee

After the check-in, the achievement mentor shows the most recently completed WRF to the student and calls attention to one or more instances of positive school engagement noted thereon. (Again, see Figure 11.1 for a sample of a completed WRF.) Experience shows that even the most disengaged students will have an interest in this as soon—however surreptitious at first—as they learn that it is positive in nature and will not initiate criticism and immediate suggestions from an adult about how to fix the problems. Achievement mentors need to be careful not to respond to students as many caring adults would, either by projecting a positive result into the future or by offering a contrast with the past, or both, such as saying, "Look at that. You had a perfect attendance record last week. Why have you not done that before? Be sure to attend school every day from now on." Disengaged students may not see the value of perfect attendance; and even if they do, they may have made resolutions to have good attendance in the past and failed to meet their goals. Thus, they may not see themselves as capable of that achievement, or they may even become so discouraged and convinced of their lack of agency that they no longer see any use in trying to improve. In addition, reminders to students of past negative behavior, such as poor attendance, may often lead them to escape or avoid the "messenger."

WRFs are shown to mentees by achievement mentors weekly because most of the minimum necessary components of school engagement that are listed there are expected from students by most school personnel. These include (1) attending school every day; (2) arriving on time; (3) abiding by school rules; (4) having necessary materials; and (5) doing homework and handing it in on time. Achievement mentors understand that many disengaged students do not have the academic, behavior, cognitive, or affective skills and habits necessary to meet those minimum expectations.

Disengaged students often have many different competing contingencies in their environments that provide immediate "payoffs" for behavior other than that expected in school. For example, a student with an ailing grandmother may need to fill a prescription or to purchase medicine when the pharmacy opens at 9. Even if the student arrives at school immediately after getting this needed item to the grandmother, school personnel typically will chastise the student for being tardy and not concern themselves with the cause of the tardiness—that the student had performed a praiseworthy act for a family member. In fact, the student may be punished with assigned detention. In order to learn components of school engagement, students must receive immediate payoffs for engaged behavior, such as attending school. Thus, an achievement mentor will praise the student. Accordingly, disengaged students can learn gradually that it "pays off" (gets them praise from their mentor) to make the effort to come to school, even though they must be late. By providing this information, the WRF serves as the basis for disengaged students to receive recognition from their mentors for praiseworthy efforts on their part that may be taken for granted, overlooked, or even punished by other school personnel.

Step 3: Praise Specific Instances of School Engagement

When reviewing the WRF with the student, the achievement mentor starts by focusing on the praiseworthy feedback, reading each positive accomplishment selectively aloud while simultaneously pointing to the entries so that the student may follow along. The tone in which this document is read is important and should convey pride and respect. When praising the students for attendance, the mentor may begin, "You attended school every day last week" and then list the days in sequence, "Monday, Tuesday, Wednesday, Thursday, and Friday." Repeating the days of the week may seem unnecessary, but this specificity is helpful for disengaged students who are often in the habit of thinking "out of sight, out of mind," and fail to connect their absences to the consequence of having missed instruction and assignments. Another illustration of the need for specifics is that more general praise may be misinterpreted. For example, if a mentor states "Your teacher also was pleased that you had the materials you needed to have in class—a notebook and a pen," the student could not construe the word "materials" as something unrelated, such as wearing the uniform.

Achievement Mentoring praise goes beyond the recitation of the praiseworthy actions and behavior. It is important to emphasize that the student himself or herself is responsible for this achievement, as disengaged students who do not feel efficacious in school often do not see themselves as agents of their actions and thus may attribute praiseworthy behavior to some outside force (Turk & Bry, 1992). To communicate the message that students are in charge of their lives and to make sure that the students hear themselves taking credit for their instances of school engagement, achievement mentors will follow up each positive instance of school engagement by asking the student, "How did *you* do it?"

If mentees do not report on something that they personally did, thought, or felt, the mentor keeps asking the question and supplies possible answers, until the student finally acknowledges his or her role in the praiseworthy action. For instance, in response to the question, "How did you manage to get to school on time on Tuesday," the mentee might say, "I don't know," or give credit to another person, that is, "My mother said she did not want to get phone calls again because I was late," or "My friend's father gave me a ride." Because a major goal of Achievement Mentoring is to enable disengaged students to learn that they can take charge of their lives, the mentor will continue to probe, "Yes, but what did *you* do to get yourself ready?" If the mentees persist in refusing to give themselves any credit for their promptness, mentors may suggest some answers based on their knowledge of the student's life. "Perhaps you asked your sister to wake you up," or "How did your friend's father know you needed a ride?" After the initial question, "How did you do it?," is repeated each week during mentoring, disengaged students learn self-efficacy beliefs when they hear the answers as more reflective of the knowledge that they have made their lives better through their own actions.

Step 4: Read Aloud Other Teacher Observations on the WRF

After mentees experience recognition for what they did well during the past week, they then are given a *choice* about what to focus on for the following week based on the mentor reading aloud feedback on the WRF that is contrary to school engagement. It is essential that the mentor communicate this feedback in an objective and empathic manner, and that the feedback be characterized as constructive so that the mentee is aware that it can be changed. It should be expressed in a way that acknowledges the mentor's realization that the feedback may hurt the mentee's feelings. Mentors should not assume or report this feedback as the "truth," but rather in terms of "what the teacher saw" or "the teacher's impressions." Learning theory suggests that just as students can learn to think differently, so can teachers. The mentors know that at present teachers have learned to believe the negative behavior to be true; however, if they have repeated experiences that point to other conclusions, this "truth" will be adjusted to reflect the new reality.

For instance, achievement mentors could read the rest of the WRF in Figure 11.1 this way: "Although Mrs. B. was pleased that you arrived on time on Monday, she reported that you were not on time on the other days of the week. And while she was happy that you had your materials for class, there are other areas she is less happy about. She would like to see you hand in assigned class work and homework. She said that she could give you higher grades if you handed in assignments. Finally, she would like to see you paying more attention to her in class. It's her impression that you are too busy looking at your cell phone to look at her." Achievement mentors then should be quiet and look up at the student with a sympathetic, inquiring gaze. If the mentee offers reactions at this point, achievement mentors should proceed with active listening. During this process, mentors would listen, repeat a few of the mentee's words, and perhaps ask brief questions for the purpose of understanding, and showing that they understand the mentee's perspective—that is, what it is like to be in their mentee's shoes.

Step 5: Motivational Interviewing

The next step in Achievement Mentoring sessions, motivational interviewing, is probably the most difficult for achievement mentors to follow because it is counterintuitive to the instincts of most caring adults who try to help adolescents (Miller & Rollnick, 2012; Naar-King & Suarez, 2011; Rollnick, Kaplan, & Rutschman, 2016). The primary purpose of Achievement Mentoring in general is the same as the primary purpose of this step: for at-risk adolescents to learn that they can succeed in, be efficacious at, and take charge of their "job" as adolescents, which is to be engaged in school. This section describes the application of motivational interviewing to Achievement Mentoring at this stage of weekly sessions. (For an extensive discussion on motivational interviewing, see Chapter 12.)

After the mentor reads objective, behaviorally based ("What did the teacher see?"), constructive feedback about the mentee's past week in the classroom from the WRF, the mentor asks, "What do you make of this?" and later, "What are you thinking?" Then the mentor stops talking and waits for the mentee to respond. This aspect of the weekly Achievement Mentoring sessions is counterintuitive because most caring adults automatically make suggestions to adolescents about how to solve problems, such as, "Well, you certainly could look at the teacher when she talks, right?" or "You could put a note in your purse about homework," or "How about if you left your cell phone in your locker during school?"

These suggestions are well intentioned and certainly sensible; however, when the goal is actual change, motivational interviewing has shown that such changes are more likely if individuals choose the area for change themselves and then generate possible ways to change themselves (Miller & Rollnick, 2012). Achievement mentors have found that a useful image for them to keep in mind during the motivational interviewing stage of the session is obtaining water from a well. The bucket is lowered; it fills up with water, and it is then brought up. While the mentee studies a teacher's feedback on the WRF, the mentor sits still and remains quiet, resisting any temptation to suggest either an *area* for change or a *method* of change. As this process unfolds, the mentor can envision a bucket slowly descending into a well, reaching the water, and even more slowly, bringing water up to the surface.

If mentors envision this process for a sufficient duration, the mentee will often interject with what motivational interviewing calls a "change statement." An outright commitment is not necessary to qualify as a change statement. Thus, a statement hinting at an area where the mentee would consider changing would suffice, as would the student stating that he or she *could maybe* set an alarm or raise his or her hand before talking in class. The mentor must keep in mind that the overall purpose of Achievement Mentoring is to allow disengaged youth to believe that they can problem-solve, make decisions, and improve their lives through their own actions. Thus, the mentor must be prepared to accept the student's choice for an area of change even if it is entirely different from what the mentor or a teacher would have suggested. This learning will inevitably involve some trial and error for the mentee, but if caring adults intercede on their behalf by making suggestions for them, students will not have the experiences that teach them that they themselves can take charge of their lives.

If a mentee does not generate a "change statement" while the mentor envisions the bucket going down and slowly coming up from the well, the mentor can ask, "Is there anything you might do so you can get more 'yes's; next week?" If mentees say, "No," the motivational interviewing method requires that mentors accept this refusal to choose a weekly goal for change, irrespective of the difficulty it may cause the caring adult. For at-risk adolescents to learn that they can make decisions themselves, they must have the chance to decide not to set a goal. The following week's WRF may reveal the consequences, if any, of the student's choice.

Step 6: Refine the Mentee's Goal for the Week

If, during the motivational interviewing step, mentees generate a "change statement," the mentor helps them refine the goal, no matter how tentative, vague, general, or implausible it may seem initially, so that it realistically could be accomplished during the subsequent week. The point of this step is to increase the probability that mentees will be successful in achieving a weekly goal. It is fine if the goal is small, such as remembering to bring pens to school on Friday for the weekly spelling test instead of borrowing someone else's. The acronym "S.M.A.R.T." (Specific, Measurable, Achievable, Realistic, and Time-bound) (Meyer, 2003) represents the attributes of a goal that is appropriate for this step.

The goal refinement process requires that mentors be aware of the life circumstances of individual mentees and what it is feasible for them to accomplish in a week, given their daily resources and supports. When the refinement process yields a goal that is so small and discrete that mentees (and mentors) believe it will be simple to achieve, it must be measurable as well so that the mentee will easily be able to ascertain whether or not it has been accomplished. For instance, if mentees with past attendance problems declare that they will attend school every day the following week, mentors can help them set a goal instead to attend one additional day—perhaps the day they are most often absent, such as Monday. If mentees are far behind in math homework assignments, they should be helped to choose one assignment to complete and hand in, instead of all of them. If mentees have a habit of fighting when they are threatened, a mentor could help them decide to experiment once by remaining in school after the final bell instead of racing out immediately to continue the confrontation.

Step 7: Plan and Practice Implementation

In this step, achievement mentors and mentees anticipate any barriers that they can imagine that might block mentees from attaining the weekly goal. Then they discuss plans on how to overcome each potential barrier. Once again, this step, as was the case with step 6 ("refine the mentee's goal for the week"), necessitates the mentor's thorough knowledge of the mentee's life circumstances because impediments toward achievement of even small goals may often arise from the unique situation of each mentee. Barriers might be focused on relationships with others—mentees find it difficult to talk to a teacher or a parent; or barriers might originate with the mentees—they have to stop themselves from performing impulsive, habitual acts, or they have to remember to do something in a timely manner, because they often forget until it is too late. Once barriers are identified, mentors and mentees either practice the new skills that might be necessary to overcome the predicted barriers, which may take the form of role-playing; or mentees may implement a plan that will serve to remind them about their goals, such as setting cell phone alarms or tying a ribbon to possessions.

Step 8: Students Write the Following Week's Goal on Their WRF and Return to Class

Achievement Mentoring sessions end with mentees writing what they will do to meet their S.M.A.R.T. goal for the following week in the designated box at the bottom of the WRF (see Figure 11.1). The goal is written on the WRF so that the mentor can review it before the next mentoring session. It is important for the student, rather than the mentor, to record the goal, so it is in the student's words and he or she is more likely to remember. An additional option to promote remembering the goal is for mentors to have blank cards on hand for students to record their weekly goals and take with them (although this measure is not always reliable, as students may misplace these cards). Mentors should remember that learning theory posits that learning new skills takes time and multiple repetitions in different environments. Thus, mentors must be careful not to show disappointment if students lose the card, do not remember their goal, or when goals are not attained. Mentees may need several weeks of discussion and planning of the same goal before it is achieved.

Step 9: Mentor Documents Mentoring Session

At the end of every Achievement Mentoring session, mentors record what was done. Because mentors often have full-time jobs in addition to mentoring, a user-friendly record-keeping "app" was developed so that this function could take less than a minute per session. Mentors automatically receive an email each week with "Weekly Online Mentoring Survey (WOMS) Reminder" in the subject line and a link to the Achievement Mentoring record-keeping app. Once the link is clicked, a drop-down menu appears with a list of that mentor's mentees. Mentors click a name, a date, and answer eight "yes" or "no" questions (see Figure 11.2) corresponding to the Achievement Mentoring steps that had been completed with each mentee that week, input the mentee's weekly goal, and then click "Submit." Mentors have the option to record additional material too, such as difficulties in meeting with their mentees.

There is no additional "paperwork." These are the only records that mentors need to keep. Mentors can access the app at any time to review their records. Their supervisors can access the app as well, to ensure that mentors get credit for Achievement Mentoring. There is provision for the Program developer, trainer, or local coordinator to learn if mentors are having trouble implementing any Achievement Mentoring steps, so that adjustments can be made. The WOMS form can be modified and customized with additional questions if the existing questions generate insufficient information. For example, an agency that provided Achievement Mentoring to students on probation wanted mentors to answer "yes" or "no" to the question, "Did your mentee meet with their probation officer?" The WOMS form was customized so that mentors working with students on probation had this question included, but all other mentors received the standard form.

Step 10: Mentor Gives Feedback to Teachers, Achievement Mentoring Program Coordinators, and Parents

Although Achievement Mentoring is repetitive and strongly focused on learning specific school engagement skills and habits, 15–20 minutes a week with the same mentor is not a very intensive learning program. As we reviewed in Chapter 10, learning theory research has shown that skills learned in one social environment at a specific time are more likely to generalize to other environments if they are reinforced, that is, if they are followed by positive consequences, or if they generate "payoffs," in other environments and at other times (Mayer et al., 2013). Thus, mentors at the end of each weekly session consider who in their mentees' environments other than the mentor (e.g., teachers, guidance counselors, coaches, the local Achievement Mentoring Program coordinator, and/or the school principal) might notice signs of school engagement and praise mentees for this effort. A note in their mailbox, or a text or email to any of these individuals, asking them to praise mentees if they see designated behaviors will aid generalization. Mentors, of course, can acknowledge

Weekly Online Mentoring Survey (WOMS)

Mentee	**Sue D**	
Week of	**October 16**	
No Mentoring this week (comment why below.):	☐	
Did you:		
1. Have Feedback to Show Mentee?	☐ Yes	☐ No
2. Talk to Your Mentee Individually?	☐ Yes	☐ No
3. Praise Something?	☐ Yes	☐ No
4. Discuss an Area for Improvement?	☐ Yes	☐ No
5. Get Student Views?	☐ Yes	☐ No
6. Help Student Generate a Small Step to Take?	☐ Yes	☐ No
7. Plan Together a Realistic Implementation?	☐ Yes	☐ No
8. Contact a Parent This Week? (Required only once a month)	☐ Yes	☐ No

Comments (include any goal for the week):

Submit Save

SAVE YOUR ANSWERS IF YOU NEED TO FINISH LATER,
or SUBMIT COMPLETED SURVEY.

FIGURE 11.2. Weekly Online Mentoring Survey (WOMS).

any indications of a student's school engagement they witness in school during the week as well.

Communication is always a two-way street. As it is common for mentors to become discouraged by slow progress, lack of progress, or a downhill slide in mentees' school engagement, they need the support of their supervisors and peers. Thus, they should speak briefly after mentoring each week with their Achievement Mentoring coordinator and/or other mentors in their school who understand the process of Achievement Mentoring. Mentors need to be reminded that they are doing a good job and can be having a positive impact even if mentees' behavior, attendance, and grades remain the same or decrease slightly. Fellow mentors and a Program coordinator can point out that, without Achievement Mentoring, their mentees' indices of school engagement would probably have decreased even more markedly (Bry, 2001a; Bry & George, 1980). (See Chapter 15 for a discussion of the research documenting this phenomenon.)

One of the strategies of Achievement Mentoring is for the parents to reinforce the youth's school engagement. Parker and Bry (1995) have shown that parents of high-risk adolescents, despite their best efforts, often feel powerless to guide their children away from conduct problems and school failure. These parents' good intentions may often be overwhelmed by the pervasive internal and external stressors of their existence, such as poverty, social and cultural isolation, depression, physical illness, poor communication and persuasion skills, a high-crime environment engendering fear, and a lack of knowledge of their children's high-risk activities (Parece, 1997). Research has shown, however, that parents feel partnered and less alone when their youth is receiving Achievement Mentoring (Alexander, 2001). This may lead parents to feel less helpless and more efficacious themselves. It is very important that achievement mentors contact the mentees' parents or caregivers monthly. Apprising them of the student's positive school behavior will allow for at-risk adolescents to be praised for their efforts by their family as well as the mentor and other school personnel.

As discussed throughout this book, it may be very difficult to reach parents during the school day, particularly those who may not be in a position to make or receive phone calls at their jobs. Notes may be sent home or messages left on parents' voice mail, but it is best if the mentor and parent agree on a convenient time and method to talk. One very concerned single father instructed the mentor to tell his foreman that this was an important call from the school so that he could be informed regularly about his son's progress. Evidence has demonstrated how critical it is to involve parents in this intervention. Achievement Mentoring may not have any positive impact in the absence of parent contact once a month (Bien & Bry, 1980).

CONCLUSION

The evidence-based Achievement Mentoring Program is elegantly simple and makes common sense to professionals and nonprofessionals alike.

Its practical nature assures feasible implementation during school days and brings satisfaction to implementers. Because program methods have been employed for many years in schools in multiple, different types of communities and locations, mentors know that the program is "tried and true" and that they are benefiting from solid experiences of myriad past mentors. Ample guidance and structure are given to achievement mentors on how they can gain access to and improve school engagement among at-risk youth. Close support and troubleshooting is provided to mentors while they mentor.

The Program lasts long enough to have a permanent versus temporary effect on at-risk students. Achievement Mentoring involves at least two of the multiple systems in youths' lives—school and parents. If mentees receive Achievement Mentoring during at least two school years, research shows that they will have fewer behavioral problems and better academic records than they would have if they had not had mentoring (see Chapter 15).

FORM 11.1.

Weekly Report Form (WRF)

WRF	**Teacher:** ----------------------	**Subject:** -------------------	**Date:** -----------	

Details about the YES's/NO's refer to behaviors—actions the teacher sees the child doing

	Monday	Tuesday	Wednesday	Thursday	Friday
In School	YES NO	YES NO	YES NO	YES NO	YES NO
On Time	YES NO	YES NO	YES NO	YES NO	YES NO
Materials for Class		YES NO	**Did Classwork**		YES NO
Satisfactory Behavior		YES NO	**Did Homework**		YES NO
			Marks/Grades		

Details about the YES's:	**Details about the NO's:**

Goal for this week generated by pupil	

CHAPTER 12

Communication Skills
for Achievement Mentoring

The primary purpose of Achievement Mentoring is to help at-risk students to become engaged in school and to take advantage of education. Youth often become disengaged when past experiences have taught them that their efforts to succeed in school will not "pay off." Thus, Achievement Mentoring must provide contrasting experiences that will teach these students that there will be a "payoff"—that they *can* succeed in school.

Learning theory research shows that self-confidence is not developed through external sources—for example, being told by others that you can succeed. Rather, self-confidence is built by repeated experiences of receiving payoffs when taking specific actions (Bandura, 1997). Gradually, these repeated experiences of taking actions that have positive effects—being efficacious—can lead to a belief in one's self-efficacy. Disengaged students have learned the opposite in their school experiences. Their assumption that they cannot bring about positive results by making efforts has resulted in "learned helplessness" (Peterson et al., 1993).

Babies do feel efficacious. They kick a noise-maker in their crib and succeed at producing a sound. They cry and get fed or changed. They smile and get smiled at. Young children are enthusiastic and inquisitive learners. Thus, disengaged students may have entered school with optimism and a growth mindset. Furthermore, disengaged students may still experience self-efficacy outside of school. Achievement Mentoring is designed to re-teach academic self-efficacy so that at-risk students can re-develop a competent identity around school engagement and can re-learn that they can succeed in school.

A major source of youth's identities is social feedback from others—feedback following everything they say, show, think, and do (Naar-King & Suarez, 2011; Tsai et al., 2009). As was discussed in Chapter 11, achievement mentors are important people to at-risk youth. Thus, moment-to-moment feedback from achievement mentors in response to what mentees say, show, think, and do has significant influence on mentees' identities and on what they will say, show, think, and do in the future. Given this level of influence, Achievement Mentoring can be positively life-changing for at-risk youth. However, it can also operate as a two-edged sword and cause harm. Skillful adherence to Achievement Mentoring communication skills will promote the former outcome. If, however, moment-to-moment feedback from achievement mentors maintains disengaged students' assumptions that they cannot succeed in school, it is irrelevant whether this may have been unintentional or inadvertent. The result is the same: such mentoring can actually reduce the chances that students will graduate. This chapter details the communication skills that achievement mentors must learn, hone, and continue to practice in order to mentor proficiently and prevent negative outcomes.

Achievement Mentoring communication skills are different from those used to engage in normal communication, in which all participants share equal responsibility for the result. In contrast, as in all professional interviewing (Ivey, Ivey, Zalaquett, & Quirk, 2012), achievement mentors have the primary responsibility for the result. Achievement Mentoring communication skills differ from teaching skills as well. Educators determine the content that will be taught and focus on providing information and the skills that need to be learned. Alternatively, achievement mentors do not determine what content will be taught or what skills need to be learned. Instead, achievement mentors must be skillful in *listening* to youths' reactions, values, and choices, and in *waiting* for the youths to generate goals to work on and strategies to meet those goals themselves. Well-intended adults usually find that latter skill most difficult, as discussed in Chapter 11. Having had experience in solving their own problems, adults instinctively offer possible solutions before adolescents have a chance to generate their own possible solutions, thus depriving youth of the chance to learn to problem-solve. It is very challenging for educators who mentor to switch their communication styles from teaching to mentoring and to wait for students to generate their own goals and strategies. In addition, the skills that youths will practice during mentoring are determined to a significant extent by the youths themselves, not by the mentor alone, during the process of troubleshooting the strategy that the youth has chosen as a possible solution.

To be able to help determine what skills an individual at-risk youth may need to learn, a mentor needs to be able to imagine walking in the mentee's shoes, while that mentee is trying to meet his or her goals. For instance, instead of assuming a student already has the skill to find out what the homework assignment is by asking another student, a mentor may realize, when putting her- or himself in the mentee's shoes, that the mentee needs to practice that skill. Another example is assuming mentees can exert some control over how they spend their time at home. Having imagined being in the mentee's shoes, a mentor may realize that the mentee needs to practice assertive communication skills.

DESCRIPTION OF SKILLS AND RATIONALE

Open-Ended Questions

Before achievement mentors can imagine what it is like to walk in their mentees' shoes, mentors must be knowledgeable about their mentees as unique individuals. All adolescents, particularly disengaged youth, have learned not to share significant life details with adults (Naar-King & Suarez, 2011). Answers to specific questions tend to be "yes" or "no" without elaboration—for example, "Weren't you absent yesterday?" "Yes." "Did you study?" "Yes." "Have you thought about getting a job?" "Yes." "Do you want a mentor?" "No." Answers could be short and factual but not necessary satisfying, such as "Who gets you to school?" "Joe."

On one hand, when interviewing someone who talks too much, asking closed-ended questions with "yes" or "no" or factual answers is a way to make the process more efficient. On the other hand, if one wants an interviewee to give more informative answers, it is most effective to ask open-ended questions that cannot be answered in a few words, such as questions starting with "What" or "How." Asking "Could you tell me more?" is also effective. Avoid both closed-ended questions that can be answered in a few words and questions with "yes" or "no" answers, such as queries that start with "Did" or "Do" or "Have" or "Was" or "Is," and those with "right" or "wrong" answers (Ivey et al., 2012). When they are not sure how to frame an open-ended question when seeking information from their mentees, achievement mentors are trained to begin questions using words such as "How" or "What." Mentors often want to help the mentee out by suggesting a couple of possible answers. They must be careful, however, not to add a closed question to the end of an open question. For instance, a useful open-ended question is, "How did you get yourself to school on time today?" Mentors must quell an impulse to say, "Did you remember to set your alarm, or did your Mom wake you?"

While it is important when asking open-ended questions for achievement mentors to hear the answers themselves, an even more significant function is for mentees to hear their own answers. Open-ended questions generally cause mentees to think about something in a new way. Thus, they hear themselves say something that they have not thought before. Mentees are more likely to remember these new thoughts if they generate them themselves and then say them out loud, instead of just answering "yes" or "no" to options given to them by mentors. Mentors who discipline themselves to ask as many open-ended questions as possible report two other advantages: (1) open-ended questions prevent mentors from inadvertently conveying negative judgments or evaluations of mentees, and (2) as open-ended questions are easier to generate, mentors also experience less pressure to form precise closed-ended questions.

Mentors should also avoid asking mentees "Why" questions as they often engender unreliable responses. We constantly ask ourselves and hear others ask us why we did something. Our answers tend to be incomplete at best and inaccurate at worst. When we give an *incomplete* answer, it often stems from the misguided view that we understand our motivations; however, we are really unaware (unconscious) of most moment-to-moment triggers and "pay offs" that motivate our thoughts, actions, and feelings. Answers to "Why" questions may be *inaccurate* because we have learned from people's reactions to distinguish which explanations are acceptable to others and thus do not bring negative consequences, and which explanations are unacceptable and thus bring negative consequences. For instance, when asked "Why" they hit another child, preschoolers learn to say, "She hit me first," or "He took my toy." Such explanations often succeed in moving negative attention away from the first child to another child. Such explanations "pay off." Adolescents and adults give analogous, effective explanations to avoid or escape punishment. For example, if adolescents are asked "Why" they were absent, they have learned to say, "I was sick." If adults are asked "Why" they were late, they have learned to say, "There was a traffic accident."

Children learn the "explanation-giving" habit very early in life, which is well entrenched by adolescence and adulthood (Ramnerö & Törneke, 2008). Thus, explanation-giving often is a learned habit instead of a pathway to the "truth." The more often mentees hear themselves answer "Why" questions with automatic avoidance or escape excuses, the more entrenched excuse-giving will become as a habit. Mentors should not give mentees more reasons to practice incomplete or inaccurate "explanation-giving." Open-ended questions that require individuals to have to think in more detail about what they do and what happens to them, such as, "How does this affect your day?" or "What does that mean for you?" do not lend themselves to being answered with habitual explanations. Instead, the answers could initiate valuable "change talk" (Miller & Rollnick, 2012).

Active Listening

The goals of Active Listening Skills are for the listener, that is, the mentor, to fully understand what it is like to be in the mentee's shoes and make the mentee aware that the mentor understands. There are many ways to engage in active listening. Minimally, mentors look at mentees when they talk, and they give them their full attention. Mentors can indicate this attention by nodding in response to what mentees say with congruent expressions on their faces. Mentors may also encourage their mentees without interrupting or changing their mentees' focus with limited vocalizations that denote presence in what is essentially, for now, a one-sided conversation. Mentors may vocalize a simple "Mmm-hmm" and repeat one or two words of their mentees that reflect the mentees' experiences, such as "scared" or "hard" or "relieved" or "excited."

Mentors listen selectively—not only for expressions of emotions on the part of mentees, but also for all aspects of mentees' thoughts, behaviors, and reactions. If mentors are not sure that they fully understand their mentees, they can paraphrase mentees' language in the form of a tentative question, such as, "Am I sensing that you feel hurt about being ignored?" Thus, not only repeated words, but also paraphrases of mentees' words, constitute active listening. Asking open-ended questions can also be part of active listening—particularly prefaced by, "I really want to understand"; "What was it like for you to be taking care of your mother?"; "Could you tell me more about that?"; "What do you mean by that?"

Note that mentors particularly listen for emotional words to repeat, as opposed to thoughts. There is an easy way to distinguish between an emotional word and a thought. The structure of the reflection of a feeling word is, "You feel . . . ," where the feeling word replaces the dots. Another sign that it is a reflection of emotion is that it makes sense if you replace "feel" with "am" or "are" or "is," such as "You are relieved." If, instead, it makes sense to say, "You feel *that* . . . ," a thought instead of a feeling is being reflected, such as, "You feel that she is unfair." Silence and thinking are yet another part of active listening. During silence, mentors focus wholly on attempting to experience what it is like to be their mentees. They are not focusing on their next agenda item or on their own reactions to or judgments about what their mentees are saying. Nor are they thinking about solutions to their mentees' struggles.

Another essential aspect of active listening is its focus on the mentees themselves instead of on other people, social institutions, or features of environments that they might discuss (Ivey et al., 2012). There are several reasons for this focus. Mentoring sessions are brief, and the goal of Achievement Mentoring is to help individual mentees. Not only is changing others or organizations outside of the Program's mandate, but mentors do not have regular, direct access to individuals other than mentees. The paramount reason that mentors focus on mentees, however, is that mentors want mentees to see themselves as the source of their own solutions. Time spent focusing on others or institutions is not only a poor use of limited resources, but it also may communicate a message to mentees that at-risk youth are helpless because solutions lie elsewhere. This message is diametrically opposed to the one Achievement Mentoring was designed to convey.

Certain habits that well-intentioned adults display in normal conversation can work against active listening's goal of making mentees aware that mentors know what it's like to be in their shoes (Princeton Center for Leadership Training, 2012). Achievement mentors should try to avoid (1) giving their own opinions ("If it were me, I would . . . "), (2) making generalizations ("It's common for teens to feel that way . . . "), (3) interjecting their own story ("When I was a student, . . . "), (4) agreeing or disagreeing with mentees' judgments ("I agree that that was not fair . . . "), and (5) giving advice ("You should consider doing . . . "). Some of these adult communication habits (2, 3) negate the unique individuality of each mentee, and others (1, 4, 5) negate the Achievement Mentoring message that the mentees can solve their own dilemmas.

Finally, active listening is an effective skill to use when parents or teachers criticize mentees (Bry, 2001b; Logan & Bry, 2013). Once mentors have developed a positive relationship with mentees, it is difficult for them to hear teachers and parents criticizing these students. Instead of arguing with parents or teachers and defending the mentees, however, mentors can use Active Listening Skills with these individuals and focus on understanding what it is like to be in the parent's or teacher's shoes. As teachers and parents feel understood by mentors, they are then more likely to soften their criticism of the mentee; be open to acknowledge positive steps made by the mentee; and want to take advantage of the mentor's good listening skills by telling their own story.

Interviewing Teachers about Mentees in Their Classrooms

As highlighted in Chapter 11, a unique aspect of Achievement Mentoring is that one of each mentee's teachers is briefly interviewed before every weekly mentoring session. This component of Achievement Mentoring serves multiple functions. The interview provides the most direct and accurate way for mentors to prepare for their sessions with mentees. The written record of the standardized interview is the basis of the WRF (Figure 11.1), which provides predictable, reliable content for mentor–mentee meetings. The presentation of the WRF by the mentor signals the purpose of the meeting to the mentee: they are there to talk about the student's schoolwork. (Interestingly, after mentors gain pictures of their mentees' lives through open-ended questions and active listening, they often realize that they are the only persons in many students' lives who discuss schoolwork with them. Thus, it falls to the mentor to recognize students' efforts and help them to meet the challenges they face in school.)

Another function of the interviews and the resulting WRF is to educate students about what schools value. For disengaged students, schools are like foreign countries with unknown customs and rules. School employees often think that the customs and rules are obvious and that every student should know them. This misperception can be quite challenging when students' experiences do not conform to the vision of an orderly environment that such rules and customs are meant to convey. In most schools, some written rules are enforced sporadically and others not at all. For instance, the written rules may indicate that students should go to their assigned rooms when they hear the warning bell. However, some employees tell the students to go to their homerooms before the warning bell rings; other employees let them stay in the hall after the warning bell; and/or some employees enforce the rule differently on different days. The same confusion befuddling disengaged students exists within classrooms: one teacher encourages students to share educational materials with each other, and others forbid it; some teachers announce when homework should be submitted, and other teachers expect homework to be put in a designated place without reminders. With WRFs as guides, mentors and mentees can discuss the school's rules and customs and how, where, and when they are enforced.

A further function of the teacher interview is to enable teachers to communicate their explicit expectations to at-risk students effectively through the mentor. Experience shows that teachers themselves tend to communicate expectations in characterological terms or in broad generalizations. Common comments by teachers on quarterly report cards, warning notices, and discipline referrals are not detailed enough for a student or mentor to know exactly what the student needs to do differently, for example, "Student is immature"; "Student needs to take more responsibility"; "Student is rude"; "Student is unprepared"; "Student is distractible"; "Student needs to try harder"; "Student is disrespectful"; "Student is an attention-seeker"; "Student is underachieving"; "Student won't listen"; "Student is unmotivated"; "Student is in danger of failing for the year." Teachers may assume that students are aware of what they should do differently, but as each classroom has its own customs and rules, it may not be clear at all to these students what is expected of them. Unless mentors sit in classrooms and observe, the mentors do not know either. Thus, mentors must ask teachers specific questions during the interviews until the mentor can visualize exactly what is expected of students in a particular teacher's classroom and the ways in which the mentee falls short of meeting such expectations. If the mentor has not asked enough questions so that the mentor can visualize what the teacher sees and wants to see in the classroom, then it is difficult to help the mentee.

As teachers answer the questions asked during each interview, they learn the information mentors will convey during mentoring and come to view the WRF as supportive of their educational goals with the mentored students. When asked to generate at least one positive observation about the mentee to be recorded on the WRF, most teachers also learn to think of the student in a new way. The question prompts them to look for something positive that mentees do and to let the mentees know that they noticed something positive that they did. This process reminds the teacher that positive reinforcement increases positive behavior. Although Achievement Mentoring does not target teacher behavior, one consequence of the interviews may be teachers' incorporating the inclination to catch a kid doing something good today. Teachers may also see mentors struggling to characterize negative feedback in a constructive fashion on the WRF and be prompted themselves to frame negative feedback in more constructive ways when speaking with students.

The WRF guides the mentor to ask the teacher first about attendance and promptness because these habits are essential for school success. Whereas honor students aim for perfect attendance and are therefore aware of their absences, disengaged students, as discussed in Chapter 10, tend to treat absences as "out of sight, out of mind" and often do not monitor their attendance and promptness. Thus, the mentor must find out such information from the teacher or the school records in order to speak accurately with mentees about the days in the prior week they attended school and were in class on time.

The remaining questions on the WRF were developed from teacher responses to open-ended questions during the Achievement Mentoring Program developer's initial weekly interviews with them (see Figure 11.1). Teachers indicated that it would be easier for them to describe briefly what at-risk students were doing in class if the mentor asked specific questions. A review of the responses that teachers had given to open-ended questions during the program's first year showed that, in addition to attendance and promptness, teachers viewed the following signs of school engagement as the most valued: (1) having the necessary educational materials (e.g., pencil, textbook); (2) doing whatever was expected during class (e.g., taking notes, watching a video, doing desk work); (3) exhibiting satisfactory behavior (e.g., raising hand before talking, staying seated at desk, letting other students work uninterrupted), and (4) turning in completed homework. If mentees met these expectations, teachers would be satisfied with their progress. The WRF also asks teachers about recent grades. This way the mentor and mentee are alerted if the student is failing the course and will not be surprised if it happens. It is also useful for a teacher who may expect that a particular student is failing to notice that this student has been improving and is getting passing grades.

Once all of the questions are answered with a "yes" or "no," mentors need to ask teachers to elaborate on their answers, giving details about what the *teacher saw* and what mentees' behavior *looked like* in class during the prior week. The point is to enable the mentors to visualize precisely what the students did to earn "yes" answers (exactly what materials are needed in that class and/or exactly what class work was being done in the class the prior week) and precisely what the students did to earn "no" answers (e.g., the teacher saw the student's head on his desk when the teacher was teaching, or the student did not pick up her pencil to begin the desk work for 5 minutes). When teachers use characterological or broad descriptions, mentors can probe further with questions such as, "What exactly does the student do when she is being rude?"; "How does the student show his immaturity?"; "What would I see my mentee doing if I were in your class?"; "What would the student do if he were more motivated?"

Once the feedback is expressed in behavioral terms, the mentor writes notes about the details on the WRF, phrasing it in such a way that it is constructive feedback for the mentee to see. For example, if the feedback was about the student's not taking notes, instead of writing "The teacher never sees you taking notes," the same underlying message is written in a constructive manner, namely, "The teacher would like to see you taking some notes." Asking a teacher for behavioral observations of mentees receiving negative feedback, being able to reframe this on the spot as constructive feedback consisting of positive alternative behaviors, all the while writing it down on the WRF, are necessary skills in Achievement Mentoring that require challenging, active thinking during the teacher interview. Achievement mentors eventually develop the habit of automatically translating negative feedback into positive possibilities. They learn how important the skill is when they read WRFs out loud to mentees. Mentees will ask what a teacher means by characterological or broad descriptions, for example, "What does Mr. Brookins mean by unmotivated?" In addition, if the feedback is not written in a constructive manner, mentees may revert to learned helplessness, saying "I can't do that," and shut down.

The teacher interview can also impart information to the teacher—as long as it does not negatively affect the teacher's view of the student—that will help the teacher understand the student's circumstances. Such information as "This foster child is living in a home with no computer or colored markers" may help the teacher understand a student's failure to complete map assignments that required students to have a computer and markers at home. As was discussed earlier, the mentor can assure the teacher that the mentor and student plan during mentoring sessions how the student might be better able to complete assignments and that the student wants to learn what the teacher is teaching. When teachers are given such information, they will see that they are not alone in trying to solve the mentee's multiple challenges and will often become more willing to offer help to mentees in class.

Praising

During training, many mentors report that the skill of praising does not come naturally to them. Some harbor the common belief that praise will lead to complacency and that further efforts to improve will cease. Some assume that "intrinsic motivation" will be reduced by immediate praise for progress; whereas research actually shows that it is "controlling" types of incentives that reduce "intrinsic motivation" (Deci & Ryan, 1985). Controlling types of incentives do not offer choice, for example, "You can leave after you draw the rose," as contrasted with, "You can leave after you either draw the rose or another flower of your choosing." Some worry that praising a small step toward a goal will not be fair to other students who already have the good habit. ("How can you praise a seventh grader for getting to school on time one day when all of the other students have to be on time every day?") Coaches know, however, that learning starts where the learner is (Cleary, 2015).

Others believe that the best way to help individuals improve is to point out what is wrong with what they are doing now. While it is true that criticism gets immediate attention for the criticizer, it also often leads to anger, rebellion, and avoidance of the criticizer in the long run (Mayer et al., 2013). Research shows that long-term improvement comes from immediate acknowledgment of small "successive approximations" of mastery (Cleary, 2015). As criticism does not teach the small steps that are necessary to do things differently, a disengaged student is brought back to the state of "learned helplessness" (Peterson et al., 1993) when a teacher says, "You are failing this course."

Effective praise involves looking directly at the mentee and including a specific description of what the mentee did that is being praised (Webster-Stratton, 2006). Thus, instead of "You did well this last week," praise should be stated as, "You got to school on time Monday.

Great." Fitting praise into this format increases the behavior that is being praised. A caveat is to make sure not to add qualifying phrases to the praise that might neutralize it, introduce a negative evaluation, or express overwhelming expectations, such as, "What took you so long?" or "How come you were late on Tuesday?" or "Now you can have perfect promptness for the rest of the year!" Mentors must practice making praise short and specific.

The final component of praise in Achievement Mentoring is asking the student, "How did you do it?" Remember that the feeling of self-efficacy is the most powerful protective factor for a successful adult life (Finn & Zimmer, 2012). Thus, the most helpful effect that Achievement Mentoring can have on mentees is to increase their awareness of and confidence in their ability to succeed at life's tasks through their own actions. If mentees answer the question, "How did you do it?" by giving credit to someone or something other than their own actions, as discussed in Chapter 11, the mentor should ask the question again until the mentee hears him- or herself taking credit for the praiseworthy behavior as a result of the mentee's own actions. Because some mentees may not be in the habit of taking credit for successes, the mentor may need to suggest some specific actions that the student might have taken to bring about the good result in the beginning of mentoring, such as, "Did you choose your clothes the night before?" or "Did you tell your Dad you needed to sleep at your grandma's?" or "Did you set an alarm?" or "Did you ask your Mom for a ride?" or "Did you tell a friend you would walk with him?"

Reporting Teacher Feedback

After praising the positive aspects of the WRF and stimulating the mentee's acknowledgment of his or her role in the praiseworthy results, the achievement mentor must know how to deliver feedback from a teacher about areas for improvement. The feedback is not presented as "the incontrovertible truth," but as "impressions" or "perceptions" of others, such as, "The teacher said . . . ," or "The attendance records showed. . . . " In relating the constructive feedback, the mentor holds up the completed WRF for the mentee to see (or lets the mentee hold it if he or she wishes) and points to and reads aloud the details given by the teacher when not answering "Yes" to the question. If the teacher uses the word "problem," the mentor replaces it with more optimistic and less pejorative terms when writing this feedback on the WRF, such as "concern," "issue," and "challenge."

First, the mentor reads the days of the week when absences were reported. Then the mentor reads the days when the student was present but was marked tardy. The mentor does not say, "Your teacher gave you a 'No' for. . . . " Instead, for each area where a "No" was recorded, the mentor reads the details about that "No," such as, "Ms. Ng would like to see you looking at her when she is teaching math." If the student objects to the feedback and says, "I *do* look at Ms. Ng when she is teaching. I don't know what she's talking about," then the mentor looks puzzled and says slowly, "Well, it's her *impression* that you do not look at her when she teaches. I wonder what makes her think you are not looking at her?" By attributing feedback to "impressions," achievement mentors do not get into arguments about whether or not feedback is the truth. This strategy is applicable to nonmentoring situations as well—for example, when parents or teachers (or your own children) disagree with feedback from others.

Motivational Interviewing

As discussed in Chapter 11, the most difficult mentoring skill for achievement mentors to employ is Motivational Interviewing (MI) (Miller & Rollnick, 2012; Naar-King & Suarez, 2011; Rollnick et al., 2016). The purpose of MI is for interviewees—in our case, mentees—to generate their own ideas on how they could change. Mentees' beliefs that they can change their lives through their own actions increase self-efficacy and combat disengagement, rebellion, and "learned helplessness." The spirit of MI is Carl Rogers's client-centered and choice-providing approach (1959).

MI is a gentle, respectful method of communication about a person's life, taking into consideration their difficulties as well as their values and goals. Individual mentees' values and goals are reflected in their "life dreams" (see Chapter 11), so referring to mentees' life dreams is instrumental in facilitating MI in Achievement Mentoring. As discussed earlier, this communication skill is difficult for some teachers or counselors to employ because their training and experience are oriented toward their generating solutions to students' issues. Thus, constant deliberate practice and feedback from trainers are needed over a considerable length of time (Simon & Ward, 2014). As Naar-King and Suarez (2011) pointed out, the natural instinct of adults, teaching young people to navigate the world and automatically correcting ideas that they perceive as wrong, results in "premature problem solving and advice giving" (p. 19). Premature problem solving and advice giving can squelch the development of intrinsic motivation and leave adolescents with the expectation that others will solve their challenges.

The stimulus for MI in Achievement Mentoring is the completed WRF (see Figure 11.1). It is common in Motivational Interviewing for interviewers to show nonevaluative information to interviewees about their behavior without judgment or analysis (Naar-King & Suarez, 2011; Rollnick et al., 2016); the interpretation and the meaning of the personalized feedback are left up to the interviewee. Achievement mentors read aloud the details about the "No's" from the most recently completed WRF and then ask mentees, "What do you make of this?"; they hand them the form and, as discussed in Chapter 11, *mentors wait*. They remember the image of the water bucket slowly going down into the well, collecting water, and slowly coming up again. If mentees remain silent a very long time, the mentor can ask, "What are you thinking?" Once mentees begin to respond, mentors employ Active Listening Skills.

Mentees often begin with what Miller and Rollnick (2012) called "sustain talk"—determination not to change, reasons why not to change, advantages of the status quo, or pessimism about change. Mentors must genuinely allow mentees to show no motivation to change during mentoring sessions. Mentors are also listening for any hints of what Miller and Rollnick (2012) called "change talk"—consideration of change, reasons to change, disadvantages of the status quo, and efficacy beliefs about change. To prompt "change talk," mentors might say, "Can you think of anything you could do so that Ms. Ng gives you more yes's next time I interview her?" Or, the mentor can use another Motivational Interviewing strategy—developing discrepancies. For instance, a mentor could ask, "How does Ms. Ng's impression that you do not look at her relate to your basketball coach's impression when he is coaching you?" Mentors can ask how teachers' observations relate to the mentee's life dream—for example, "How do your grades in math relate to your goal of running your own beauty salon?"

Helping Mentees Shape a Small, Feasible Step to Take

When mentees express any "change talk," open-ended questions can help a mentee move toward a decision, such as, "What might you do to figure out how to do a math assignment?" Even though the mentor "knows" many solutions for a teacher's "No" on a WRF, mentors must remember that the highest priority is for mentees to choose their own area of change and experience, doing their own problem solving and decision making. The student's choice might surprise the mentor. For instance, the student who does not do math homework assignments may decide to ask at home if he or she can move out of a sibling's bedroom. Given what the mentor knows about the student's life, the mentor then can help the student hone the decision to a weekly goal that seems manageable to both the mentor and mentee, and that has a high probability of success. The acronym S.M.A.R.T. (Meyer, 2003) represents the common, current definition of a goal that is specific, measurable, achievable, realistic, and time-based. Once goal setting has been completed, implementation can be planned.

Planning Implementation

This mentoring skill involves imagining all of the small steps that will incrementally advance the mentee toward meeting the goal, and seeing all the possible obstacles and barriers that might be encountered along the way. A skilled achievement mentor will realize that a weekly goal may seem deceptively simple but involve multiple steps, the fulfillment of which may require some habits and skills that a mentee does not have. For example, the goal to "Hand in math homework tomorrow," involves at least 10 steps:

1. Learn what the homework assignment is.
2. Have the assignment in writing.
3. Remember to take the written assignment home.
4. Have the necessary resources at home (textbook, colored pencils, calculator, etc.).
5. Remember to do the assignment at home.
6. Find the time to do the assignment.
7. Get help if needed.
8. Put the completed assignment together with other things that are taken to school.
9. Remember to take it to school.
10. Turn in the assignment so you receive credit.

Role playing can be used to rehearse potential communication challenges. Brainstorming can enhance flexible thinking to overcome barriers. If the weekly goal still seems doable after anticipating the steps, practicing necessary communication skills, and brainstorming new strategies, then the mentee is asked to write the weekly goal in his or her own words on the completed WRF (see Figure 11.1).

CONCLUSION

Merely following the Achievement Mentoring steps described in Chapter 11 is not enough to bring about positive outcomes. Those activities must be accompanied by Achievement Mentoring communication skills. These skills differ somewhat from usual conversational skills. They deliberately teach at-risk youth self-efficacy—that they can make their lives better through their own actions. Specifically, in addition to providing school-based efficacy experiences for youth, mentors use Achievement Mentoring communication skills to increase at-risk adolescents' beliefs that they can succeed in school.

CHAPTER 13

Achievement Mentoring

A Case Example

Erik Howard, a White, 14-year-old seventh grader, lived with his mother, Ruthie, his 13-year-old sister, Sonia, and his 3-year-old brother, Vinnie, in a low-income, formerly industrialized, small town with predominantly White residents. Erik's failing grades and excessive absenteeism made it doubtful that he would be promoted to eighth grade in June. At the end of January, Erik entered the Achievement Mentoring Program and was assigned to Mr. Morris as his mentor. Mr. Morris had been hired by a county agency to do Achievement Mentoring in the middle school.

Erik's current issues with academic performance and attendance were consistent with his prior school history. He had failed his classes in the sixth grade and had received a "social promotion" to seventh grade because of his age—he was one of the oldest students in his class because he repeated kindergarten—and because of the feared impact that his being in the same grade as his younger sister would have on his self-image. He had been absent for 50 days in the sixth grade and was on track to match his record this year, having already been absent for 24 days. Erik had been evaluated by the district's Child Study Team the prior year, and no learning or emotional problems were found that would have interfered with his academic performance. In fact, Erik showed above-average verbal and quantitative reasoning skills. Results also indicated knowledge deficits; for example, he did not know math facts such as the multiplication tables.

Erik showed little interest in academic achievement and took no initiative in completing in-class or homework assignments. When given an in-class assignment, he would compliantly take out a pencil and write his name on the paper. He refused teachers' offers to help him get started when they would stop by his desk. Erik would either submit assignments and tests with only a few questions answered or not submit them at all. When teachers asked him questions in class, he would answer with one or two words or say he did not know. He often looked tired. Although teachers reported no disruptive behavior on his part, they observed his isolation in the classroom. His only social relationship in school appeared to be with his sister, whom he accompanied to and from school and seemed to protect. Sonia's school performance was acceptable, but she appeared to share her brother's difficulty with peer relationships. Whereas her classmates sat with each other in groups during lunch, she ate with the school nurse.

THE SCHOOL'S KNOWLEDGE OF ERIK'S FAMILY

The achievement mentor assigned to Erik, Mr. Morris, had had no prior contact with Erik or his family because of his recent placement in the school by a county agency. As Erik was at least a third-generation family member to attend the local public schools, his family history was well known by the guidance counselor and the teachers who had worked in the school for a long time. Both Erik and Sonia had been born while their mother, Ruthie Howard, was still in high school. Their father, Chad Robinson, had been her classmate and played on the high school football team. It was common knowledge that while in high school he and Ruthie used drugs and "partied" on weekends. They never had a committed relationship—they neither married nor lived together at any time—but their weekend "partying" pattern persisted to the present time. Although both Ruthie and Chad had attended high school for four years, neither had graduated with a diploma.

Erik's maternal grandmother, Bea Howard, had given birth to Ruthie's two older sisters while she was still in high school. Neither Bea nor her oldest three daughters had graduated from high school. Bea had "partied" a lot herself while her three oldest daughters were growing up, but she was now in recovery for alcoholism and was the only member of the Howard or Robinson families who was employed full time (as an assembly-line worker for a small manufacturer) and owned a car. Bea's youngest daughter, Margie, was experiencing a much different life trajectory from that of other family members. Being a talented basketball player, she had been mentored by the high school's girls' basketball coach and was now attending a local college on a basketball scholarship. (See Chapter 2 for a discussion of the transformative power a key adult can have on the life of an at-risk youth.) Thus, Erik's Aunt Margie was his only relative with a high school degree.

Erik's father, Chad, lived a few blocks away from him with his 72-year-old adoptive mother, Emma Robinson. Emma, who had always loved children and had not been able to have her own, "informally" adopted Chad as an infant when his birth mother, unable to care for him, "handed" him to Emma. (See Chapter 4 for an extensive discussion of informal kinship care.) Although Emma was not employed full time, she worked for a number of families who lived in an adjacent upper-income town helping out with housework, such as laundry and ironing, and babysitting. She did not drive, so she would be picked up and dropped off at her home by the families she worked for. In addition, Emma took care of Ruthie's children when Ruthie and Chad "partied" on weekends. Chad was not Vinnie's father, but Emma gave Vinnie the same love and attention as she did to the two children Ruthie had with Chad. Thus, the children spent at least a third of their time each week with Emma, whom they called "Grandma" Emma.

LEARNING THEORY CASE CONCEPTUALIZATION

Erik exhibited three out of the four components of school disengagement (see Chapter 10):

1. *Academic component:* He was inattentive in class, showed little motivation to learn, refused help with schoolwork, and displayed no academic initiative. He apparently had not learned mathematical skills. He did not have the habit of regular school attendance.
2. *Affective component:* Erik displayed no affective connection with school. He did not expect or look for acceptance from teachers or fellow students. He spent as little time in school as possible, and he participated in no extracurricular activities. Erik did not seem to value education or connect success in school to future benefits.
3. *Cognitive component:* Erik showed no belief in his academic competence. There was a strong indication of "learned helplessness" in that Erik exhibited (1) no academic self-efficacy, (2) no problem-solving competence, (3) no help-seeking, and (4) little belief that he was in charge of his life.

In a nutshell, Erik showed no attention to, investment in, or effort to do schoolwork. He exhibited little future orientation, and he lacked the habits and skills that would enable his success as an independent adult. It seemed as if Erik had learned how to avoid facing challenges and to escape working hard to overcome them. Prior experiences may have included making such efforts but not deriving any payoffs from them, or being punished or facing other negative consequences when he attempted to take charge of his life and to overcome challenges. Perhaps he had learned to fear what would happen if he asserted himself. In addition, he could not do much "observational learning" of benefits from educational achievement because no adults in his households could serve as educated or successful role models. He also did not appear to have any friends who achieved in school.

Because Erik waited quietly instead of doing schoolwork, perhaps taking initiative had been trained out of him. Or perhaps his refusal to do schoolwork was a way he had learned, in his otherwise disordered world, to exert some control over his life—by quietly not following adults' instructions and not responding to their requests when they were not looking. It was not clear whether Erik had assertive communication skills, but he at no time exhibited this behavior. It appeared that somehow the enthusiasm and curiosity that Erik must have had as a baby had not "paid off" for him and/or had brought negative consequences. On the positive side, Erik showed control over himself while he sat quietly in class doing nothing. He was polite and compliant. He seemed respectful and aware of ways to go unnoticed in school.

ACHIEVEMENT MENTORING PROGRESS

The aims of the achievement mentor in working with Erik were (1) to acknowledge Erik's good habits and skills; (2) to listen actively and learn about his thinking and feelings about himself, his life, and school; (3) to show him role models who were getting payoffs for school engagement; and (4) to wait for him to express "change talk." Then decision making; problem solving; improving skills, such as math competence (e.g., multiplication tables); and taking charge of his life could be modeled, practiced, and acknowledged.

The First Achievement Mentoring Session

Soon after the school assigned Erik to him, Mr. Morris took Erik out of class and conducted their first 20-minute meeting in an empty guidance counselor's office. Mr. Morris explained to Erik that he had been chosen for mentoring because school personnel had seen him as someone who could do better in school. Mr. Morris asked Erik to describe his experiences in a typical day—how he woke up, got to school, and, with the help of a printed copy of Erik's class schedule, what each class was like for him. Then he asked about what he did after school, in the evening, and in preparing to go to sleep. Erik was polite, compliant, and pleasant to interview. He described his life inside and outside of school credibly; however, he did not volunteer any information beyond short answers to Mr. Morris's questions.

Before taking Erik back to class, Mr. Morris asked how he could contact Erik to remind him about their meeting the following week. School personnel had been unable to contact Erik's family to discuss his school performance, as the phone number on school records had been disconnected and letters sent to the address on file were returned stamped "Addressee unknown." Erik explained that his family had just been moved out of a motel into a house. There was no phone, but he gave Mr. Morris their current address. Mr. Morris also informed Erik that he would be talking to one of his teachers to ask about the teacher's observations of what Erik was like in class. Mr. Morris asked Erik to predict what his teacher would say, and he responded that a teacher would say that he did not do schoolwork.

Erik seemed to accept Achievement Mentoring as another school experience over which he had no control. He seemed pleased to be taken out of class, and he was cautiously happy to hear that this would happen regularly. That was the extent of his emotional reaction to mentoring. He remained emotionally detached from the mentor as well, conveying a "take him or leave him" attitude. As a result of his Achievement Mentoring training, the mentor had learned that detachment might be due to Erik having been disappointed in the past by adults who had made promises but did not keep them.

During their brief first meeting, Mr. Morris learned that Erik did not have the "typical days" of most students whose parents or caregivers constructed a daily routine focused around their children attending school. On some school days, he and his sister would wake up early if their grandmother Bea came to their house before her shift at work started so that Ruthie could do her hair. On those days, everyone woke up early enough for the children to get to school on time. They did not take school bus transportation because Ruthie had never informed the school of where they lived, and Bea could not drive them to school because she had to be at work much earlier than students were allowed to arrive at school. As the means by which most students got to school were not available to them, Erik and Sonia had to walk. Neither had winter coats, so on those days when it was too cold outside to walk, they did not go to school. When Bea did not come to the house before she started work, Erik and Sonia would wake up too late to go to school. Interestingly, Ruthie only appeared motivated to get her children to attend school if her mother stopped by and woke up the household. Then, Ruthie would yell at the children to get themselves ready to walk to school and threaten that child protection services would take them away from her if they did not go to school.

On days they did not go to school, they often accompanied Ruthie in the hospital van to her drug rehab program and watched Vinnie while Ruthie received treatment at the hospital. Vinnie's father had died a year earlier in the same hospital. Ruthie also said the children would be taken away if she missed too many days of rehab. One day a week, Grandmother Bea picked up Erik and Sonia after her shift ended at work so that they could help her with her second job—cleaning an office building. This activity allowed them to learn some job skills. Erik's other activities when he was not in school were to explore wetlands in town with some older boys until it got dark when he would return home to watch TV.

Although Erik reported his experiences without much emotion, Mr. Morris sensed that Erik's home life was dominated by fear and regular threats of negative consequences. Because the focus of Achievement Mentoring is solely on the mentee's experiences, Mr. Morris did not ask for details about the threats from child protection services or about Erik's mother's or Vinnie's father's illnesses, although he guessed they stemmed from drug addiction. When Erik was asked, "If your life goes well, what will you be doing at 25 years old?" Erik said that he had not thought about it. Mr. Morris inputted the following observations on his WOMS (Figure 11.2): "Erik answered questions politely and gave no elaboration. He reported no 'life dream.' He does not seem to have habits or skills to get to school regularly because his home life does not have routines. He guesses that teachers will report that he does no schoolwork."

Weekly Report Forms

Even though different teachers were interviewed, Erik's WRFs (Figure 11.1) were consistent week after week. Erik was correct that teachers would report that he did not do class work or homework. Mr. Morris had inquired of the school and learned that Erik was eligible for school busing at his new address. He then arranged for this transportation, at which point Erik's attendance and promptness improved. Mr. Morris praised Erik for this improvement. Erik initially gave the school bus all of the credit for his improved attendance. When Mr. Morris persisted, asking what Erik himself had done, Erik finally reported that he hurried more in the morning now to "get away from my mother's yelling." Erik still typically missed school on Monday, though, because he slept overnight at "Grandma" Emma's house. Mr. Morris also arranged for the nurse to help Sonia and Erik pick out warm winter jackets from the school's donated clothing closet. They also were able to obtain gym clothes—both had been failing physical education (PE) because they did not change clothes—and locks for their gym lockers. Mr. Morris also praised Erik for his good behavior reports in class. When asked how he did that, Erik looked surprised that his behavior was praiseworthy and eventually offered, "None of my friends are there?" with a shrug. When Mr. Morris persisted and asked what Erik himself did, he said, "I think about last night's basketball game on TV."

When Mr. Morris asked Erik what he made of the teachers' reports about class and homework assignments that they did not see him do, he shrugged again, and said, "I don't do schoolwork." When asked if he could do anything to get more "Yes's," he would say, "I don't know." This pattern was repeated week after week. Mr. Morris would then talk to Erik about the latest sports that Erik saw on TV. On Erik's WOMSs (see Figure 11.2), Mr. Morris would write "no change talk" and "perhaps sports could be a life dream."

One component of Achievement Mentoring, monthly parental contact (see Chapter 11), proved helpful. Mr. Morris needed to inform Ruthie of something praiseworthy Erik had done. Mr. Morris also wanted to have Erik accompany him to the local high school one day after school. Mr. Morris had to deliver reports to the school and hoped that a visit might engender in Erik a positive view of the high school and of continuing his education, and might spark more of a future orientation for him. Mr. Morris told Erik that he planned to visit Ruthie at the family home to inform her of Erik's improved attendance and to ask her permission to take him to the high school. Mr. Morris asked if Erik would tell his mother that he was coming. He also asked Erik if there was anything he would like Mr. Morris to say to her. Erik agreed with the first request but said, "Not really," to the second question.

Although Mr. Morris heard the TV and voices inside when he arrived at Erik's home, no one answered the door for a significant length of time. Eventually, a scared-looking Sonia opened the door. Mr. Morris respectfully waited outside until an anxious Ruthie appeared and invited him in. He saw some mattresses on the floor, a couch with Vinnie in the corner eating cheese puffs, a blaring TV, large plastic bags of clothes, and Erik peeking around the corner. Mr. Morris delivered his praise for Erik, inquired how Ruthie had gotten him to school on more days, and how she had taught him to be polite in school. Then Mr. Morris asked Ruthie's permission to take him on the high school visit. Ruthie said, "Erik never listens to me, and you don't need my permission; just take him." He stressed that he needed her permission because she was the parent. When Mr. Morris initially heard Ruthie's criticism of her son, his first instinct was to be protective of Erik, but then he tried to imagine what it was like to be Ruthie and communicated empathically that it must be hard to be a mother of three. "It is hard," she agreed; then she added that she was glad that Erik was polite in school.

Acquiring a "Life Dream"

On the way to the high school, Mr. Morris learned, in response to open-ended questions, that Erik never wanted to go to high school. Erik's older friends said the teachers and principal were mean and that the only good thing about high school was playing football. His mother would not let him play football because she believed he would get hurt and that would result in medical bills that she could not pay. This entirely negative view of high school probably helped to explain his otherwise puzzling refusal to do schoolwork. At the high school, Mr. Morris and Erik set out to deliver some papers to Mr. Morris's summer school colleagues, a writing teacher and a physical education teacher. The regional high school contrasted starkly with the small, dated, dark, local middle school. They passed bright, open, airy classrooms with computers, TVs, tools, a house under construction, music, and dancing on their way to find the PE teacher who was in the gym, supervising basketball practice. Erik's eyes opened wide. Mr. Morris suggested they sit down and watch for a while. When the teacher was introduced to Erik, he asked if he might be related to Margie Howard, the basketball player. When Erik said, "She's my aunt," the coach said, "I hope to see you on my team when you get to high school, too." After that visit, Mr. Morris inputted on the next WOMS (see Figure 11.2), "Erik now has a 'life dream'—to be a basketball player!"

When Mr. Morris interviewed Erik's seventh-grade PE teacher for the WRF (see Figure 11.1), the teacher had positive observations about the student who, prior to Achievement Mentoring, was failing this class because he did not change into gym clothes. Mr. Morris informed the teacher that Erik's life dream was to be a basketball player. The teacher expressed surprise that Erik did not participate in the middle school's evening intramural basketball program. Mr. Morris explained Erik's mother's lack of a car. Because the teacher/coach saw Erik's promising potential and good behavior in class, the teacher said he would invite Erik to play basketball in the evening and offered to drive him home.

More Coordination with Others in Erik's Environment

Despite some positive changes, Erik still did not do class work or homework, or take standardized tests. He had begun to express some "change talk" when Mr. Morris asked during Motivational Interviewing about the discrepancy between his life dream of being a wealthy basketball player and not doing math. (See Chapter 12 for an extensive discussion of the Motivational Interviewing component of Achievement Mentoring.) Mr. Morris decided to arrange a teacher conference between Erik's mother and his math teacher so that Ruthie could hear that he had homework each night and might communicate to Erik the need for him to do it at home. After some hesitation, she agreed to attend, but when the time came for the conference, she took so long to get herself and her children ready when the mentor picked them up that Mr. Morris was afraid that the school would be empty and locked up before they arrived. Ruthie reluctantly followed Mr. Morris into the school, carrying Vinnie, but refused to go into the math teacher's room, remaining in the hallway instead.

Mr. Morris substituted for Ruthie in the teacher conference, but the teacher had gotten a glimpse of Ruthie standing in the hallway and realized that they had attended this middle school at the same time. When Mr. Morris hypothesized that Erik's past poor school attendance resulted in his not knowing enough math facts to do his assignments, the teacher's impression of him as "stubborn and trying to upset her" changed to seeing him as concerned about embarrassment and failure. She also became more sympathetic to him given what she knew of his mother's history. From then on, she did not wait for Erik to ask a question or to seek help. She devised ways of surreptitiously providing him with the multiplication tables during class so that he could have the needed tools to begin to think about how to solve math problems. Mr. Morris was so impressed with her sensitivity to Erik's history and her success in opening him up to learning that he wrote a laudatory letter to her principal for her file, which later contributed to her earning tenure.

Despite the positive involvement of more adults in Erik's life, such as the mentor, the gym teacher, and the math teacher, Erik's seventh-grade report card still showed mostly failing grades, and he had not taken the required standardized tests to be promoted to the eighth grade. The principal was firm in his decision that Erik would have to repeat seventh grade, despite the same concerns that had resulted in his social promotion the previous year, that is, his age and being in the same grade as his younger sister. Mr. Morris tried to change the principal's mind by advocating for summer school for Erik and felt badly when he did not succeed. Mr. Morris stopped by Erik's house to inform the family of the principal's unfortunate decision that Erik's summer school attendance would not be sufficient to overcome his poor grades and thus earn a promotion to the eighth grade. Mr. Morris assured them that he nevertheless would continue mentoring Erik for a second school year.

Grandmother Bea was in the home, as this was the day she picked up Erik and Sonia to help her clean the office building. Bea, like her daughter Ruthie, tended to yell at the children instead of problem-solving with them. However, Mr. Morris had praise for Bea as well. He told her how her youngest daughter Margie's good reputation had helped Erik's gym teacher choose to include him in the intramural basketball team. Mr. Morris asked Bea what she had done to support Margie's success. Unbeknownst to Mr. Morris, Bea soon called Margie and told her to visit the principal and persuade him to let Erik earn his way into eighth grade by attending summer school. Margie did just that and succeeded. It is apparent that the family involvement component of Achievement Mentoring, coupled with praising adult family members for their efforts, accomplished what the mentor was unable to accomplish on his own.

Erik took math and language arts classes every morning during summer school. Fortunately, Mr. Morris was able to continue to mentor Erik as his county agency also placed him at the summer school. When Mr. Morris interviewed Erik's summer school math teacher for the WRF and mentioned that Erik apparently had not learned math facts because of his excessive school absences, the math teacher took improving Erik's math skills as a personal mission and tutored him individually every day from noon to 1 P.M. As a result of the math teacher's gentle coaching, Erik was able to answer questions on math tests and pass math for the first time, earning a C–. No bus transportation was provided for summer school students, but Mr. Morris was willing to drive Erik to and from school. Erik had to wait in Mr. Morris's office for 2 hours until he finished work at 3 P.M. for the ride home.

When Mr. Morris noticed Erik with an interesting-looking book of short stories, he asked Erik about his language arts homework assignment. Erik told him he was supposed to answer questions about Toni Cade Bambara's (1996) story, "Raymond's Run," which they had read aloud in class. When Mr. Morris asked what the story was about, Erik told him that it was about a girl who took care of her brother and whom no one liked. Then the girl won a race and made a new friend. Together, Mr. Morris and Erik reviewed the assignment and found the answers to the homework questions. Erik used a pad in Mr. Morris's office to write the answers. Mr. Morris reminded him to put his name on the paper and asked where Erik would put the paper so that he would have it with him to hand in during class the next day. (See Chapter 12 for an in-depth exploration of the steps involved when at-risk youth learn the skill of completing and submitting homework.)

With Mr. Morris's encouragement, Erik began completing more language arts homework and turning it in. On another afternoon, after Mr. Morris had to leave Erik alone in his office during a staff meeting, Mr. Morris noticed more writing on his pad. The mentor asked Erik if he could read what he had written, and Erik agreed. It was an engaging short story about a boy who lived with his grandmother and was jailed after stealing candy from a store. Then the boy's mother came to get him out of jail and took him to live in another town with her. Mr. Morris was amazed that Erik could craft a short story so well. The sentence structure and grammar were good, and there were only a few minor spelling errors. When Mr. Morris asked Erik where he got the idea for his story, Erik said he had been looking out the window at the other students and thought about a friend of his who had moved to another town. Erik also passed language arts class that summer and, as he passed both summer school classes, he was promoted to eighth grade.

By the end of summer school, Mr. Morris was no longer picking Erik up and dropping him off at Erik's mother's house as the children were now living with "Grandma" Emma. One day Emma whispered to the achievement mentor that she was now taking care of Sonia and Erik full time because their mother and father were in jail. She was also helping out with Vinnie while Bea was at work. Emma had been informed that she would get no financial assistance for taking care of Sonia and Erik and asked Mr. Morris to call child protection services (CPS) and find out why. Emma said that she had a sixth-grade education and did not understand the rules denying these children support simply because she had "raised their father."

Mr. Morris learned that CPS's policy at that time was to provide no funds for "kinship foster care." (See Chapter 4 for an extensive exploration of the financial challenges faced by informal kinship care providers.) When Mr. Morris explained to CPS that Erik and Sonia's father was not biologically related to Emma, CPS agreed to provide her with minimal monthly financial support but added that they could offer a larger stipend if she attended foster care training. Emma, however, refused to participate in the training. Although the children were enrolled in Medicaid, Mr. Morris discovered that they had not received any preventive medical care in years. Emma put the children in charge of calling doctors' offices to find providers who would accept Medicaid. After many rejections, they finally got dental work, vaccinations, and hearing and vision tests. Erik was prescribed glasses, which enabled him to see math examples on the blackboard for the first time.

Emma was a fastidious housekeeper. This was advantageous in the event of foster care inspections, but her neatness had one extremely negative aspect. Emma's overzealous house cleaning involved throwing out virtually anything that she did not need to maintain the household, including the children's school-related items—pens, pencils, colored markers, and texts. She had even thrown out library books that Erik had borrowed from the town library to complete his homework projects. As

Erik could not pay the resulting library fines, he was no longer allowed to borrow books from that library.

Given Emma's tendency to dispose of items Erik needed for school, the achievement mentor guided Erik, when he set weekly goals, to either ask teachers if he could stay after school to complete projects when he needed special supplies, or to make sure that he bring back to school the next day any supplies he took home overnight before Emma had the chance to "clean the house" the following morning. Mr. Morris also helped Erik and his science class partner keep and monitor an ant farm in school instead of at home. The two students subsequently won a science fair award for daily recording and charting the length of the ant tunnels.

A Behavioral Problem from the Past

Erik's academic, affective, and cognitive school disengagement decreased after he moved to "Grandma" Emma's. His attendance and promptness continued to improve, and he was handing in some classwork and passing some tests. He played Pop Warner football in Emma's neighborhood, and the coach saw him as an asset to the team. Erik now believed he could do schoolwork and wanted to earn grades that would make him eligible to play football in high school. Erik still did not appear to have friends in middle school. In their small town, he believed that everyone knew his parents were in jail, and he once described feeling ostracized because of this situation. Erik was, however, taking more initiative in his life. For instance, one day Mr. Morris came to class to pick him up for a mentoring session. But Erik told the teacher that he did not want to leave his class that day because they were dissecting frogs. While Mr. Morris initially felt rebuffed, he realized that Erik's refusal meant progress for Erik, who now felt empowered to determine, to some extent, his school experience.

In the midst of all this progress, a behavioral problem from the past now surfaced. Erik was absent from school one day because of a court date for a past arrest. Apparently, when Erik was living with Ruthie, he and his older friends burglarized houses and sold the items they stole in order to have some cash. Because Erik was the youngest of the group, attended school regularly, and had no other criminal record, he was given community service while the older boys were put on probation or given prison sentences. Mr. Morris, who had consistently praised Erik for his better attendance, promptness, and class work completion, could now point out how those improvements "paid off" for Erik when he went to court, and would continue to pay off in the following year by making him eligible to play football in high school. Mr. Morris stayed in regular phone or face-to-face contact with "Grandma" Emma, who was committed to monitoring the children in her care. Because Emma only left home for occasional ironing and babysitting jobs and to shop for groceries once a week, she was able to pay close attention to where Erik was at all times and she began to get to know the people he spent time with. (See Chapter 2 for a discussion of the importance of parents and/or caregivers monitoring adolescents and the case example in Chapter 8 for an example of the value of parents knowing the peers with whom adolescents associate.) She and Grandmother Bea compared notes about the children every day when Bea came to pick up Vinnie after work.

End of the Second School Year

In the check-in segment at the beginning of a May mentoring session (see Chapter 11 for a discussion of the mentoring session steps), Erik reported that he had taken the eighth-grade standardized tests. Because Erik had refused to take such tests previously, Mr. Morris was pleased to hear that Erik had gone ahead and taken these tests on his own initiative. When Mr. Morris praised him and asked how he had done it, Erik said simply, "I wanted to get it over with." If Erik passed most of his eighth-grade courses, his taking these standardized tests would mean that he could go on to high school. His standardized test results would have no bearing on his promotion, but he had to complete the tests before he could leave the school because they were used to evaluate the school's performance.

Mr. Morris had already done a considerable amount of "prep work" with the high school to ease Erik's adjustment. He had met with the basketball and football coaches with whom he had preexisting professional relationships, and also with the director of the creative writing program. Mr. Morris had shown her Erik's short story about his friend, and she considered Erik sufficiently talented to qualify for the small, selective creative writing program at the high school. This four-year program of daily classes, which provided students with a supportive community within the large regional high school, substituted for the standard language arts curriculum. When Mr. Morris informed Erik's middle school guidance counselor, who was in charge of scheduling the eighth-grade students for ninth-grade classes, she objected, stating that she could not endorse Erik for the creative writing program because of his borderline academic record in middle school. When Mr. Morris reported the guidance counselor's position to the creative writing program director, she stood up for Erik and assured Mr. Morris that Erik's schedule would include creative writing.

Mr. Morris's final advocacy for Erik was to help him and his foster grandmother gather documentation and fill out the necessary forms so that he would qualify for a municipal summer work program designed for low-income students. Mr. Morris followed up with program administrators to make sure that Erik's application would not be overlooked. Under the tutelage of job coaches, Erik helped custodians clean the schools during the summer for which he was paid a salary. When Mr. Morris checked in with him in the middle of the summer, Erik confided proudly that he no longer needed to steal because he now had another way of getting money. Although the 2-year mentoring commitment was formally completed, Mr. Morris assured Erik that he would continue to be a presence in his life and promised to check in periodically with Erik in high school.

DISCUSSION

This account illustrates many of the common strategies, competencies, conceptualizations, challenges, and rewards of Achievement Mentoring. When Erik was chosen for the mentoring program in seventh grade, he already had spent 13 years learning his customary habits of school disengagement. It is not surprising, therefore, that it took almost 2 years of Achievement Mentoring before those ingrained patterns began to change. To continue mentoring Erik for that duration, Mr. Morris needed (1) good training, (2) belief in the program's effectiveness, and (3) ongoing acknowledgment and support from his peers. (This was especially important as Mr. Morris did not get much positive feedback about his mentoring from Erik or Erik's teachers during much of that time.)

Mr. Morris also needed a consistent conceptual framework to explain Erik's puzzling presentation. Because Erik did not explain himself well, Mr. Morris often had to guess about Erik's perspectives, expectations, and the "payoffs" for his habits. Learning theory provided hypotheses that did not pathologize Erik. Achievement Mentoring also provided regular steps to follow and communication skills to use with Erik. Breakthroughs and turning points in mentoring evolved from repeated applications of Achievement Mentoring skills. Furthermore, Mr. Morris did not help Erik all by himself. Mentoring functioned well in large part due to coordinated, extensive, and supportive multisystems environments. Although Mr. Morris played a primary role in initiating the process, coordinating the efforts, and empowering the contributors, Erik's extended family; teachers and other personnel in the middle school, summer school and high school; child protection services; and the juvenile justice system all made invaluable contributions to changing Erik's life trajectory.

Two-Year Commitment

With support and encouragement from his fellow achievement mentors, his local Program coordinator, and his ongoing Achievement Mentoring trainer, Mr. Morris remained patient and respectfully persistent during the two school years of mentoring. A particularly discouraging period occurred when Erik's promotion to eighth grade at the end of the first year of mentoring was in serious doubt. Mr. Morris's WOMSs about his work with Erik (Figure 11.2) communicated to his local Program coordinator and to his ongoing trainer the difficulties he was experiencing. Each week he would input virtually the same comments: "Attendance better, but WRF shows no schoolwork done. Erik chose no weekly goal." During regular Achievement Mentoring staff meetings, troubleshooting and problem solving was done regarding all mentoring challenges, including Erik's.

A concern that Mr. Morris often asked the group to consider was the power differential between himself and Erik and his families. Because the families had not invited Mr. Morris to mentor Erik and because they passively complied with most of Mr. Morris's requests, he understood that the situation could lend itself to the more powerful individual (Mr. Morris) abusing that power and causing harm. Mr. Morris checked often with colleagues to make sure that this was not the case. His colleagues and trainer considered each proposed step and suggested that he continue to inform Erik and his family members and ask permission, when appropriate, to carry out mentoring activities. That they would compliantly agree in the face of his "power" was not in any way harmful to them or Erik. In fact, learning theory suggests that family members could learn that they had power themselves through observing him. In actuality, Bea, Emma, Erik, and Margie each took empowered actions on Erik's behalf while Mr. Morris was mentoring. Because each action brought positive consequences, the probability of their repeating such actions in the future increased. It is interesting that most of their empowered actions occurred after Mr. Morris made clear that he would continue mentoring Erik during a second school year. The promised continuity apparently communicated to those family members that they would not be acting alone and gave them hope that their efforts could be effective.

Learning Theory Conceptualization

After getting to know more about Erik and his family circumstances, Mr. Morris was able to construct a more complete explanation of the probable sources and maintaining factors in Erik's school disengagement than school personnel initially could provide. Mr. Morris's understanding of

Erik's life was so comprehensive that Mr. Morris realized that, given the same circumstances, he might have developed Erik's coping habits himself. They indeed were not pathological; they were adaptive.

When the mentor visited Ruthie's house to get permission to take Erik on the high school visit, he felt the fear of negative consequences that dominated the atmosphere. He sensed that his praise was not really heard by the family members because they had learned to respond to threats and criticism instead. He experienced Ruthie's sense of powerlessness and saw the dearth of opportunities and material resources, including shoes and winter jackets: pictures are worth a thousand words. Despite the inability of family members to acknowledge praise, Mr. Morris persisted in commending them for praiseworthy actions and showing respect so that Erik would witness ways to influence people that were different from what he heard from the adults in his home environment—yelling and threats. Erik needed the one-to-one, face-to-face aspect of Achievement Mentoring in part because he had learned "social distrust" so thoroughly that he needed repeated, individual experiences with a consistent person to up-end his expectations.

After visiting Erik's homes, Mr. Morris sensed that Erik had never been able to exert much control over what happened to him. He would be moved from home to home, given meals or not, and ordered to do this or that regardless of what he himself did. He could not win. He seemed to have learned that the best way to avoid punishment was to remain as quiet, inactive, and invisible as possible. A component of Erik's learning that there were things he could do that would bring positive consequences was the WRF (see Figure 11.1). The consistent criteria offered opportunities for him each week to earn the praise of teachers who were looking to "catch him doing something good today." Erik, who had learned to tell adults as little about himself as possible, evidenced change when he confided in the mentor that he had been engaging in chronic stealing. Now he felt comfortable trusting at least one adult with information about himself.

A turning point in mentoring came when Erik visited the high school. Prior to that time, his only sources for information about high school had come from negative stories he was told by his older friends and parents, none of whom had graduated. There were no males close to him who had thrived in high school, graduated, and subsequently found regular jobs and stable family lives to serve as role models. His father was in and out of jail. Vinnie's father, whose life experiences were similar to those of Erik's father, was already deceased. Erik's visit to the high school introduced him to expanded life possibilities and to adults who valued and welcomed him. This gave him the incentive to meet middle school teachers' criteria on WRFs and get passing grades. He learned for the first time that attending school could be a path to gaining pleasure rather than a chore to "get out of the way" to avoid negative consequences.

Achievement Mentoring Techniques

Because of Erik's habit of saying little about himself, open-ended questioning and focusing on the mentee were important Achievement Mentoring techniques for working with him. Answering open-ended questions required that Erik do some thinking about himself and his life that he was not accustomed to doing. Focusing the questions on Erik's *experience* (e.g., "How was your walk to school yesterday?"; "What do you make of this WRF?"; "How is it for you to sit there quietly while others copy math notes from the board?"; "What kind of stories do you like?"; "How does it feel to leave the house while Vinnie is crying?"; "What do you like about Spiderman?"; "What do you do when a map assignment is given?"), instead of asking questions that Erik was used to answering concerning details that related to others in his life (e.g., "Where are you parents tonight?"; "Has Vinnie had supper?") or the circumstances of his life (e.g., "Where do you live?"; "Why were you absent from school?"), prevented tangential talk. When answering Mr. Morris's questions, Erik probably heard himself saying things he had never said before. Simultaneously, Erik's mentor learned more about what it was like to be Erik. He learned of Erik's need for a winter jacket and for glasses, his difficulty with multiplication, and his rejection by the library. Erik's answer to the question, "What do you look forward to in high school?" surprised Mr. Morris the most but also may have been the most enlightening. Erik's declaration that he did not want to go to high school allowed Mr. Morris to put Erik's middle school disengagement into perspective and realize the logic underlying his otherwise puzzling behavior.

Motivational Interviewing also was important in Erik's development. Erik was very skilled at avoiding and escaping from teacher influence. It was very consistent with his habits, most notably his habit of refusing to do school assignments, for him to avoid and escape setting weekly academic goals. After Erik was enabled to recognize the concept of a life dream as relevant for him, he acknowledged the discrepancy between needing good grades to play football and his doing no schoolwork. Erik was then open to Mr. Morris's help in completing a language arts assignment that interested Erik.

Multiple Coordinated Environmental Influences

It is true for all achievement mentors that Achievement Mentoring is never done in a vacuum. It is effective only when it activates and coordinates other influences on students. Learning theory posits that behavior is determined by one's environment (Biglan, 2015). Mr. Morris came to understand Erik's total and puzzling disengagement from school as a manifestation of Erik's adaptation to his past environment that may have served him well in other circumstances but was self-defeating and threatening his future ability to live a stable and productive life as an adult.

As the mentor was in Erik's immediate environment for a short period of time each week, it was necessary that other aspects of Erik's social environment had to become involved for his behavior to change. These new aspects also had to offer "payoffs" for Erik's school engagement to continue and hopefully increase.

Mr. Morris's knowledge of the town, school system, and school personnel aided his efforts to influence and coordinate Erik's broader environment. The involvement of *multiple systems,* such as those related to the school (e.g., the school busing system, the school's "clothes closet," intramural basketball, after-school homework sessions, tutoring, summer school) and the community (e.g., the summer job program) complemented one another. Mr. Morris's work made teachers' lives easier by augmenting their work with Erik. Once Erik's teachers learned more about Erik and about Mr. Morris's methods and goals through the WRF interviews, they became proactive in helping Erik to achieve the goals, thus making the intervention more comprehensive and powerful. In return, Mr. Morris praised the teachers' efforts and acknowledged one particular teacher's sensitivity in reaching out to Erik when he wrote a letter that helped her earn tenure.

The mentor's advocacy facilitated the student's ability to access opportunities. It should be emphasized that it was *Erik himself* who overcame his learned habit of passivity to take advantage of the opportunities. The achievement mentor empowered *family members* to overturn negative school decisions by informing them about how such decisions were made. The family had its most powerful advocate, Margie, intervene, and this initiative had the desired outcome. Finally, Erik obviously came to mentoring with certain strengths that school personnel could easily overlook in light of his disengagement. Through the members of his extended family, he had learned not only to be polite and compliant, but also to experience what it felt like to be loved and cared for.

CHAPTER 14

Achievement Mentoring Implementation in Schools

with Mina Yadegar

It is common for schools (Green, 2014) and other organizations (Real & Poole, 2004) to adopt new programs and methodologies with high hopes for their success. Despite diligent investigations before decisions to adopt and extensive training of staff after decisions to adopt, difficulties in implementing new programs nevertheless can prove insurmountable to even the most inspired, well-intentioned, and motivated employees. In a study of the implementation of an evidence-based, depression prevention program designed to be conducted in schools, Mendel (2016) interviewed middle and high school guidance counselors from six school districts who had volunteered to undergo training and to implement the program in their schools.

Of the 33 counselors who had been trained to competence, none had been able to implement the program as designed. Only one counselor was able to implement the program within 6 months of training, and only after significant modifications had been made. Two counselors had attempted to implement the program together but were not successful. The other 30 counselors reported that their efforts to implement the program were thwarted before they could even begin. They attributed

Mina Yadegar, PsyD, is a Postdoctoral Psychology Fellow at New York–Presbyterian Hospital/Weill Cornell Medicine.

the barriers to implementation to the following: (1) not enough time, (2) little support from their school communities, (3) incompatibility with their schools' priorities and needs, (4) difficult logistics, (5) their lack of readiness to implement, and (6) their uncertainties about the program's effectiveness. Even though their implementation efforts ultimately proved unsuccessful, the three counselors who reported being able to achieve some progress acknowledged the following as helpful to their efforts: (1) support from their school communities, (2) feasible logistics, (3) their readiness to implement, (4) their beliefs in the program's effectiveness, and (5) their determination to "make it work" (p. 30).

How can school and agency professionals avoid the barriers cited by the 30 counselors unable to implement the intervention and build on the supports cited by the other three counselors to learn to do Achievement Mentoring proficiently and implement the program consistently and competently in schools? Our experience (Boyd-Franklin & Bry, 2000) and implementation science (Fixsen, Naoom, Blase, Friedman, & Wallace, 2005; Wiseman et al., 2007) have provided guidelines. Excellent staff training (Stage 1 of training) is a necessary prerequisite, but it is not sufficient (Henggeler et al., 2009; Webster-Stratton, Reid, & Marsenich, 2014). The immediate requirements, incentives, and resources of trainees' work environment—both structural and human—take over as soon as staff members return from training. Thus, organizational supports need to be in place.

A new program such as Achievement Mentoring can be implemented by line workers only if their institution regards it as consistent with organizational goals and as meeting current organizational needs. Otherwise, supervisors or the school principal will not prioritize Achievement Mentoring tasks, and mentors will be called away from interviewing teachers concerning a mentored youth, meeting with mentored youth, or attending Achievement Mentoring Program monthly meetings (Stage 2 of training) to perform duties considered to be of greater importance. Mentors also need school resources, such as (1) access to a working computer to comply with Achievement Mentoring record keeping (e.g., submitting WOMSs) and (2) permission, access, and time to copy blank WRFs. (The blank version of the Achievement Mentoring WRF reproduced at the end of Chapter 11 can be photocopied for readers' use, and an enlarged version that can be downloaded and printed is provided online—see the box at the end of the table of contents.) In addition, Achievement Mentoring trainees face personal consequences if they do not have organizational support. Staff members who attempt self-initiated projects within an organization that has assigned them other responsibilities can feel lonely, unacknowledged, frustrated, and, in the end, thwarted, as was apparently the case with 30 out of 33 of Mendel's (2016) school counselors, who were unable to implement the program for which they had received training.

Clearly, school administrators need to negotiate and agree on organizational supports for achievement mentors before training begins. A school must be prepared to provide achievement mentors the time, space, materials, personal acknowledgment, promotion within the community, initial Stage 1 training days, local logistics facilitation/coaching/feedback/troubleshooting, and ongoing Stage 2 skills training (Fixsen et al., 2005). Ongoing Stage 2 training is as necessary as initial Stage 1 training, as Blase, Schroeder, and Van Dyke (2014) have reported that, even with good organizational support, it takes newly trained agency staff 2 to 3 years to become proficient in a new methodology. Thus, schools must be willing to commit to this period of learning time for mentors.

SCHOOL COMMITMENTS BEFORE ACHIEVEMENT MENTORING ADOPTION

The Achievement Mentoring Program targets issues often faced by schools, such as low achievement, absenteeism, behavior problems, and dropout. School administrators typically hear about Achievement Mentoring from one of three sources: their school district, a governmental agency, or an employee who has learned about the program. Although occasionally specific funds designated for mentoring become available to schools, which allow for program implementation, more often schools must make difficult decisions about allocation of resources in order to fund Program adoption. Whatever the circumstances, the school principal must understand how offering a high-quality service, such as Achievement Mentoring, to eligible students should be a point of pride for the school. School administrators who are in charge of determining professional staff job descriptions and day-to-day task assignments must become knowledgeable about the program's functioning and requirements. Other administrators who also need to "buy in" before the program is adopted in some districts may include vice principals, curriculum supervisors, directors of guidance, directors of special services, community school directors, superintendents of schools, and, in Ireland, school completion program directors. If such officials do not become invested in Achievement Mentoring, it is doubtful that staff trained in the intervention will receive the necessary resources and administrative supports needed to implement the Program as designed. As Mendel's (2016) investigation demonstrated, training without support is a recipe for failure.

Initial Conversation between School Official and Training Representative

An early step toward adoption of Achievement Mentoring is a detailed phone or face-to-face conversation between the school principal (or the principal's delegate) and a representative of the agency that provides schools with Achievement Mentoring training, consultation, and ongoing support. (For schools in the United States, the training agency is the Center for Supportive Schools in Princeton, New Jersey, at *www.supportiveschools.org/achievement-mentoring*. For schools in Europe, the training agency is Archways in Dublin at *www.archways.ie/our_programmes/mentoring_for_achievement_programme/*.) The conversation serves three primary purposes: (1) for the training agency representative to explain the benefits to the school of adopting Achievement Mentoring (see Chapter 11), (2) for the agency representative to educate the school principal as to the organizational commitments that need to be made and their underlying rationales, and (3) for the Achievement Mentoring training representative to get a sense of whether or not the school will be able to make the necessary organizational and training resources available to achievement mentors. To assess whether the intervention is an appropriate fit for the school, the conversation is structured so that the following questions, drawn from the authors' experiences (Boyd-Franklin & Bry, 2000), Bosworth's *Protective Schools* (2000), and Wandersman's *Getting to Outcomes* (Wiseman et al., 2007), are addressed to the principal (or delegate):

1. Are there professional staff members (e.g., teachers, guidance counselors, child study team members, nurses) who will want to do this program as part of their jobs? Which professional staff members will you encourage to do Achievement Mentoring?

2. As each achievement mentor will need a total of 90 minutes a week (time estimates are for two mentees per mentor) to accomplish the required mentoring activities, when in the school day will members be free to do these tasks, and how will each mentor have time in the school day to do these tasks?
   a. 10 minutes—Interview one mentee's teacher, and write comments on a blank WRF (see Figure 11.1).
   b. 10 minutes—Perform the functions listed in (1) above for the second mentee.
   c. 25 minutes—Find and mentor one mentee.
   d. 25 minutes—Find and mentor the second mentee.
   e. 10 minutes—Open email from the Achievement Mentoring

website on a computer, click link, and complete two WOMSs (see Figure 11.2).

    f. 10 minutes—Find or be found by the Local Achievement Mentoring Program coordinator for a weekly update, consultation, and troubleshooting. Leave notes for mentees' teachers.

3. Where can weekly mentoring sessions take place?

4. How will each mentor have time to participate in the following necessary Achievement Mentoring periodic activities, training, and ongoing training/consultation/technical assistance (b and c below)? And when would you schedule the training days on the school calendar (a)?

    a. 3 full training days (7 hours/day).

    b. 20 minutes/month—a conversation or a note with a parent of each mentee.

    c. 40 minutes/month—Achievement Mentoring ongoing training/consultation/technical assistance.

5. Where can day-long Achievement Mentoring Stage 1 training workshops and monthly ongoing Stage 2 training/consultation/ technical assistance meetings occur?

6. What regular duties can achievement mentors be relieved of so that they can spend an average of 1½ protected hours/week doing Achievement Mentoring, plus another protected hour for Achievement Mentoring activities once a month?

7. What acknowledgment and incentives can achievement mentors receive for bringing consistent and competent mentoring into the school?

8. Each school must have a local Achievement Mentoring Program coordinator to (a) be trained as an achievement mentor; (b) help select students for the program; (c) provide mentors with logistics, resources, such as blank WRFs, information, and other help, such as reminders to complete WOMSs (Figure 11.2); (d) review program mentoring record keeping; (e) meet briefly with every mentor each week for guidance, support, and troubleshooting; (f) report mentor/mentee demographic information, progress, and challenges to the principal and to the Achievement Mentoring trainer; and (g) arrange achievement mentor staff meetings for ongoing training/consultations/technical assistance. Who among your administrative staff could serve in this capacity?

    Total time every week (for six mentors): 90 minutes

    Additional 1 hour Achievement Mentoring staff meeting time once a month

9. Can the school commit itself to these resources, protected personnel time, and effort for 2 school years?

10. What needs does the school have for Achievement Mentoring? What school success indicators are you hoping mentoring will affect?

11. What might be the reaction of the nonmentoring staff to having Achievement Mentoring in the school, to being interviewed by achievement mentors, and perhaps to having mentees taken out of class for 20 minutes of mentoring each week?

12. How can the nonmentoring staff be informed and ask questions about Achievement Mentoring? (This usually occurs at a regular faculty meeting.)

13. What accountability feedback about the Program would be helpful for the principal and the local Program coordinator to receive from the training agency, and how often would they want this scheduled—monthly?, yearly? How would the information help the principal? To whom would the principal report such information?

14. How would students be chosen for the program? (See Chapter 11)

15. What plans would be made for the program to continue after the 2-year training period?

If, as a result of this conversation, the principal becomes invested in the implementation of Achievement Mentoring in the school and indicates that the school is willing to undertake the necessary commitments and, additionally, if the training agency representative senses that the school will be able to meet those commitments, an Achievement Mentoring trainer will be selected to work with the school and hold further decision-making meetings with the principal and additional school personnel (e.g., administrators, guidance counselors, and potential mentors) whose cooperation is essential to successful implementation. At these meetings, the Achievement Mentoring trainer describes the methods by which other schools have been successful in implementing Achievement Mentoring, and the principal considers such recommendations and determines what is feasible for that particular school within the context of its competing needs, priorities, and logistics. The overarching principle of Achievement Mentoring—that by addressing challenges such as absenteeism, failing grades, behavior problems, or low graduation rates, adoption of the Program should make the school's work easier in the long run, not harder—needs to be communicated by the trainer and understood by school personnel during the planning and decision-making stage.

Steps that the principal and other school personnel need to take before Achievement Mentoring training begins are to (1) select the school professionals to be trained as achievement mentors; (2) decide on the other school-related weekly tasks mentors will be relieved of so that they can devote the necessary time (1½ protected hours a week) to mentoring activities and training; (3) make the logistical arrangements relating to the 3 days on which Stage 1 training will occur (e.g., the dates, the location of training, and coverage for mentors' duties for those days); (4) brainstorm and determine where and when the mentors can meet for the monthly Achievement Mentoring meeting with their ongoing Stage 2 trainer; and (5) identify, on a tentative basis, the at-risk students to be mentored.

Before Achievement Mentoring training begins, a document is prepared that delineates the decisions and commitments made during the planning meetings. This memorandum of understanding (MOU) is signed by the school and training organization. Prior to or during the course of implementation, changing circumstances may dictate the modification of some of these initial decisions; youth chosen for mentoring may transfer to schools that have not adopted Achievement Mentoring or may move out of the district entirely, or one of the selected mentors may become unavailable to do mentoring.

During implementation, the ongoing achievement mentor trainer visits the school regularly to meet with the mentors for Stage 2 training. At the same time, the ongoing trainer (1) reviews and monitors the school's compliance with the commitments listed above; (2) meets face to face with the principal and local Achievement Mentoring Program coordinator during each visit to address any questions, misunderstandings, difficulties, and requests that may have arisen since the last visit; (3) advocates with the principal when mentors need more resources or protected time to mentor each week; and (4) informs the principal about the positive efforts of the mentors and the promising progress of the mentees.

SUPPORTS FOR MENTORS DURING
ACHIEVEMENT MENTORING IMPLEMENTATION

After organizational structures are put in place to support the adoption of any new initiative, effective methods to help employees learn and practice the innovation must be applied. As Henggeler et al. (2009) pointed out, training experienced professionals to adopt a new methodology is unlike teaching new practice skills to university students, who by and large offer a *tabula rasa*. Incorporating new ideas and methods into old scripts is difficult no matter how motivated employees are to be more effective. As anyone who has tried to keep a New Year's resolution may attest, changing ingrained habits and routines may even be painful. We have been shaped by evolution to avoid pain and respond automatically when we can. This is especially salient in the case of professionals selected to become achievement mentors, whose experience often has allowed them to establish automatic ways of handling most situations, a process that has imbued them with increasing confidence in their routine day-to-day competence. The training process often decreases professionals' hard-won sense of competence when they are confronted with the need to recognize that their usual response could be improved and the need to replace automatic actions with new methods. In addition to posing these challenges, trying to incorporate new skills takes more time and brings uncertainty—uncomfortable feelings for busy, responsible professionals. Motivated professionals may face an additional barrier to learning Achievement Mentoring if they have undergone prior training in new methodologies for working with high-risk youths that failed during the implementation process. Such experiences often result in professionals' fears that history may repeat itself.

To address such concerns, the following recommendations are indicated. These recommendations are based on the authors' experiences (Boyd-Franklin & Bry, 2000), adult learning theory (Forman, 2015), and implementation science findings (Fixsen et al., 2005; Meyers, Durlak, & Wandersman, 2012): (1) careful trainee selection, (2) thorough theory- and skill-based training, (3) long-term ongoing training/coaching/consultation/technical assistance and peer support for mentors in the workplace, and (4) continual implementation quality measurement and feedback. The confidence of achievement mentors' in their competence will increase as they practice the steps and skills of mentoring and demonstrate their mastery of this intervention through their qualification for Achievement Mentoring certification (see below).

ACHIEVEMENT MENTOR SELECTION

Schools that do not allow for personal choice but rather assign staff to perform Achievement Mentoring as a component of their position (e.g., guidance counselors or teachers) find that a substantial percentage of the trainees fail to implement the program. We have learned that trainees must be personally motivated and have an investment in improving their ability to work with disengaged students in order to (1) put themselves back into the painful position of being an "unskilled trainee," so that they may learn a new intervention method such as Achievement Mentoring, and (2) do the hard work of changing their own past habits.

Mentors should possess the following qualifications and qualities: (1) they should be professional employees of the school (e.g., teachers, counselors) or employed by a community agency that places them in the school to provide student services for a set amount of time each week; (2) they need to have knowledge of and feel comfortable with school procedures and personnel so that they can help disengaged students learn to feel more knowledgeable and comfortable in the school; (3) they should be adults who are interested in and have both respect for and confidence in at-risk youth; (4) they need to be good listeners; (5) they are patient; (6) they are able to see and celebrate small, fleeting signs of progress; (7) they do not take personally students' failures or ambivalences about having a mentor; (8) they are good team players with other teachers (and mentors) in the school, as the cooperation of such staff members is instrumental to the effectiveness of Achievement Mentoring; and (9) they have the required protected time to devote to this activity.

It should be an honor to be invited to serve as an achievement mentor. An individual invitation from an authority figure in the school, such as a curriculum supervisor, a director of student services, a vice principal, or a principal, will communicate recognition of and respect for the staff member's motivation and commitment. When professional staff members are being selected to mentor, administrators may already have someone in mind to invite to be the local Achievement Mentor Program coordinator. Alternatively, school administrators may wait to make this decision after Program implementation has started, so that they can assess which of the trained mentors has demonstrated the motivation and leadership ability most appropriate for this responsibility.

TRAINING ACHIEVEMENT MENTORS

Achievement Mentor Initial Day-Long Stage 1 Trainings

The most important outcome of day-long training in Achievement Mentoring is that mentors acquire necessary competencies. Accordingly, the majority of time is spent on Achievement Mentoring steps and skills. Some trainers conduct training days at interspersed intervals during the school year, while others provide training on consecutive days. The adult training literature uniformly holds that skilled practitioners of any method will be most proficient if they also understand the method's theory of change (Forman, 2015). Such understanding of the assumed mechanisms of change will enable them to have the flexibility to personalize their work and optimize a method for each individual and circumstance rather than functioning by rote. A final area that should be introduced during initial training is the projected long-term effects of

Achievement Mentoring. This discussion of expected long-term effects will facilitate mentors' ability to identify, focus on, and encourage relevant signs of progress in mentees.

Topics and Methods in Stage 1 Training Days

  I. Overall description of Achievement Mentoring
 II. Advantages of the intervention being conducted within the school day
III. Anticipated joys and fears of Achievement Mentoring
 IV. Goals of Achievement Mentoring
   - Reawaken academic self-efficacy
   - Reconnect the youth with the school
   - Reduce school failure
   - Reduce behavior problems
   - Increase autonomous problem-solving skills
  V. Achievement Mentoring theory of how to bring about change
   - Provide a supportive nonparental adult
   - View adolescents' problems as habits that can be changed
   - Reframe what they are not doing as skills that are not yet learned
   - Explain student behavior using learning theory:
     □ Achievement Mentoring has an optimistic orientation, as illustrated in the use of terms such as "habits" and "skills" to talk about student behavior. Habits can change and new skills can be acquired. Trainees are told that Achievement Mentoring assumes that students can change their maladaptive behaviors through the process of learning, just as they learn multiplication tables and how to ride a bicycle. Achievement Mentoring does not label students with personality characteristics, such as "lazy," "aggressive," "self-defeating," or "unmotivated." That is a very pessimistic way to think. Trainees may need to refamiliarize themselves with the concepts of learning theory they studied in their undergraduate education, as learning explanations may have been supplanted by the more prevalent societal view of ascribing other people's behavior to personality characteristics (Jones & Nisbett, 1971).
     □ Learning occurs when choice is present through setting goals, breaking them down into small steps, problem solving, and practicing repeatedly with positive feedback. Learning does not occur when someone is told to do something.

VI. Weekly Steps of Achievement Mentoring (see Chapter 11).
- Mentor interviews a teacher and writes teacher's observations on a WRF
- Mentor meets with mentee for 20 minutes:
  - Checks in
  - Gives positive feedback from WRF
  - Reads other feedback on WRF
  - Does Motivational Interviewing regarding teacher's observations on the WRF
  - Focuses on "change talk" and selects small weekly (S.M.A.R.T.) goal
  - Practices skills needed to reach goal
  - Mentee writes goal on WRF
- Mentor documents mentoring session online by submitting WOMS
- Mentor reports mentee progress to a teacher or parent
- Mentor briefly discusses weekly mentoring with local Achievement Mentoring coordinator

VII. Achievement Mentoring Communication Skills
- Asking open-ended questions
- Engaging in active listening
- Focusing on the youth, instead of others or situations
- Praising
- Reporting teachers' feedback as nonjudgmental, objective observations
- Doing Motivational Interviewing
- Helping mentee choose a small, feasible (S.M.A.R.T.) step/goal for the week

VIII. • Planning details of the step's implementation
Certification procedures that trainees eventually can use to show mastery of Achievement Mentoring.

Training methods include (1) role-play demonstrations by the trainers; (2) breaking Achievement Mentoring skills down into simple, explicit, behaviors; (3) practicing each small skill repeatedly in the trainee group until trainers can be confident that trainees perform this skill correctly; (4) practicing several activities and skills together in trainee triads with printed protocols that can be easily consulted while trainers watch; and (5) reviewing audio recordings of the practice sessions using interpersonal process recall, a method that guides trainees to recall and share unspoken, moment-to-moment thoughts and feelings that they had during the practice sessions (Kagan & Kagan, 1991).

During the course of program implementation, it was discovered that trainees often have a fear of the certification process. Thus, activities were developed to include practice for Achievement Mentoring certification as part of day-long training. In this exercise, trainees audio record a role-play situation, review the audio and write examples of the prescribed skills that they used, and complete a page in the certification booklet about their role play.

In summary, Achievement Mentoring Stage 1 training days include (1) two or three chances to see trainer demonstrations; (2) opportunities for trainees to practice the essential skills needed to carry out Achievement Mentoring activities; (3) trainer coaching toward trainee proficiency, including completing WRFs and WOMSs; and (4) preparation for Achievement Mentoring certification procedures.

Ongoing Stage 2 Training, Consultation, and Technical Assistance

Research shows that new behaviors are learned fastest when they are positively reinforced frequently (Mayer et al., 2013). Being told about and successfully performing Achievement Mentoring activities and skills one or two times in a controlled environment does not result in automatic new competencies; there is no one-trial learning of Achievement Mentoring. It requires the same repeated conscious drill and feedback from both trainees and trainers that all learning does. As Stage 1 training workshops have been designed to provide positive experiences with mentoring, trainees typically feel confident that they can perform the new skills they have been taught.

Training workshops, however, often function as only an introduction to the learning of the program that occurs "on the job." Training workshops cannot be expected to prepare mentors for the unique individuals they will work with or the specific circumstances they will encounter in various school environments. In addition, research has shown that trainees typically absorb only 10% of the material presented at a workshop (Webster-Stratton, 2016), and even that must be used right away or it is forgotten. Thus, close supports for the mentors are necessary. Ongoing Stage 2 training must be done by someone skilled in both Achievement Mentoring methodology and consultation (Henggeler et al., 2009). Without this support in the mentors' work settings to facilitate accurate implementation, mentors could actually harm at-risk students. For instance, Jones and Nisbett (1971) found that people naturally tend to explain others' troubling behaviors in terms of unchangeable personality traits, such as laziness, rebelliousness, and aggressiveness. Newly trained achievement mentors need long-term practice in the presence of Achievement Mentoring experts before the skill of conceptualizing at-risk youth's behavior in terms of habits and skills becomes automatic for them. Achievement Mentoring Program staff meetings with the ongoing trainer or the local Program coordinator are scheduled monthly, either in an hour-long small-group format of three mentors or individual sessions of 20 minutes. Mastroleo, Magill, Barnett, and Bosari (2014) found that counselors' new skills improve to a greater degree with a combination of individual and group ongoing training meetings than with group meetings alone. Therefore, it is suggested that both individual and group meetings be incorporated into ongoing Stage 2 training. These meetings should follow specific steps in much the same way as mentoring sessions with at-risk students follow specific steps.

Initial meetings will cover all of the activities necessary before mentoring begins, including (1) making the final assignment of mentees; (2) informing parents or getting parent permission if required by the school; (3) planning a Program Launch Luncheon for all of the new mentees and mentors; and (4) providing mentors with a copy of the protocol for the first mentoring session. Once mentoring begins, the local Program coordinator will give each mentor a folder with the protocol for each ongoing mentoring session stapled inside the front cover and a supply of empty WRFs.

Before each Achievement Mentoring staff meeting, the meeting convener prepares by reviewing online the mentors' WOMSs for the prior 2 weeks. Because the WOMSs reveal any difficulties mentors may have with execution of the Achievement Mentoring Program, completion is essential to successful implementation. Mentors who have not submitted their WOMSs prior to the meeting are asked to fill them out before discussions of each mentee's progress commence. After the discussions, the meeting convener collects completed WRFs from mentors for the prior 2 weeks. These forms indicate whether further coaching on interviewing teachers and/or completing WRFs is in order for mentors to reach competency.

The first half of group meetings focuses on reviewing each mentee's progress. When indicated, coaching and role playing are done to increase proficiency. The second half focuses on enhancing mentors' skill development. For example, if one mentor has achieved success with a mentee (e.g., the first time a mentee has met a S.M.A.R.T. goal), this is discussed so that other mentors might gain insight into how they might be more effective with their own mentees. For skills that are especially difficult for mentors to learn, such as Motivational Interviewing, handouts may be distributed and role playing in individual or small-group meetings may be helpful. Meetings also include distributing blank WRFs for mentees for the next few weeks. Once the convener is satisfied that mentors have achieved mastery of Achievement Mentoring competencies, the next step is to help mentors prepare for certification by submitting Achievement Mentoring certification workbooks to the Program developer.

Implementation Quality Measurement and Feedback

Weekly Online Mentoring Surveys

Consistent with the goal of making work as easy as possible for mentors, a user-friendly, recordkeeping "app" has been developed so that they can take less than a minute to document each mentoring session. After trained mentors have held their weekly mentoring sessions, they automatically receive an email each week with "Weekly Online Mentoring Survey (WOMS) Reminder" in the subject line and a link to the Achievement Mentoring record-keeping app. Once the link is clicked, a dropdown menu appears with a list of that mentor's mentees. Mentors click a name, a date, and click "yes" or "no" to eight questions that correspond to the Achievement Mentoring steps that had been completed with each mentee that week; input the mentee's weekly goal; and then click "Submit." There is also a comment box in which mentors have the option to record additional material, such as difficulties in meeting with their mentees (see Figure 11.2). Completed WOMSs reveal all of the work mentors have done to their local Program coordinator and ongoing trainer, who will report aggregate data about their Achievement Mentoring to their principal and/or community school director.

In addition to the benefit of receiving credit for their work, utilization of the WOMS app offers an important record-keeping benefit to mentors. The retention online of previously submitted WOMSs makes relevant information (e.g., the timing of meetings with mentees, showing them a WRF, the mentee setting a weekly goal, contacts with a parent, and additional comments) readily available, as opposed to having to rely on memory or locating pieces of paper. Emailed reminders to fill out and submit the WOMS make their lives easier by structuring their weekly record keeping.

The ability to review WOMSs offers significant benefits to the Program developer as well as other individuals, such as mentors, trainers, ongoing trainers, local Program coordinators, and records coordinators. In addition to learning about problems and barriers that achievement mentors encounter implementing the program, the Program developer also has an interest in ensuring that the program is implemented as planned. (These indicators are called Quality Improvement measures by MST.) As mentioned earlier, a long-term, adult-implemented program such as Achievement Mentoring can do harm if the mentor does not follow protocol. It is important for the Program developer to be aware of, and be able to correct, mentors' use of negative procedures, such as labeling the students with negative personality characteristics, and/or engaging in misguided attempts to motivate high-risk students by telling them what they "should" do and/or setting goals that are too large or unrealistic for them to attain. To facilitate feedback analysis, charts and reports that reflect the frequency and fidelity of Achievement Mentoring in the schools are extrapolated from aggregated data, with identifying information of mentors and mentee removed. It cannot be forgotten, however, that the Achievement Mentoring Program's highest accountability, of course, is to the youth.

Achievement Mentoring Certification

Certification in Achievement Mentoring requires that a trained mentor complete an application process showing that he or she can perform essential Achievement Mentoring skills and competencies with proficiency. Mentors demonstrate this mastery by:

- Submitting to the Program developer audio *recordings* of one mentoring session with each of two different mentees and accurately identifying from these recordings examples of Achievement Mentoring steps and skills in a *certification workbook*.
- Describing mentees' behaviors in school and how mentors explain (conceptualize) these behaviors in the *certification workbook*. (Mentors are expected to use learning concepts and the terms "skills" and "habits," instead of long-term personality characteristics or unobservable attitudes or beliefs. The certification workbook includes explicit instructions and definitions of "behavioral explanations" so that mentors can evaluate their explanations to verify that they are behavioral.)
- Completing and submitting associated WRFs based on interviews with teachers.
- Completing all WOMSs.

After the Program developer and one of her staff members review and approve the certification materials, the Program developer transmits a document to the mentor acknowledging the mentor's status as a certified achievement mentor.

CONCLUSION

Research and experience reveal that excellent Stage 1 workshop training alone is not enough to enable professional employees to implement a new program such as Achievement Mentoring in schools. All levels of school administration must have policies and procedures that support trained employees as they learn and practice Achievement Mentoring. Achieving high-quality implementation of new methods in a worksite can take up to 2 years. Details about all of the organizational supports that are necessary for employees to master Achievement Mentoring can be agreed upon before employees are trained in a signed MOU.

Employees who are learning new methods in the workplace also need reliable face-to-face Stage 2 training, coaching, and guidance from experts in the methods. Achievement Mentoring ongoing trainers visit the schools regularly to meet with mentors and oversee the schools' compliance with their MOUs. Once mentors have mastered the program methods, these ongoing trainers will help achievement mentors prepare applications for certification in Achievement Mentoring.

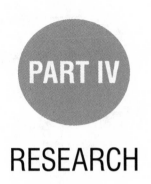

RESEARCH

CHAPTER 15

Relevant Research for Home-Based Family Therapists and Achievement Mentors

Numerous randomized controlled trials (RCTs) have demonstrated that the two interventions that form the basis of our approach with at-risk youth, multisystems home-based family therapy and Achievement Mentoring, reduce issues faced by at-risk adolescents and improve life outcomes for this population. The best standards of evidence support the effectiveness of these two types of interventions, whether provided separately or together, for at-risk adolescents.

This chapter is intended to make research results accessible to practitioners, home-based family therapists, other clinicians, program directors, achievement mentors, and educators (teachers, counselors, principals, and school administrators). It draws on existing research to address common questions and concerns that clinicians and educators may have in seeking to implement these interventions with adolescents, such as:

- For what types of *youth* are these interventions effective?
- What specific *problems* do these interventions change?
- What is the *duration* of the effects of the interventions?
- What are the necessary *tasks* practitioners must accomplish for each intervention to succeed?
- What seem to be the *reasons* that each intervention works?
- What are *characteristics* of successful clinicians and mentors?
- What *working conditions* facilitate the successful delivery by professionals of these interventions?

- What types of *settings* have hosted successful implementations?
- How do professionals, youth, and parents *evaluate* these interventions?

HOME-BASED FAMILY THERAPY

Multisystemic therapy (MST) has been the home-based family therapy intervention subjected to the most rigorous investigation (Henggeler & Schaeffer, 2016; Schoenwald et al., 2016). In the 30 years that researchers have investigated MST's effectiveness with youth, a total of 100 studies have been conducted, including 25 randomized clinical trials plus numerous surveys of the reactions of youth, parents, therapists, and supervisors (Henggeler, 2016; Henggeler & Sheidow, 2012). By far, more is known scientifically about MST than about any other youth intervention, documenting MST's effectiveness as an evidence-based intervention for serious behavior problems in this population (Henggeler, 2016; Schoenwald et al., 2016).

Who Is Helped by MST?

MST has been found to be effective for adolescents with serious antisocial behavior and delinquency problems. The original studies (Borduin et al., 1995; Henggeler et al., 1986; Henggeler, Melton, & Smith, 1992) were conducted with juvenile offenders, many with chronic and violent behavior problems, who ranged in age from 11 to 17 (average 14 years).

The majority of the participants (70–80%) were male and were also of low-income, lower-socioeconomic status. The youth were evenly divided between those who lived with a single caregiver and those who lived with more than one caregiver. These initial studies were conducted with youth from various geographical locations in the Southeast and Midwest of the United States—specifically Memphis (Henggeler et al., 1986), rural Missouri (Borduin et al., 1995), and South Carolina (Henggeler et al., 1992). As the participants were drawn from diverse geographical locations, wide disparities existed among the racial composition of the populations studied. For example, the rural Missouri youth were 76% White and 22% African American; the Memphis urban youth were 65% African American and 35% White; and the South Carolina youth were 81% African American and 19% White.

By the start of treatment, the youth had been arrested an average of 2 to 4 times, including for violent crimes such as assault, and the majority of the youth had been previously incarcerated and were currently in danger of being placed outside of their homes again. The participants had an average age of 11.7 at the time of their first arrest. With the exception of psychosis or dementia symptoms—the only exclusion criteria in the original MST studies—the juvenile offenders exhibited the multisystemic and multigenerational issues their families typically present in treatment, including school difficulties, drug and alcohol abuse, family conflict, and parenting problems. Moderation studies have shown no consistent type of juvenile offender who is more likely to benefit from MST than any other therapy (Sawyer & Borduin, 2011). However, one recent study has suggested that current gang members are less likely to complete treatment than non-gang-involved youth (Boxer, Kubik, Ostermann, & Veysey, 2015). Longer-lasting, community-wide MST interventions have been investigated by Swenson et al. (2005) for the most challenged youth (e.g., gang members), as the usual 4 months of intensive home-based family therapy may be insufficient to achieve success with this population.

Since the time of the original scientific tests of MST, this home-based family therapy has been made available to an extensive number of youth from a wide geographical area both in the United States—from urban New York City to rural Arizona—and around the world, from Norway to New Zealand to Chile. Among the 11,958 youth whose clinical MST was completed during 2014, 71.5% of the youth were treated within the United States and 28.5% were treated abroad; 66.4% were male, averaging 15 years of age; 40.9% were White, 28.8% were Black, and 17.2% were Hispanic (MST Services, 2015). Caregivers were predominantly English speaking (80%), although 13 different primary languages were spoken.

What Specific Problems Does MST Change?

MST's stated goals are to keep at-risk juveniles at home, in school, and out of trouble (Henggeler, 2016). Twenty-five studies have compared outcomes of youth with serious behavior problems who were randomly assigned by a coin toss to MST with outcomes of youth who were randomly assigned instead to usual community services (typically, individual treatment provided by Master's-level community, fee-for-service practitioners). These RCTs used "intent to treat" designs, meaning that the outcomes of all of the youth who started treatment were included, whether or not treatment had been completed for reasons such as the youth being placed out of the home or having voluntarily dropped out of treatment. The studies consistently showed that youth who were assigned to MST showed fewer behavior problems, fewer average arrests, fewer days per year (33 vs. 70 days) of incarceration (Henggeler et al., 2009), and fewer out-of-home placements one to two years after treatment than did youth who were assigned the usual community services. As statistical testing revealed that these differences could not be explained by chance, the differences in outcomes were attributed to the greater effectiveness of MST.

As MST interventions have been adjusted to be responsive to diverse populations within the United States and around the world, outcomes have continued to improve over time (Brunk, 2016a). MST Services, the organization that supports MST teams across the United States and around the world, reported the following examples of improved outcomes: from 2009 to 2014, the percentage of youth who were still in their homes when their cases were closed increased from 86% to 90%, the percentage of youth who were in school or working increased from 84% to 86%, and the percentage of youth who had had no new arrest increased from 82% to 86% (MST Services, 2015).

Do MST Outcomes Last?

Given that the youth's serious behavior problems and the families' multisystemic challenges have developed over a period of years, it is reasonable to question how well youth and families sustain MST's positive outcomes once therapists no longer visit the homes of youth and families after the usual 4 months of intensive MST have been completed (MST Services, 2015). Do youth continue to improve, or do they backslide? Most therapists do not have the opportunity to see long-term results of their efforts once treatment is complete. The long-term outcomes of youth and families who have participated in MST, however, can be more easily envisioned because this intervention has been studied for a more extensive period of time than have other treatment interventions. This research has been conducted and includes comparisons to youth who were randomly assigned the usual community services instead of MST.

Although the serious nature of the initial youth and family problems—the predicate for youth entry into MST or usual community services—continued to have ramifications for many of the youth in both groups, the positive outcomes of MST-treated youth have been found to last into early and middle adulthood (Sawyer & Borduin, 2011; Schaeffer & Borduin, 2005). When examined 22 years after treatment, MST-treated youth showed statistically significantly improved outcomes in comparison to the youth assigned to usual community services (Sawyer & Borduin, 2011). As with the short-term outcome studies, the long-term follow-up investigations had "intent to treat" designs, including all youth who began treatment, even if they did not complete it. Sawyer and Borduin's 22-year follow-up study found that participation as a youth in MST not only improved one's chances of staying out of trouble as an adult—felony re-arrests were considerably lower for the MST participants than for the usual community services participants (35% vs. 55%)—but also improved other indices of the youth's adult life adjustment, such as family issues that would manifest in legal proceedings. For example, youth who had participated in MST were involved in significantly fewer civil lawsuits that reflected family instability (divorce, paternity and/or child support suits). Lowering the probability of the occurrence of those stressors in adulthood is definitely life changing.

In another study, a 25-year follow-up, Wagner, Borduin, Sawyer, and Dopp (2014) compared the adult criminal records of closest-in-age siblings of the at-risk youth in the MST group with those in the usual community services group. The investigators found a direct preventive effect of MST on closest-in-age siblings, as follows: (1) a 40% reduction in arrests for MST siblings compared to usual community service siblings (43% vs. 72%), and (2) a 56% reduction in felony convictions in the 25-year span for MST siblings compared to usual community service siblings (15% vs. 34%). As the MST intervention treats the entire family, it stands to reason that the siblings who participated in family treatment would have an altered life course.

Although MST has been shown to have a considerable positive impact, decision makers may wonder if the cost of MST outweighs its benefits. For example, each family is in treatment for an average of 130 days (MST Services, 2015), during which time therapists are available to families 24 hours a day, 7 days a week. As the demands on MST therapists also include travel to and from home visits as well as attendance at school and other meetings—which would not be common in traditional office-based therapy—an average of 60 hours is spent treating each family (Schaeffer, McCart, Henggeler, & Cunningham, 2011). Training, supervision, and consultations result in even more personnel time, limiting the ability of MST therapists to treat more than four to six families at a time.

Given these demands, researchers have explored whether MST is cost effective. Schoenwald, Ward, Henggeler, Pickrel, and Patel (1996) compared short-term direct costs for treating delinquents and substance abusers with MST versus the direct costs of usual community services, and found that within a year the higher costs of providing MST were nearly offset by the costs incurred by the increased number of out-of-home placements for youth treated with usual community services.

A later study by Dopp, Borduin, Wagner, and Sawyer (2014) explored the financial impact of MST treatment over the long term (25 years) when compared to usual community services. In addition to treatment costs, the costs associated with re-arrests of juvenile offenders and their closest-in-age-siblings were examined. These costs comprised those borne by taxpayers (e.g., community supervision and incarceration) and those borne by crime victims (e.g., property damage, medical expenses, lost income, and pain and suffering). The researchers found that during the 25-year period subsequent to treatment, taxpayers and victims derived a $5.04 benefit for every $1.00 that had been spent on the youth offenders' MST when compared to the costs associated with those youth assigned usual community services. The authors acknowledged that the long-term cost benefits analysis of MST versus usual community services might not be decisive in agencies' decision making, as year-by-year budgets govern funding decisions more often than long-term perspectives do. They pointed out, however, that public funding sources would not have a seemingly interminable wait before recapturing the costs of MST, as MST has been shown to reduce recidivism and thus subsequent expensive out-of-home placements, such as hospitalization, detention, and incarceration. In fact, it was likely that those funding sources would recapture their costs for MST during the first few years of the program, given that most recidivism occurs within 2 years after treatment (Schaeffer & Borduin, 2005).

What Are the Essential Components of MST?

As a result of the extensive body of research investigating this model, the components necessary for the successful implementation of MST are well established, (Henggeler & Borduin, 1990; Henggeler et al., 2009). They are:

1. *Support from MST Services.* Program developers discovered, repeatedly, that when at-risk youth are treated by MST therapists who are not simultaneously receiving organized MST support, the youth's criminal behavior is not reduced (Smith-Boydston, Holtzman, & Roberts, 2014). This finding underscores the importance of specific back-up from MST Services for effective MST of youth with serious behavior problems and their multisystemically stressed families.

2. *Full family participation in home-based therapy.* Although other family therapies have incorporated home-based treatment, some models permit a focus on one person. MST researchers found that family participation is not only necessary, but the degree of that participation is directly proportional to the magnitude of youth improvement (Gervan, Granic, Solomon, Blokland, & Ferguson, 2012).

3. *Family/therapist collaboration in goal setting.* Following an initial assessment of the referred adolescent's problems and the family's strengths that could influence change, the MST therapist and family

discuss and agree upon a list of MST goals to reduce the youth's behavior, community, and school problems.

4. *Therapist/supervisor systemic functional analysis.* The therapist and supervisor meet to perform a systemic functional analysis in which hypotheses are developed about how factors in and outside of the home may be contributing to the youth's targeted problems (Borduin, 2016).

5. *Therapist/family generation of action plans.* With the overall goal of empowering the family, the therapist brainstorms with them as to how they together can change factors in and outside the home that have been hypothesized to contribute to the youth's presenting problems. MST therapists are expected to do "whatever it takes" (Henggeler et al., 2009, p. 18) to empower families to reach the youth's treatment goals.

6. *Therapist persistence, intensity, and availability.* Unlike many other treatment modalities, MST therapists engage in outreach to other systems that impact the life of the youth and family, such as school, home, peers, the probation department, and the community. Therapists' clinical notes show that they intervene in a minimum of two different systems for each MST case (Sawyer & Borduin, 2011). MST therapists have to be available to the families on a 24-hour-a-day, 7-day-a-week basis. As the goal is to complete treatment in an average of 4 months, much must be accomplished in a limited time frame.

7. *Evaluation and quality assurance processes.* On a regular basis, parents, youth, and therapists complete measures designed to assess the degree to which MST strategies are being implemented. Once a week, local supervisors and MST expert consultants talk to therapists to review MST implementation and each family's progress toward their targeted goals. In addition, local supervisors provide resources, knowledge of community institutions, and specialized expertise. The feedback helps the therapists to be as effective as possible each week (Schoenwald, 2016).

8. *Highly structured clinical supervision processes.* MST does not expect any one therapist, supervisor, or consultant to be an expert in all youth problem areas. Therapeutic success is a team effort, involving the youth, family, therapist, local supervisor, and telephone consultations with an MST expert (Schoenwald, 2016).

What Are MST's Mechanisms of Change?

There typically are so many multisystemic problems in families of at-risk youth that therapists must constantly make choices about what to pay attention to and emphasize. Their decisions should be guided by whatever research says are the changes in youth and families that are associated with improvements in problem behavior, ability to live at home, and school/work involvement. Answers to these questions can influence the priorities of MST therapists.

Almost every MST study that explored what brought about improved youth outcomes identified changes in the family. As mentioned earlier, the amount of family involvement and participation in treatment brings about change (Gervan et al., 2012). That is, how many family members spend how many hours contacting schools and probation officers of the youth, writing and implementing a youth safety plan, monitoring and examining weekly data, implementing short- and long-term rewards for good behavior? How persistent and resilient are they in the face of barriers? These research findings support Henggeler and Borduin's reminder that the primary goal of MST therapists is to empower families to address multisystemic barriers to their youths' positive development both during therapy and afterward.

A qualitative study further supported Henggeler's (2016) and Borduin's (2016) emphases on empowering youth's caregivers. Kaur, Pote, Fox, and Paradisopoulos (2015) found that MST-treated youth attributed their positive outcomes to their families' increasing resilience in facing difficulties. A family's adoption of a multisystemic approach will in the short term help not only the youth, but the entire family as well. The skills they develop to advocate for their youth in schools and other systems will serve to empower them to solve problems whenever and wherever they occur. Additionally, a multisystemic approach will help them to identify sources of support for themselves, such as neighbors and other community members. Furthermore, parental persistence and resilience in the face of barriers will model these qualities for youth as well as affect the change needed for their positive outcomes.

Other family changes that research consistently finds to be associated with youth improvement are parenting practices. The parenting practice changes cited by researchers include (1) effective parental supervision and monitoring of their youth's activities (Robinson et al., 2015) and (2) more reliable follow-through with disciplinary practices (Henggeler et al., 2009). Improved parent monitoring and follow-through can lead to the final change that is associated not only with short-term improvements in at-risk youth, but also with long-term positive changes into their adulthoods. When MST therapists manage to empower parents to help their youth to replace delinquent peers with prosocial peers during therapy, youth outcomes at the end of therapy and short-term follow-up are better (Fain, Greathouse, Turner, & Weinberg, 2014). When Schaeffer and Borduin (2005) found that the positive effects of peer group change were still evident 14 years after treatment, they hypothesized that the removal of deviant peers might have allowed the youth to begin experiencing previously unattainable success in school, work, and other important developmental arenas, such as healthy romantic relationships, both during adolescence and adulthood. A recent qualitative study of at-risk British youth (Paradisopoulos, Pote, Fox, & Kaur, 2015) seems to support their speculation, as the participants reported that the removal of negative peer influence in their lives led to their actively working toward positive future goals.

Who Are the MST Therapists and Where Do They Work?

The initial studies investigating MST were conducted with graduate students trained in family therapy by the program developers, Henggeler and Borduin, and supervised by them (Borduin et al., 1995; Henggeler et al., 1986). Subsequently, MST research has included community therapists with master's or doctoral degrees who work in psychiatric, psychological, social services, and juvenile justice settings. The agencies are predominantly private with public funding (Henggeler et al., 2009).

All MST therapists work on teams of at least two therapists and a local supervisor, who meet every week to review MST cases (Henggeler et al., 2009). Therapists also have a weekly phone discussion with an expert MST consultant. Brunk (2016a) reported that the average therapist stays in a work setting for about 2.5 years. Thus, MST teams are continually training and orienting new MST therapists.

What Conditions Support MST Therapist Effectiveness?

Adherence to the MST model is challenging. It requires individualized, systemic functional analyses of the unique problems of each youth (Borduin, 2016). The nexus between reduced effectiveness and low adherence to the MST model has been supported by numerous studies that compared outcomes with adequate treatment adherence to outcomes with low treatment adherence. For instance, Sundell et al. (2008) showed that low MST therapist adherence was associated with MST youth continuing to be arrested.

In response to the repeated research evidence that well-trained, well-intended MST therapists found it difficult to sustain adherence to the MST model and thus to maintain effectiveness in treating at-risk youth, Henggeler and Borduin drew on their experiences during the initial MST trials when, as professors, they provided continuing supports for their graduate students on campus. Henggeler et al. (2009) tested a structured system of providing comparable long-term supports to MST therapists and supervisors working in communities, specifically a weekly telephone consultation for the group with a regional MST expert.

After the weekly phone calls from expert MST consultants were instituted, Schoenwald, Sheidow, and Letourneau (2004) showed that therapist adherence and consequent better youth outcomes resulted, but only to the extent of consultant competence. As consultant competence was shown to be a factor in the successful implementation of MST, such consultants (or regional MST experts) also became subject to supervision, continuing training, and oversight. Regional MST experts are supervised by an MST coach, who listens to a random selection of consultation sessions, conducts quarterly reviews of consultants' development, and holds biannual booster training sessions for groups of expert consultants. All of their work is guided by a web application that shows therapist adherence data, supervisor ratings, and regular progress regarding youth's goals.

Despite the MST organization's efforts to provide ongoing comprehensive support services, agencies that provide MST treatment may find that budget constraints limit their ability to continue their relationship with the MST organization. An implementation study by Smith-Boydston et al. (2014) designed to assess the effectiveness of MST therapists over a 6-year period showed the need for ongoing MST organizational support for MST therapists. All MST therapists in Smith-Boydston et al.'s (2014) study had received training, supervision, and support for 3 years, which consisted of 5 days of MST orientation training, biannual 1.5-day booster sessions at their worksite, and a weekly expert phone consultation provided by the central MST Services organization. However, 3 years after initial implementation of the MST program, that source of support was withdrawn when the agency could no longer continue to fund its association with the MST organization. The effectiveness of MST therapists faded over the next 3 years. The reduced effectiveness was probably due to drift from the MST model that the local therapists and supervisors did not notice.

Indeed, implementation data showed that the number of meetings with each family during treatment decreased during that second 3-year period by 50%. The number of families that met treatment goals decreased from 46% during the first 3-year period to 16% during the second 3-year period. Thus, even after 3 years of intense, systematic training and feedback, MST therapists still had the need for MST organization support. Therapists apparently need ongoing support from MST experts to effectively manage home-based family therapy for youth with serious behavior problems. A complete MST team, including both local and central MST Services support, is necessary for MST effectiveness. And the need for this support does not end—even after 3 years of intense, systematic training and feedback.

In addition to continuing support from the MST organization, MST therapists require initial and continual support from the administrators at their worksite. As Ghate (2016) stated, "eventually the highest quality evidence-based program can be constrained in its effectiveness by an unaccommodating, inflexible, or impoverished systems context" (p. 814). Research has shown that MST therapists have difficulty adhering to the MST model and thus have difficulty being effective in reducing youth's antisocial behavior when their agencies do not institute policies and practices that are necessary for MST therapists to be effective. These include (1) assigning therapists no more than four to six families at any time; (2) supplying technological and practical resources, such as work cell phones, insurance, vehicles, and workspace; (3) providing timely cost reimbursement; (4) imposing no limits on number of sessions per week or number of weeks of treatment; (5) enforcing MST-determined discharge policies; (6) granting training, supervision, consultation time, and space; (7) having a 24/7 on-call system; (8) negotiating interagency agreements that the MST therapist controls the course of treatment; (9) ensuring confidential information sharing; (10) arranging appropriate referrals for MST; and (11) managing short wait-times to reduce treatment refusal.

As therapists would not be able to implement or sustain these administrative practices themselves, the MST Services organization sends a representative to meet with administrators to set up policies and practices. In addition, in response to quality assurance and clinical outcome data, which are collected weekly on the MST website, an MST Services representative conducts a semiannual review of administrative supports and barriers to MST adherence with administrators. Collaborative problem solving and specific strategies are planned so that identified issues may be addressed (Schoenwald, 2016).

These ongoing, highly structured supports for MST therapist adherence and effectiveness account for the yearly improvements from 2009 to 2014 in clinical outcomes for MST-treated youth and their families. The current average international posttreatment figures are as follows: 90% of each MST team's youth were living at home; 90% were in school or working, and 86% had no new arrests (MST Services, 2015).

What Do Parents, Youth, Practitioners, and Referral Sources Think of MST?

Positive reactions of youth, parents, supervisors, and referring agencies to MST have been documented in research. This is important because no matter how effective and long lasting the results of a therapeutic intervention may be, if the interested stakeholders—clients, therapists, and the community service organizations responsible for referrals—do not find such treatment acceptable, it will not be adopted and sustained. As indicated earlier, in order to implement effective MST treatment, the

MST organization has instituted multiple layers of feedback and over-sight. One such mechanism is a brief quantitative instrument in which youth and caregivers rate their MST therapists every month during the course of treatment. The scale ranges from 0–1.00, with .61 being the lowest average rating that is empirically associated with treatment effec-tiveness (Brunk, 2016a). Brunk (2016b) reported that the actual world-wide average client rating of MST in 2015 was .76, with 80% of parents rating their therapist above .61.

In a quantitative study conducted in Norway, Norwegian research-ers compared caregivers' satisfaction with MST versus caregivers' sat-isfaction with usual community services. This particularly stringent randomized controlled trial, completed independently from MST devel-opers, offered a compelling testament to the satisfaction with MST treat-ment. In Norway, usual community services, which form the basis for comparison with MST, are governed by the "best interests of the child" standard, even when the child is a serious youth offender. These ser-vices include wraparound supports and, if indicated, psychotherapy. In contrast, in the United States the focus is on punishment (detention or incarceration) and protection of the public from serious youth offenders. Although to a lesser degree than their U.S. counterparts, Norwegian caregivers in this study nonetheless rated MST higher than their compre-hensive usual community services (Ogden & Halliday-Boykins, 2004).

Qualitative studies of clients' perspectives on MST yield more infor-mation. The caregivers interviewed attributed positive changes during MST to (1) a good therapeutic alliance, (2) a focus on interpersonal rela-tionships, and (3) increases in family resilience (empowerment) in the face of life difficulties (Kaur et al., 2015). Youth credited their MST positive outcomes to (1) a therapeutic alliance, (2) a focus on awareness of them-selves and others, (3) the removal of negative peer influences, and (4) their working toward positive future goals (Paradisopoulos et al., 2015).

Another source of evaluation of MST is found in the instrument MST therapists complete every 2 months to assess their view of the sup-port they receive from their supervisors. With a quantitative rating range of 0 to 100, therapists reported high or very high satisfaction on the fol-lowing measures: (1) supervisors' guidance in MST principles (average 0.90), (2) supervisors' help in generating functional analyses of youths' behavior problems (average 0.90), and (3) supervisors' structure and process (average 0.84). Therapists also showed satisfaction with supervi-sors' focus on clinician professional development (MST Services, 2015).

Given the increased costs that providing MST treatment incurs in terms of time, effort, and financial expense, the number of at-risk youth consistently referred for MST treatment is a strong indication of how the community views this intervention. Research conducted in various countries outside the United States found increased satisfaction rates with MST when compared to other modalities among referral sources. For example, in a study of referral rates in Norway, Ogden et al. (2012) found that more youth with serious behavior problems were referred to MST than to a similarly targeted, evidence-based treatment over a 10-year period. In a qualitative study conducted with Australian child protection workers, questions were designed to identify the advantages the professionals saw in referring at-risk youth to MST rather than other treatments. Responses included (1) the 24/7 availability of MST therapists to families; (2) the MST staff's greater communication, collaboration, and partnership with the child protection workers; (3) MST's more intense and effective treatment of families' complex issues, rather than only addressing surface issues; (4) the improved perceptions of child protection workers by families who had received MST; and (5) MST's ability to reduce barriers to the families' participation in MST (Hebert, Bor, Swenson, & Boyle, 2014).

ACHIEVEMENT MENTORING PROGRAM

Research has been done since 1973 on the effects of providing Achievement Mentoring in schools to youth at risk for juvenile delinquency, substance abuse, and failure to graduate from high school. The program has been called different names, but the procedures and principles have stayed the same. Past names are Early Secondary Intervention Program (ESIP), Preventive Intervention, and Behavioral Monitoring and Reinforcement Program (BMRP).

Six randomly controlled trials (Bry, 1982; Bry & Witte, 1982; Clarke, 2009; Holt et al., 2008; Taylor, 2010) and one quasi-experimental study (Bry, 2001a) have tested outcomes, and three implementation studies have examined which mentor supports promote program effectiveness (Bry & Yadegar, 2013; Kelly, Butler, McDonnell, & Bry, 2013; Yadegar & Bry, 2014). In addition, the reactions of youth, mentors, teachers, principals, and parents to Achievement Mentoring also have been investigated. All outcome studies have shown that Achievement Mentoring is more effective than the usual school services in preventing behavior problems among at-risk youth. Achievement Mentoring research has addressed the following questions.

Who Does Achievement Mentoring Help?

Achievement Mentoring has been shown to help primary school sixth graders, middle school seventh and eighth graders, and high school ninth and tenth graders whose teachers and other school personnel have identified as having an increased likelihood of failing to remain in school and graduate from high school. These students are so identified because of (1) poor grades (average grades for Achievement Mentoring nominees were D+ for middle school students and D for high school students, with a range of B– to F), (2) excessive absenteeism (average number of annual absences is 15 for middle school nominees and 22 for high school nominees), and/or (3) behavioral problems (many nominated students had several discipline referrals prior to nomination).

The student populations studied by Achievement Mentoring researchers show considerable demographic variability: these youths lived in small towns, suburbs, and urban areas; in various states in the United States (e.g., Maine, New York, and Maryland); and in numerous locations in Ireland (e.g., Dublin, Wexford, Cork, Galway, and Sligo). Within the United States, the majority were male (60% boys and 40% girls). Mentored youth in the United States are representative of the country's three largest racial/ethnic groups, White, African American, and Hispanic. A moderator study revealed no preprogram characteristic of nominated at-risk youth that predicted greater Achievement Mentoring effects than any other preprogram characteristic (Russell, 1979).

What Specific Problems Does Achievement Mentoring Help Prevent?

As the experience of having to repeat grades or receive multiple suspensions can be life altering, the goal of Achievement Mentoring is to prevent the negative outcomes associated with school disengagement. Because the Program is designed to prevent problems, the only way to determine the potential problems that may have developed if at-risk youth had not been assigned an achievement mentor is to look at the problems that developed for youth who were otherwise qualified for Achievement Mentoring but did not enter the program owing to a random selection process (e.g., a coin toss). Six randomized controlled trials tested this precise situation, all of which showed that at-risk youth who had been assigned an achievement mentor developed significantly fewer behavior problems at program completion than at-risk youth who received the usual school services (Bry, 1982; Bry & Witte, 1982; Clarke, 2009; Holt et al., 2008; Taylor, 2010). This disparity existed over a range of measures, such as school discipline records and self-reports of negative school behaviors, juvenile delinquency, and substance use. As statistical tests showed that these group differences would not have occurred by chance, the prevention of behavior problems could be attributed to Achievement Mentoring.

The Achievement Mentoring outcome studies also show the prevention of other aspects of school disengagement, as measured by attendance, grades, sense of alienation, decision making, and school dropout before graduation, for mentored youth (Bien & Bry, 1980; Bry, 2001a; Bry & George, 1980; Bry & Witte, 1982; Clarke, 2009; Holt et al., 2008). In most of the studies, the nonmentored students' pre–post measures showed significantly greater increases in school disengagement than did those of the mentored students. Essentially, Achievement Mentoring helped mentored students maintain a degree of school engagement, while nonmentored students became more disengaged. While nonmentored at-risk ninth graders' perceptions of teacher support decreased from September to June, the mentored students maintained the same degree of perception of teacher support from September to June (Holt et al., 2008). While the nonmentored high school students' GPAs decreased from 1.5 to 1.2 (D = 1), mentored students' GPAs rose slightly from 1.5 to 1.6 (C = 2) (Bry, 2001a). For middle school students, the GPAs for the nonmentored group decreased significantly, from 1.8 to 1.2, with the result that several of those students had to repeat eighth grade; mentored students' GPAs decreased only slightly, from 1.8 to 1.6, with the result that all mentored youth were promoted to high school (Bry & George, 1980). Sixteen percent of nonmentored students left high school after their sophomore year, as compared to only 2% of mentored youth (Bry, 2001a). It should be noted, however, that while the mentored students tended to maintain their preprogram levels of school engagement, there was also evidence of decreased school engagement for some mentored students, albeit on a lesser scale than for nonmentored students. For example, while both samples showed decreases in school attendance, the average number of days in school decreased 13% for nonmentored high school students as compared with 4.5% for mentored students (Bry, 2001a).

Do Achievement Mentoring Preventive Effects Last?

Although achievement mentors are an active presence in mentees' lives for a recommended 2 years and although they maintain contact in the subsequent year for booster sessions, the intervention is brief each week and low in intensity (see Chapter 11). As the research findings discussed in the previous section indicated, the effects of Achievement Mentoring can be seen primarily in the prevention of worsening behavior and academic performance. Although there are examples of Achievement Mentoring having a pronounced positive effect on a student's achievement level (see the case example in Chapter 13), the Program does not often turn students with marginal behavioral and academic records into honor students and award winners. In fact, in the absence of the RCTs described earlier, the positive effects generated by Achievement Mentoring may have remained unknown to mentors, teachers, and principals. Given the lack of a sharp and visible contrast between pre- and postmentored student performance, it is legitimate to question whether the lives of at-risk mentored students are any different than they would have been if they had not had an achievement mentor.

Again, the only way to know the answer to this question is to compare the records of mentored youth with those of similarly situated youth who, owing to random selection, had not been mentored. In the county in which this study was performed, young people's names were recorded at the probation office only if their offenses were serious, such as armed robbery, or chronic, such as more than two instances of shoplifting. When county probation records were accessed 7 years after at-risk youth had been randomly assigned to Achievement Mentoring or usual services, it was found that 10% of the mentored youth had files in the county probation department but three times as many (30%) of the nonmentored youth had files (Bry, 1982). Thus, the mentored students were statistically less likely to have been arrested and under the jurisdiction of the county probation department than nonmentored students. The prevention of being arrested and having to report to the county's probation department is another life-altering effect of Achievement Mentoring.

What Are the Essential Components of Achievement Mentoring?

In an initial outcome study with component analyses, Bien and Bry (1980) explored components of Achievement Mentoring that mentors need to perform in order to have a positive impact on at-risk youth.

Teacher Consultations

The first in a series of sequential components is the weekly consultation that mentors have with teachers during which mentors discuss the selected at-risk student's classroom behavior. During the initial experimental phase of Achievement Mentoring, teachers requested that this interview be guided by a standardized set of questions (Bry & George, 1980). In response, the WRF was created, supplying achievement mentors with a list of questions to ask teachers. Teachers' responses are recorded by mentors in constructive behavioral terms (see Figure 11.1). While this consultation process was necessary, research data showed that merely discussing at-risk students' classroom behavior with their teachers was not enough.

Student–Mentor Meetings

Next, Bien and Bry (1980) added brief weekly meetings during school hours with the at-risk students selected for Achievement Mentoring. During this meeting: (1) positive responses on the WRF were praised; (2) the student chose one area needing improvement to address; and (3) the achievement mentor and student together planned one small S.M.A.R.T. goal for the week and its implementation. These meetings were with students individually or, if there were significant time constraints, in small groups. In both formats, the achievement mentor spoke with each student individually concerning the WRF feedback and planning for the next step. In the group format, the other students listened while mentors spoke to each youth in turn. Despite difficulties in scheduling these meetings during the school day when other school activities such as assemblies and fire drills competed for limited time, or the student was absent, the importance of the regularity of these weekly meetings was shown by Holt et al. (2008). These authors compared the outcomes of students whose achievement mentors conducted a session with them at least half of the weeks of the school year with outcomes of students whose mentors met with them less frequently. They found that *all* of the mentored students experienced decreased discipline referrals and maintained expectations of teacher support and their good decision making when compared to nonmentored at-risk students, but the mentored students who were seen more regularly also increased their sense of belonging in the school.

Adding brief weekly meetings with at-risk youth to consultations with their teachers improved these students' GPAs more than was the case for students whose sole intervention was teacher consultations. However, the mentored students' GPAs were not higher than the GPAs of at-risk students who were randomly assigned to usual school services (Bien & Bry, 1980).

Mentor–Parent Contact

As a method by which mentoring could be reinforced at home and thus have the potential to increase students' GPAs, Bien and Bry (1980) added monthly parent contacts to the weekly teacher and student meetings. Parents, contacted by telephone or mail, were praised for their contribution to at least one sign of progress their child had shown during the past month. For instance, an achievement mentor would say, "Shawn has gotten to school on Mondays for 2 weeks in a row now! Whatever you are doing to get him there, keep it up." Once the parent contact component was added to the weekly teacher and student meetings, the randomly assigned, mentored, at-risk students' GPAs improved to a level that was statistically significantly higher than the GPAs of the similarly situated students who had been randomly assigned to usual student services. Thus, all three program components are essential.

Two-Year Achievement Mentoring Program Duration

Mentoring the at-risk students for at least 2 years is the final essential component of Achievement Mentoring. Although some mentees can benefit from only 1 year of mentoring (Bry & Witte, 1982; Holt et al., 2008), researchers (Bry, 2001a; Bry & George, 1980; Clarke, 2009) have repeatedly shown that Achievement Mentoring during 2 school years is necessary for reliable, lasting prevention of negative academic and behavioral outcomes among at-risk students.

What Are Achievement Mentoring's Mechanisms of Change?

The following questions are addressed in this section:

- What, according to mediation research, brings about sustainable prevention of at-risk youth's academic and behavioral problems during 2 years of Achievement Mentoring?
- What changes in the youth are associated with maintaining school engagement and staying out of trouble, in both the short run and the long run?
- What Achievement Mentoring research findings should guide mentors' priorities?
- Which mentee skills and habits, among the myriad typical at-risk student characteristics, does research suggest achievement mentors should target for the greatest payoff?

Achievement Mentoring is based on the original proposition that at-risk youth would be less likely to become involved in behavior problems, including drug abuse, if they reengaged in school—both cognitively and affectively. It was hypothesized that school reengagement would enable them to experience efficaciousness through the moment-to-moment accomplishment of the usual tasks of adolescence (e.g., getting to school on time, abiding by the rules, and doing schoolwork). A final element involved the peer group. It was assumed that if at-risk youth reengaged in school and experienced effectiveness in these realms, they would be less likely to engage in unacceptable behaviors to feel efficacious with antisocial friends, such as thwarting authority, fighting, stealing, damaging property, or getting high (see Chapter 11).

Achievement Mentoring research has supported the original assumptions that increasing the cognitive and affective aspects of school engagement would eventually result in the prevention of behavioral problems and school dropout. The cognitive and affective effects of mentoring associated with reduced behavior problems are as follows:

1. Holt et al. (2008) found that high school freshman mentees maintained their views of themselves as *good decision makers* from September to June, while, during the same period, nonmentored students' beliefs that they made good decisions decreased. By June, nonmentored students reported that they were less likely to agree with the statement that they often "stop to think about options before you make a decision."

2. At-risk middle school students randomly assigned to Achievement Mentoring increased their beliefs in internal *locus of control* of their school behaviors during their first year of mentoring. At-risk students assigned to usual school services, however, remained convinced that their school behaviors were caused by external forces, endorsing statements such as, "Schools are run by others and students can do little about it," and "No matter how hard I try, I don't seem to understand the content of my classes very well." In comparison, the mentored students reported increasing self-efficacy beliefs, reduced helplessness, and greater empowerment (Bry & Witte, 1982).

3. Middle school Achievement Mentoring mentees also reported positive *changes in self-concept*, with a greater likelihood of endorsing statements such as, "I am well behaved in school," and a lesser likelihood of reporting, "I cause trouble for my family," while the self-concepts of other at-risk students remained the same (Bry & Witte, 1982). All of the at-risk students' one-year changes in self-efficacy and self-concept correlated significantly with one-year changes in their GPA and attendance (Bry & Witte, 1982).

4. Not only does Achievement Mentoring change at-risk students' views of themselves, it also affects their *views of teachers and peers*. Mentored at-risk high school freshmen maintained positive expectations of high school teachers from September until June, while the perceptions of teachers held by nonmentored at-risk students receiving usual school services decreased significantly by June (Holt et al., 2008). Clarke replicated this finding in a second RCT in the same urban school the following year (Clarke, 2009), finding that mentees' perceptions of teachers improved from September to June of their freshman year, while

nonmentored students' perceptions decreased. Perceptions of teachers that were endorsed by Achievement Mentoring mentees in June and not by nonmentees were: "Teachers are interested in me," "Teachers respect me," and "I can talk to one teacher."

5. The Clarke (2009) study also investigated at-risk students' concept of how peers perceived them and found that mentored students' beliefs that their classroom *peers accepted them* improved statistically during their second year of mentoring versus nonmentored students' beliefs. Mentees became more likely to endorse statements such as, "Students in my classes are willing to listen to me," "My classmates want me to do well," and "I can ask my classmates for help with my homework."

Research corroborates Achievement Mentoring as a treatment intervention that can facilitate changes in students' thoughts and affect that foreshadow or accompany behavioral and academic improvement as they move toward reengagement in school and/or slow their progress toward disengagement, while nonmentored at-risk students continue to disengage. Research has demonstrated that as a result of this intervention, mentees (1) increase their beliefs that they can succeed in school through their own actions, (2) increase their self-esteem, and (3) maintain or increase feelings that teachers and classmates want them to succeed. Thus, achievement mentors should find opportunities each week to encourage the changes in mentees' perceptions by showing them that it is their own attitudes and actions, and not external forces, that account for their daily accomplishments, such as getting to school on time and finishing assignments; and by communicating that teachers want mentees to succeed and that classmates are sources of help. The rapport between mentor and mentee is an additional factor that facilitates school engagement. Achievement Mentoring research shows that high school freshman mentees who rated their relationship with their mentor at the highest level also reported the greatest sense of belonging to their school at the end of freshman year (Holt et al., 2008). And, eventually, these cognitive and affective changes reduced behavioral problems.

Who Are the Achievement Mentors and Where Do They Work?

All achievement mentors have graduated from college, and many have advanced degrees. Their ranks include men and women of diverse ethnic/racial backgrounds, including Whites, African Americans, Hispanic/Latino Americans, and Asian Americans. Research studies have shown that achievement mentors are overwhelmingly employed full time as teachers in schools, although other school professionals, such as guidance counselors, school psychologists, social workers, substance abuse counselors, vice principals, principals, and nurses, also function as mentors. Full-time teachers tend to mentor two at-risk students at a time. In Ireland, Achievement Mentoring is also performed by professionals who come into the schools weekly but are not school employees; specifically, they are community youth workers or employees of the School Completion Program.

What Conditions Support Achievement Mentor Effectiveness?

Research has shown that the future behavior and academic problems of at-risk youth are most likely to be reduced when achievement mentors adhere to the Achievement Mentoring Program, as presented in Chapters 11 and 12. As is true of MST, adherence to an intervention requires training—2 to 3 full days of introductory mentor training is provided during the first year of mentoring—and ongoing support. In the United States, Achievement Mentoring training and ongoing training are provided by the Center for Supportive Schools and in Ireland and the rest of Europe by Archways.

Ongoing Support

Research has shown that each employment site needs a *local Achievement Mentoring Program coordinator* who acts as a liaison to the site's ongoing Achievement Mentoring trainer and Achievement Mentoring records coordinator, and facilitates the mentoring process by (1) providing weekly support to mentors encountering difficulties with mentees; (2) providing resources for mentors, such as mentees' school records, teachers' schedules, and copies of blank Achievement Mentoring forms (see a blank version of the WRF in Chapter 11 and at *www.guilford. comXYZ*, which readers can photocopy for their use); and (3) reminding mentors to complete WOMSs (Bry & Yadegar, 2013). Research has also shown the importance for mentors to have meetings with *ongoing Achievement Mentoring trainers* monthly (or more often, if need be) in person or on Skype, either individually or in small groups, until mentors have obtained certification that they have mastered Achievement Mentoring (Yadegar & Bry, 2014).

These supports for mentor effectiveness were developed in response to information about how adherent achievement mentors were able to be in their weekly mentoring at their employment sites. Support provision is a dynamic process: as new information is obtained pertinent to the issue of adherence, currently offered supports are adjusted in order to facilitate the highest level of adherence.

Initially, mentors' adherence to Achievement Mentoring was observed in person and rated by the Achievement Mentoring Program developer with the assistance of a graduate student during three sequential New Jersey RCTs (Clarke, 2009; Holt et al., 2008; Taylor, 2010). Serving both as Achievement Mentoring trainers and ongoing trainers, the Program developer and her assistant visited the schools weekly and had face-to-face meetings with achievement mentors in their offices or classrooms during prep periods. During these meetings, the Program developer and her assistant reviewed the WRFs completed by the mentors about their mentees; independently completed adherence checklists reflecting mentor compliance with Achievement Mentoring steps during mentoring sessions; and discussed with the mentor, and took notes on, the mentor's most recent mentoring session. Prior to the meeting's end, plans were made with the mentor for the next mentoring sessions. After the meeting, the Program developer and her assistant compared their checklists and notes. Research revealed that the agreement between the Program developer and assistant on the mentors' adherence to the prescribed steps of Achievement Mentoring weekly mentoring meetings was very high—90% (Clarke, 2009; Holt et al., 2008; Taylor, 2010).

As discussed in Chapter 11 regarding the steps of weekly Achievement Mentoring sessions, the mentor praises something the mentee accomplished in the previous week that is reflected in the WRF. During the first RCT where adherence was noted, the Program developer's and assistant's adherence ratings showed that achievement mentors performed this step during only 57% of the weekly sessions (Yadegar & Bry, 2014). As this level of adherence was unsatisfactory, training was modified so that praise, and its theoretical function, received greater emphasis by the Achievement Mentoring trainers during day-long training and weekly ongoing training meetings. After such adjustment, adherence data showed that praise increased the following year to 72% of mentoring sessions and continued to increase over the next 10 years (Yadegar & Bry, 2014).

Adherence was also low initially for the Achievement Mentoring step of mentors asking for their mentees' views of the WRFs (Yadegar & Bry, 2014). Because of adherence data indicating that this step was followed during only 40 to 45% of the sessions, training was modified so that (1) ongoing Achievement Mentoring trainers began asking mentors specifically what mentees' views were, and (2) training day agendas included a more detailed explanation of the "spirit of Motivational Interviewing" (Miller & Rollnick, 2012) and the function of asking at-risk students for their views, instead of suggesting what the student should do about teacher feedback on WRFs. Consequently, by the third RCT where adherence was rated, a substantial increase was found in mentors asking mentees for their views. This was now generating a 70% adherence level in mentoring sessions (Yadegar & Bry, 2014). Thus, adherence data showed that trainers could not assume that trainees were proficient and would employ Achievement Mentoring communication skills after initial training was complete, but that adjustments in initial and ongoing training could elevate mentors' proficiency and use of Achievement Mentoring skills. (See Chapter 14 for a discussion of training and ongoing training.)

The dissemination of Achievement Mentoring beyond its origins in New Jersey introduced new challenges. The New Jersey-based Achievement Mentoring Program developer and her assistant could not visit trained achievement mentors weekly in their employment sites—which were now in Maine and Ireland—and coach them on Achievement Mentoring adherence. Nor could they observe mentor adherence and subsequently make observation-based adjustments to increase adherence. To support mentors' adherence to Achievement Mentoring and thus facilitate the Program's effectiveness in preventing or reducing at-risk students' future behavior and academic problems, a user-friendly, non-observational method for collecting adherence data had to be devised for long-distance adaptation. A computer application, the WOMS, was developed to address this need. An email is sent automatically to trained achievement mentors each Tuesday that contains a link taking them directly to the mentoring records of their assigned mentees. A screen appears, and they click "yes" or "no" to each of the eight mentoring steps to indicate whether they performed the step with the mentee that week. Completing a WOMS takes less than a minute per mentee. (See Chapter 14 for further description of the WOMS.)

These weekly electronic mentoring records by achievement mentors communicate to local Program coordinators, ongoing trainers, and the Program developer how well mentors are able to adhere to Achievement Mentoring procedures. Those procedures can be adjusted in response to the electronic adherence data in the same way that procedures were adjusted in response to adherence data obtained through on-site weekly observations performed by the Program developer and her assistant in New Jersey.

As might have been predicted, overall mentor adherence to Program procedures decreased when the Program developer was unable to meet face to face with the trained mentors weekly in their distant offices and classrooms (Yadegar & Bry, 2014). The rate fell from nearly 100% during the third New Jersey RCT with face-to-face adherence ratings to 80% in Maine and Ireland. Two Achievement Mentoring steps that experienced the most significant decrease in adherence were (1) collecting and writing feedback from teachers (WRFs) to show mentees and

(2) the related step of the mentor discussing with the mentee an area for improvement (Yadegar & Bry, 2014). Adherence for collecting and writing feedback from teachers dropped from 100%, when mentors were visited weekly in New Jersey, to 80–82% in Maine and Ireland, when mentors reported their mentoring session activities through a computer application (Yadegar & Bry, 2014). Adherence to the step that involved mentor/mentee discussions on areas for improvement decreased from 92 to 72% (Yadegar & Bry, 2014). If mentors failed to interview teachers each week and thus obtain the information needed to complete the WRFs to show mentees, they would lack the basis on which areas for improvement could be discussed. To the extent that goal setting was done in mentoring sessions, it would not be done with reference to teacher input, but would rather reflect the goals the mentors thought mentees should set for the next week. Alternatively, no goal would be set at all. While the decrease in adherence in New Jersey was attributable to inadequate training, decreased adherence in Maine and Ireland might have had more to do with the lack of direct contact. When the Program developer and assistant asked mentors in face-to-face meetings each week what the teacher interviews revealed, mentors did the interviews. When this face-to-face accountability procedure was replaced by clicking boxes on a computer application, mentors might not have made fitting the teacher interview into their busy school days a priority, and that step in the program drifted.

To remedy decreased adherence in the absence of weekly face-to-face meetings with the Program developer and her assistant, Achievement Mentoring trainers in Ireland and the United States experimented with different ongoing training/coaching methods, such as conference calling, texting, and Skyping. However, ongoing trainers found that the best way to prevent drift and maintain mentors' adherence to weekly teacher interviews was to replicate, as best as possible, the New Jersey model. Thus, ongoing trainers arranged to visit the schools and to have face-to-face meetings with mentors to review WRFs and their progress with mentees. Because travel distances were sometimes prohibitive for Irish trainers, they devised a plan for mentors to scan or photograph WRFs and email or text them before Skype or phone training sessions with the ongoing trainers. With all of these data-based adjustments, average mentor adherence across implementation sites increased from 63 to 93% from 2004 to 2014 (Yadegar & Bry, 2014).

Mentor completion of WOMSs presented another challenge that accompanied long-distance dissemination of Achievement Mentoring. When trained mentors do not complete a weekly WOMS for each of their mentees, the Program developer, trainers, and local Program coordinators cannot know how the mentors are implementing the Program, and so the ongoing training process becomes less effective. Bry and Yadegar (2013) experimented with different interventions to increase long-distance mentors' WOMS completion, using an interrupted time series design to track the effects of different interventions on percentage of WOMS completion in different Achievement Mentoring implementation sites.

The researchers found that the WOMS completion percentage was increased by the following methods: (1) *an email from the Achievement Mentoring records coordinator* with specific information that a WOMS was missing, the week for which the WOMS was missing, and, if the WOMS had been submitted but was incomplete, the exact items that were missing, and a link to the mentors' incomplete WOMS; (2) *a separate reminder from the mentors' ongoing trainer or local Program coordinator*; and (3) *an email acknowledgment from the records coordinator* immediately after the completed WOMS was submitted. The importance of the local coordinator reminder, in addition to the records coordinator's, can be demonstrated by the following: When the local coordinator of one site reminded achievement mentors about past-due WOMSs, a very low proportion (12%) of uncompleted WOMSs resulted. However, when all of the interventions were implemented at another site except for the reminder from the local coordinator, a relatively high proportion of uncompleted WOMSs (36%) resulted (Bry & Yadegar, 2013).

Of course, the method by which mentor adherence to Achievement Mentoring is measured by WOMS is dependent on valid self-report by mentors. Thus, Achievement Mentoring trainers emphasize the importance of valid self-reports from their first demonstration during full-day training. During this training, trainers role-play completing WOMS when some mentoring steps were not carried out, so that mentors will understand that omitting steps is an accepted occurrence. Apprising mentors that no negative consequences will ensue for indicating that some steps were not carried out, or that sessions were not held for justifiable reasons, such as mentee absences, school assemblies, or mentor illness, supports veracity as well.

At the same time, mentors' WOMS responses, no matter how valid, are no substitute for *hearing or seeing* a mentor conduct a mentoring session. Thus, to qualify for certification, a trained mentor must submit audio recordings of two sessions with two different mentees to the Program developer for review. In this way, the Program developer can determine whether a mentor carries out all of the steps of the Achievement Mentoring sessions and whether the steps were carried out skillfully. In addition, the requirements for Achievement Mentoring certification give the mentors further incentives for completing WOMs and WRFs. All WOMSs for the two mentees must have been completed, and the WRFs that were shown to the mentees during the sessions must accompany the recordings. These requirements for Achievement Mentoring certification give the mentors further incentives for completing WRFs and WOMs. Since the institution of the Achievement Mentoring certification opportunity, mentors have needed fewer reminders from Achievement Mentoring records coordinators and local Program coordinators to complete WOMSs.

What Do Youth, Mentors, Parents, and Other School Personnel Think of Achievement Mentoring?

In qualitative interviews with Irish sixth graders after one semester of Achievement Mentoring, mentees expressed very favorable views of their mentors, describing them as "cool," "the best," "funny," "a nice person," and "someone who never shouts at you like teachers" (Kelly et al., 2013, p. 65). Another mentee said he felt "lucky" to have a mentor (Kelly, Butler, Twist, McDonnell, & Kennedy, 2011). The mentees reported that their mentors helped them with school-specific endeavors, such as "spelling," "reading," and "doing homework," as well as with skills with broader applications, such as "turn-taking" and "managing emotions." The students' attributed improved performance in school to positive feedback from teachers and mentors for attempting and completing schoolwork. For example, one mentee said, "We got homework last night but I didn't want to be doing it, but I done it last night" (Kelly et al., 2013, p. 62).

A study of 392 New York City high school students conducted after one school year in Achievement Mentoring also yielded very positive responses about the mentoring experience. On a scale of 1 (a great amount) to 5 (not at all), with 2 signifying "quite a bit," mentees rated a range of answers prefaced by the phrase: "To what extent did Achievement Mentoring help you to . . . ?" The answers "care more about graduating," "care more about staying focused," and "know my mentor really cares about me" generated a 1 or 2 rating from 90% of the mentees surveyed (Center for Supportive Schools, 2016). The answers "care more about attending," "stay out of trouble," "make better decisions," "improve setting and achieving goals," and "do better in school with my mentor's help" also generated significant positive responses—85–89% of the mentees gave 1 or 2 ratings to these mentoring outcomes.

A typical response to the open-ended question, "How much did you look forward to meeting with your mentor and why?" was, "A great amount. When I meet with my mentor, she encourages me to go toward my goals." Another open-ended question, "Please describe one way that your relationship with your mentor has been important . . . ," generated responses indicating that mentors' positive influence on their mentees' lives extended to other areas in addition to school. Typical answers included, "I was going through a little family situation and—she . . . made me feel like she cared," "My mentor is one of the reasons I went from missing school to not missing a day . . . ," and "I got to express myself. My voice was heard and there wasn't any judgment."

In a study by Holt et al. (2008), high school teacher/mentors were asked to rate their experiences in the program. They reported high levels of satisfaction with Achievement Mentoring with respect to training, guidance, and support. Similarly, in Kelly et al.'s (2011) investigation of Irish community youth workers who visited schools each week to mentor sixth graders, participants reported in interviews that they liked "the simplicity and brevity" of the program and the training, and they also stressed the necessity of ongoing training, particularly for coping with practical issues and for handling emotions. They liked the frequent communication with teachers very much. The need to submit WOMSs was seen as helpful in that participants found it took them a while to understand the intervention, and the WOMS served as a reminder of what they learned in training. Another participant stated that the program required "an open mind regarding outcome" because mentee progress was sometimes so slow (Kelly et al., 2011).

A study of 40 achievement mentors in New York City high schools found that mentors credited Achievement Mentoring with improving their Active Listening Skills and their ability to help mentees set S.M.A.R.T. goals for themselves (Center for Supportive Schools, 2016). Interestingly, when mentors were asked the open-ended question, "What has been the best part for you, personally, about participating as a mentor in Achievement Mentoring?," they responded similarly to their high school students, citing a range of positive experiences that were school-related and had broader applications. Mentors' answers included: "the connections I made with students. I like that they come up to me and want to talk. They are eager to show me their progress in school," "having an active share in a student's academic and emotional growth," and "knowing that each student I mentor went from failing to passing every class with my positive feedback and praise."

One graduate student achievement mentor wrote more extensively about her experiences:

> I was often surprised by my adolescent's . . . hesitation to accept credit for good work and effort. . . . I simultaneously act as a constant—reliably and consistently guiding my [mentee] in the direction of positive academic related behaviors—and as a flexible and adaptive resource—adjusting to the adolescent's concerns, moods,

and environmental needs. . . . I also spent a substantial amount of time . . . speaking with teachers and counselors. Although the teachers are overwhelmingly busy, I was amazed with the time they were willing to spend with me, either formally during their prep period or even just passing in the hall, stopping momentarily to let me know that my [mentee] had turned in her makeup work (or not). (P.-A. Urga, personal communication, January 29, 2004)

In another study, conducted with high school Achievement Mentoring teachers and counselors in upstate New York, responses to the interview question, "What difference does mentoring make?" were: "Knowing someone is looking for them," "Just let[ting them] know you are there—available," "Step out of the role of teacher," and "Give him hope" (Bry & Attaway, 2000). Once again, those involved with Achievement Mentoring felt that their contribution was not restricted to school performance.

In an independent study of Achievement Mentoring in Ireland, where the intervention is termed the Mentoring for Achievement Programme (MAP), Kelly et al. (2011) found that the benefits of mentoring extended to primary school teachers who were not mentors themselves. These nonmentoring teachers gave positive feedback about the program in their school as they witnessed at-risk students beginning to attempt and complete academic assignments. They also saw improvements in mentees' behavior, describing some mentored students as "calmer" and "more settled" (p. 1021). The teachers considered MAP mentors to function as an "intermediary between mentees and teachers . . . sharing with teachers . . . what might help them in class" (p. 1020). Nonmentoring teachers also offered positive feedback consistent with mentors and mentees in other research studies, when they praised the effects of MAP to reach beyond the classroom. One said: "[MAP is] good for communicating between the three; the teacher, the child, and the home" (p. 1022).

In a follow-up study that included high-ranking school officials (Kelly et al., 2013), principals noted the value of MAP as not only a "fantastic support" for at-risk sixth graders (p. 65), but also as an aid in preparing youth for the higher grades as primary school teachers often found preparing at-risk students for larger, more impersonal secondary schools to be a difficult challenge. One Irish principal appreciated having MAP in his school because "some . . . teachers [are] more amenable to teaching sixth [grade] knowing that MAP will be available for the transition period. . . . MAP enhances transfer . . . to secondary school" (Kelly et al., 2013, p. 65). Results of research conducted with parents of mentored students (Kelly et al., 2011) also reflected a positive view of mentoring. One parent of a mentored sixth grader reported that her son is "more positive towards school. [He] wants to get things finished" (p. 2019). Another parent was "almost tearful" because she appreciates the MAP mentor's support (Kelly et al., 2013, p. 67).

COORDINATED ACHIEVEMENT MENTORING AND HOME-BASED FAMILY THERAPY

Once efficacy of the school-based Achievement Mentoring Program was demonstrated to prevent at-risk youth from developing more serious problems, Program developer Bry wondered whether adding a home-based family therapy component to the school-based Achievement Mentoring might help youth even more. This is consistent with multisystems theory that the more systems there are that promote youth achievement, the more likely it is that youth will achieve. (See Chapter 6 for a discussion of the Multisystems Model.) Optimally, the combination of both interventions could result in youths' *improving* overall functioning, instead of being limited to preventing future problems. Accordingly, employing the same learning principles and risk factor research that provided the structure for Achievement Mentoring, Bry and her graduate students developed the Targeted Family Intervention (TFI) (Bry et al., 1991), in which the home-based TFI family therapists either implement both Achievement Mentoring and TFI themselves or coordinate TFI implementation with mentees' school-based achievement mentors.

The findings from two sets of single-case design studies, one RCT with a 15-month follow-up, and one quasi-experimental study with a 3-year follow-up, confirmed the hypothesis that two coordinated interventions brought about more improvement than only one intervention. The at-risk youth who were provided both interventions improved their academics and reduced their risky behaviors more than when intervention consisted of Achievement Mentoring alone (Alexander, 2001; Bry, Conboy, & Bisgay, 1986; Bry & Krinsley, 1992; Krinsley, 1991).

Who Is Helped by Coordinated Achievement Mentoring and Targeted Family Intervention?

Participants in research studies on coordinated Achievement Mentoring (AM) and TFI comprised 12- to 16-year-olds who were predominantly (approximately 60%) male. In one working-class community research site, 82% of the at-risk youth were White and 18% were African American or Latino (Krinsley, 1991). Another community research site provided a contrasting demographic: 92.5% of the nominated youth were African American, 5% Latino, and 2.5% Asian American (Alexander,

2001). Most of the families in this community were low income, and 73% were headed by a single parent.

What Specific Problems Does Coordinated AM/TFI Change?

Whereas AM by itself prevents deterioration in GPAs and escalation of negative behavior, adding TFI resulted in mentees (1) achieving more passing grades in academic subjects; (2) getting higher GPAs; and (3) having fewer days in which drugs and/or alcohol were used (Alexander, 2001; Bry et al., 1986; Bry & Krinsley, 1992; Krinsley, 1991). Notably, in the Krinsley (1991) RCT, not one student in the AM/TFI group initiated or increased substance use during the 18-month period from assignment to the intervention until the end of follow-up.

In the Alexander (2001) study, the positive school engagement effects of coordinated AM/TFI did not appear until two school years had elapsed. At the end of the first year of AM/TFI, the coordinated interventions showed only preventive effects. However, the preventive effects were in stark contrast to the at-risk students who had been assigned to usual school services, 30% of whom had "extremely negative outcomes," such as (1) failing enough academic courses to be retained or "socially promoted," (2) increases in absences from one year to another of more than 35 days, or (3) a decrease in final numerical GPA (ranging from 0 to 100) from one year to the next of more than 15 points (Alexander, 1997; Bry, 1982). None of the students who were receiving both AM and TFI demonstrated an extremely negative outcome at the end of the first intervention year. It also should be noted that the single-case design studies repeatedly showed a common trend among at-risk youth in AM/TFI: grades and behavior got worse instead of better at the beginning of treatment. Family therapists should not become discouraged if a youth's behavior worsens at the beginning of treatment, as outcomes improve by the end of treatment (Bry et al., 1986; Bry & Krinsley, 1992).

Do AM/TFI Outcomes Last?

Again, the single-case design studies are instructive. Once AM/TFI is finished, grades initially tend to decrease again and drug use to increase. The first three at-risk youths studied recovered their treatment gains spontaneously during the 15-month follow-up (Bry et al., 1986). The next youth studied, however, did not—follow-up revealed that he had been expelled from school and placed in a youth detention facility. In response, booster sessions were added to AM/TFI. Subsequently, at-risk participants who continued to show some recurrence of academic and behavior problems immediately following AM/TFI termination reliably recovered treatment gains during or after the booster sessions (Bry & Krinsley, 1992).

Alexander (2001) compared long-term outcomes of middle school at-risk students who received coordinated AM/TFI with those of students who received usual school services. At the time of assignment to coordinated AM/TFI or to usual school services, the GPAs of both groups averaged 69 (D+). Reliable GPA differences between the groups did not appear until 1 year after booster sessions ended, and these differences were sustained and increased slightly through the end of the following year. These are often called "sleeper effects." Four years after interventions started, the average GPA of students who received AM/TFI during middle school was 72 (C), while the average GPA of those assigned to usual school services was 64 (D). Not only was the AM/TFI group's academic performance significantly better than that of those who received usual services, but their average GPA was actually higher than it was before the interventions. This improvement in academic performance replicates the results of the three other AM/TFI outcome studies indicating that at-risk students' grades and behavior were better at the end of follow-up than they were before intervention. Thus, the effects of coordinated AM/TFI are not merely preventive. AM/TFI actually improves academics and behavior. Service providers and administrators should remember, however, that positive outcomes may not be immediately apparent.

Another measure that confirms the long-term positive effects of AM/TFI is the contrast between the groups regarding school dropout. Four years after the study began, more than 50% of the at-risk students who received usual school services in middle school were no longer in school, while 60% of the students who received AM/TFI were still enrolled.

What Are the Essential Components of TFI?

The essential components of TFI were derived from (1) research on the factors differentiating families with adolescent problems from families without adolescent problems, and (2) microanalyses of family responses to family therapist techniques during sessions. Members of families of at-risk adolescents were found to respond to each other's conversational statements with significantly more blaming and lecturing than members of families without adolescent problems. They also engaged in significantly fewer problem-solving discussions (Krinsley & Bry, 1991), appearing helpless and disempowered in the face of problems that they see as externally caused (Parker & Bry, 1995). In addition, they were inconsistent and contradictory in their response to the negative behavior of their adolescents (Bry & Krinsley, 1990). In contrast, Greene and Bry (1991) observed that solution statements generated by families without adolescent problems are likely to be followed by agreement statements and preceded by descriptions of contingencies (if–then statements).

Communication Training

An essential component of TFI is *communication training* as a first step to problem solving. Family members are coached to break down dissatisfactions and complaints into discrete, specific "problems" that the concerned person "owns." The TFI therapist repeatedly and respectfully helps family members communicate their concerns in a nonblaming way, beginning with "if–then" statements and next identifying their evoked emotion. That is, family members are coached to start problem statements with, "When _____ happens, I feel 'worried' or 'ignored' or 'hate' or 'trapped' or 'lonely' or 'appreciative' or 'loving.'" Other family members are taught to *listen* to problem statements quietly.

Problem Solving

Once family members have learned the communication skills involved in problem solving, they are guided to *choose one member's complaint or concern to work on at a time* and, with the therapist's help, work through the steps of problem solving, including (1) brainstorming possible alternative solutions without judging them; (2) choosing the alternative that is least objectionable to the most of them; (3) planning implementation details for that solution; and (4) agreeing on how to proceed if their proposed solution does not work (Robin & Foster, 2002). The therapist leads the family through these steps during every family meeting, until families are adept at practicing communication of problems, listening, and problem solving on their own.

Contingency Management

Parents are coached in *contingency management*—providing immediate positive consequences for "catching a kid doing something good today" and providing consistent negative consequences for adolescents' negative behavior. Parents' ability to apply consequences consistently and cooperatively often requires that the therapist do some preparatory marital work until parents are able to agree on the outcomes they seek. This task is made easier when the TFI therapist models positive reinforcement of discrete prosocial family member behaviors during the therapy sessions.

Parental Monitoring

A related essential component of TFI is parental monitoring of the youth's behavior. Achievement Mentoring's WRFs can be of valuable assistance for this component, as they provide up-to-date and precise information about the at-risk adolescent's behavior and performance in school. This information can serve as the basis for parental praise of school engagement and as incentives they may offer the adolescent for more engagement. When the TFI therapist is also implementing AM with the youth, the therapist will have a completed WRF each week. If the TFI therapist and the achievement mentor are separate individuals, a copy of the completed WRF can be made available each week through coordination between the two professionals. Another benefit of utilizing the WRF in TFI is that the adolescent will not feel "blindsided" by any discussion arising out of WRF contents in family therapy, as this information has already been disclosed during the weekly mentoring session in school.

Home-Based TFI Sessions

After students begin receiving AM at school, families are contacted to meet with either the AM/TFI therapist or a coordinating TFI therapist to "discuss the family's ideas about how their at-risk adolescent can do better in school." Because families did not ask for help, it may be difficult to schedule a meeting with them. The therapist offers to come to the home to make it convenient for the family, and, if family members still seem reluctant, the TFI therapist respectfully persists in asking to schedule or reschedule a meeting. As participation in the AM/TFI program is voluntary and not mandated, and as families are not self-referred, they typically do not come to school or to a clinic for these meetings.

Once families meet for the first time with the AM/TFI therapist, they see the value in TFI and agree to further meetings. These meetings typically occur 8–12 times over a 3- to 4-month period until the family sees positive changes. In Krinsley's (1991) clinical trial of coordinated AM/TFI, 87% of the identified at-risk youth's families agreed to participate in the research, and 100% of those families eventually met with the TFI therapist once and subsequently continued to work with the therapist for 3–4 months.

Booster Sessions

When the youth has made progress, he or she continues to receive Achievement Mentoring at school for the duration of the program, but regular weekly family meetings no longer need to be scheduled. The family's involvement continues in the form of booster sessions held with the therapist so that this source of reinforcement is maintained. During booster sessions, conducted in the home, as was the case with the earlier weekly meetings, changes that the family and youth have made to support the youth's staying out of trouble and succeeding in school are reviewed and reinforced. If necessary, troubleshooting is done to sustain changes. The first booster session is scheduled for 1 month after the last TFI meeting, the next occurs two months after that, and the final booster session is scheduled 3 months thereafter. If the home-based booster sessions cannot be scheduled, extended phone calls can substitute for face-to-face meetings.

What Are Coordinated AM/TFI Mechanisms of Change?

This section addresses the following issues: (1) the changes in at-risk youth and families associated with coordinated AM/TFI outcomes; (2) the ways in which youth and families are affected by AM/TFI so that academic performance improves and negative behaviors, such as substance use, decline; and (3) the interim goals that should be the focus of AM/TFI therapists. As both at-risk youth and their parents gain knowledge in AM and TFI about the ways in which schools work and the importance of communication skills in making a difference in family functioning, they feel less helpless and at the mercy of external forces and more empowered and efficacious.

AM/TFI research has revealed several youth perspectives on both school and home that correlate with their school engagement and drug use (Bry et al., 1986). As youth become more engaged in school and less involved in negative behavior, they are more likely to endorse statements that are more reflective of school engagement, such as, "Students' ideas about how the school should be run are often used in this school," and statements that are reflective of improved communication patterns with parents, such as, "My dad listens when I need someone to talk to." Likewise, parents' views of their relationship with their child change as TFI progresses (Sternberg & Bry, 1994), and parents realize that they can make a difference to their adolescent. As a result, parents are more likely to endorse statements that reflect an enhanced ability to communicate with their adolescent, such as, "My child and I compromise during arguments." The more empowered that youth and parents feel and are, the better their outcomes will be in coordinated AM/TFI. Thus, TFI therapists should point out and reinforce instances of adolescents and parents feeling and being effective during therapy meetings.

Few families of at-risk youth enter TFI with effective problem-solving skills. During the first session, families typically generate only 0 to 5 possible solutions. The more skill parents and youth develop in generating possible solutions during problem solving, the more satisfied/pleased they are with their adolescents' improvement, and the better the outcomes will be for the youth and parents. By the final session of TFI, families can be expected to generate 33–55 possible solutions for problems (Sternberg & Bry, 1994). These findings suggest that TFI therapists will be most effective in improving at-risk youth's school engagement and in reducing negative behaviors if they notice and reinforce solution generation during family meetings. Sternberg and Bry (1994) found that therapists can increase family solution generation directly by stating "that's an idea" whenever a possible solution is mentioned during family meetings.

Who Provides Coordinated AM/TFI, and Where Do They Work?

Every AM/TFI intervention has been provided by Bry and graduate students under her supervision. In Alexander's study (1997), the therapists, all of whom delivered both AM and TFI, were 20% male and included a majority (62%) of Whites, with a third African Americans (33%), and a small number (5%) of Asian Americans. In Krinsley's (1991) study, the graduate students who provided TFI coordinated with teachers who were achievement mentors but did not provide both interventions themselves. In this sample, 50% of the therapists were male, a majority 60% was White, and the remaining therapists were divided equally among Latinos, African Americans, and Asian Americans (each group represented 13% of the sample).

What Conditions Support AM/TFI Therapist Effectiveness?

Weekly face-to-face supervision of graduate students on campus by faculty members supported adherence to manuals and protocols. An additional method of enabling therapist effectiveness was *audio recording of TFI sessions*, with the family's consent, which was reviewed by supervisors to monitor adherence and quality-of-service delivery. In Alexander's study (1997), one randomly selected audio recording of every AM/TFI therapist was assessed for adherence, using a list of TFI therapist behaviors and a coding system. Forty percent of the coded recordings were reviewed by a second independent coder. Interrater reliability was 76%. Therapists were found to have implemented an average of 72% of the activities that the TFI manual prescribes for each family session (Bry et al., 1991). For example, coded TFI activities reflected essential TFI components, such as, "Therapist compliments a family member in

some way," and "Therapist introduces information from school personnel during the session."

What Do Parents Think about Coordinated AM/TFI?

Four years after 20 middle school adolescents had been randomly
assigned to AM/TFI following teacher identification as at risk for school
dropout and behavior problems, 15 parents were interviewed in a study
(Alexander, 2001) designed to investigate parents' perceptions of this
coordinated preventive intervention. Before the start of family treatment, there was some difficulty scheduling at-home meetings because
parents who do not ask for help with their adolescent may often exhibit
some reluctance to engage in treatment. The 15 families eventually met
with the coordinated AM/TFI therapists in their homes weekly for 3–4
months. Before, during, and after the regular TFI sessions were completed, the students also saw the same therapist once a week in school for
Achievement Mentoring. During the second school year of the intervention, AM continued in the schools, and booster sessions were provided
to the families.

Eighty percent of the parents interviewed rated the coordinated AM/
TFI intervention as "quite helpful" or "very helpful," while 20% said it
was "helpful." When asked what surprised them about the intervention,
parents volunteered (1) its intensity, (2) how vigilant the therapist was
in monitoring their adolescent in school, (3) how informed the parent
became about the school, (4) how personable the therapist was, (5) the
considerable amount of time the therapist spent, and, a related item,
(6) the therapist going "beyond the call of duty"—for example, attending school meetings with the parent and interceding on the adolescent's
behalf. The parents also were surprised that the therapist counseled all
members of the family and not just the youth who was a participant in
the Achievement Mentoring Program.

When parents were then asked, "What was it like for you to have
an adolescent in coordinated AM/TFI?" the most frequent response
was that the parent felt "emotional relief" and "supported" (Alexander, 2001, p. 60). The program empowered the parents as they learned
how the school worked and how they could keep abreast of their child's
academics and behavior at school. Eighty percent of the parents said
they liked seeing the WRFs with teachers' observations written on
them. Sixty-four percent of the parents reported that they took remedial
actions for their adolescent based on what they learned from the WRFs.

When asked how the intervention affected their at-risk youth,
the most common spontaneous response was that there were positive
changes in his or her attitude or behavior. One parent said, "He wanted

to try harder and do things better, just improve a lot of areas where he was just not doing well" (Alexander, 2001, p. 72). Another said her son had become more respectful of authority both in and out of school. She said that she therefore felt more "in control" of her family because her son "began to follow rules and regulations" (p. 73). Another parent interviewed commented favorably on her son's associations with prosocial peers: "I saw the difference in his peers association, [his being with students who] were interested in doing something with their life. . . . Not like the roughneck type" (p. 73).

Finally, parents were asked for general comments about the intervention. Most said that they found family therapy to be a good experience. They appreciated that it occurred in their home instead of in an office. They believed that the program should continue to be associated with the school and be extended to include summer sessions and more families in need. Perhaps remembering that they had not asked for this help themselves, parents often said that many families in their neighborhood do not know they need help: "It takes you coming here. . . . Someone has to start opening their eyes and caring" (Alexander, 2001, p. 77).

CONCLUSION

This chapter highlights research findings that are most relevant to practitioners, educators, and organizations that work with at-risk youth. First and foremost, studies show that adolescents who are fortunate enough to receive the multisystems-oriented, home-based, family therapy—MST—and/or the multisystems-oriented, school-based intervention—Achievement Mentoring—enjoy significantly improved life outcomes. Adolescents' behavior problems are reduced; their chances of earning a high school degree are increased, and their family relationships are improved. These positive effects have been repeated with rural, suburban, and urban youth, from different racial, ethnic, and national groups, in the United States and other countries. Recent calculations also indicate that MST and Achievement Mentoring are cost effective. These interventions save more money by preventing future problems than it costs to implement the programs in the first place (Elliott & Fagan, 2017).

In addition to showing that MST and Achievement Mentoring are effective, research results offer specific guidelines for addressing at-risk youth's challenges. According to the findings, the most important change that families and adolescents must make to attain improved outcomes is to increase their sense of efficacy. Positive effects of MST are associated with parents becoming more empowered to influence their adolescents' multiple systems (e.g., schools, courts, and peers). Thus, MST therapists' first priority is to help parents remove external barriers to their adolescents' success through persistent monitoring and follow-up. To help parents do this, research shows that MST therapists must be available to families 24/7 and be intensively involved with them. Relatedly, positive effects of Achievement Mentoring are associated with adolescents feeling more engaged and competent in school. Accordingly, the first priority of achievement mentors is to increase students' successful experiences through teaching them necessary habits and skills. Studies indicate that to accomplish this objective, mentors should, during two consecutive school years, interview a teacher each week, help mentees choose a small weekly goal based on the teacher's feedback, and report progress to parents monthly. If MST therapists or achievement mentors fail to provide these essential, research-identified, program components, studies show that positive program effects fall away fairly quickly.

Research also has determined what organizational supports MST therapists and achievement mentors require so that they can deliver their necessary program components. Interestingly, studies found that frontline providers of both MST and Achievement Mentoring need regular, structured discussions about their clients or mentees with a program expert in their work settings. This is because both interventions should to be individualized for each at-risk youth within the specific program's principles. Furthermore, studies have shown that providers of each program need space, time, and instrumental supports from their employers in order to implement their interventions faithfully. Because family therapists and educators do not determine their organizations' administrative policies, implementation studies of both programs have shown that the outside agencies that deliver MST or Achievement Mentoring training must take responsibility for overseeing employer practices. Thus, it is up to the training agencies to ensure that organizations and schools provide necessary support and resources so that the interventions can be implemented as intended.

References

Abrantes, A. M., Hoffman, N. G., & Anton, R. (2005). Prevalence of co-occurring disorders among juveniles committed to detention centers. *International Journal of Offender Therapy and Comparative Criminology, 49,* 179–193.

Alexander, A. S. (1997). *The impact of behavioral family therapy on early adolescent problems: Replication and an attempt to enhance outcome through neighborhood parent meetings.* Unpublished master's thesis, Rutgers, the State University of New Jersey, New Brunswick, NJ.

Alexander, A. S. (2001). Three-year follow-up and parent perceptions of preventive school- and home-based behavioral family therapy for high-risk adolescents (Order No. 3000809). Available from Dissertations & Theses @ Rutgers University. (230795205). Retrieved from *https://search-proquest-com.proxy.libraries. rutgers.edu/docview/230795205?accountid=13626.*

Alexander, J. F., Waldron, H. B., Robbins, M. S., & Neeb, A. A. (2013). *Functional family therapy for adolescent behavior problems.* Washington, DC: American Psychological Association.

Alexander, K. L., Entwisle, D. R., & Hoorsey, C. S. (1997). From first grade forward: Early foundations of high school dropout. *Sociology of Education, 70,* 87–107.

Amber, J. (2013, July 29). The talk: How parents raising black boys try to keep their sons safe. Retrieved from *http://content.time.com/time/magazine/article/0,9171,2147710,00.html.*

Anderman, L. H. (2003). Academic and social perceptions as predictors of change in middle school students' sense of school belonging. *Journal of Experimental Education, 72*(1), 5–22.

Anderson, J. L. (2006). An evaluation of African-American adolescent health status with gender comparison. *California Journal of Health Promotion, 4*(2), 168–174.

Aponte, H. J. (1995). *Bread and spirit: Therapy with the new poor.* New York: Norton.

Aponte, H. J., & Kissil, K. (2016). *The person of the therapist training model: Mastering the use of self.* New York: Routledge.

Ayon, C., Aisenberg, E., & Cimino, A. (2012). Latino families in the nexus of child welfare, welfare reform, and immigration policies: Is kinship care a lost opportunity? *Social Work, 58*(1), 91–94.

Bachman, J. G., O'Malley, P. M., Schulenberg, J. E., Johnston, L. D., Freedman-Doan, P., & Messersmith, E. E. (2008). *The education–drug use connection: How successes and failures in school relate to adolescent smoking, drinking, drug use, and delinquency.* Mahwah, NJ: Erlbaum.

Balfanz, R., & Byrnes, V. (2012). *Chronic absenteeism: Summarizing what we know from nationally available data.* Baltimore: Johns Hopkins University Center for Social Organization of Schools.

Balfanz, R., Herzog, L., & MacIver, D. J. (2007). Preventing student disengagement and keeping students on the graduation path in urban middle-grades schools: Early identification and effective interventions. *Educational Psychologist, 42,* 223–235.

Bambara, T. C. (1996). Raymond's run. In M. Evler et al. (Eds.), *Characters in conflict* (2nd ed., pp. 162–169). Austin, TX: Holt, Rinehart & Winston.

Bandura, A. (1977). *Social learning theory.* Englewood Cliffs, NJ: Prentice Hall.

Bandura, A. (1997). *Self-efficacy: The exercise of control.* New York: Freeman.

Barkley, R. A. (2013). *Taking charge of ADHD: The complete, authoritative guide for parents.* New York: Guilford Press.

Barkley, R. A., & Robin, A. L. (2014). *Defiant teens: A clinician's manual for assessment and family intervention.* New York: Guilford Press.

Bartollas, C. L., & Schmalleger, F. J. (2014). *Juvenile delinquency.* Boston: Prentice Hall.

Basch, C. E. (2011). Aggression and violence and the achievement gap among urban minority youth. *Journal of School Health, 81*(10), 619–625.

Baumrind, D. (2005). Patterns of parental authority and adolescent autonomy. In J. Smetana (Ed.), *New directions for child development: Changes in parental authority during adolescence* (pp. 61–69). San Francisco: Jossey-Bass.

Belfield, C., & Levin, H. M. (Eds.). (2007). *The price we pay: Economic and social consequences of inadequate education.* Washington, DC: Brookings Institution Press.

Belgrave, F. Z. (2009). *African American girls: Reframing perceptions and changing experiences.* New York: Springer.

Belgrave, F. Z., Nguyen, A. B., Johnson, J. L., & Hood, K. (2011). Who is likely to help or hurt?: Profiles of African American adolescents with prosocial and aggressive behavior. *Journal of Youth and Adolescence, 40,* 1012–1024.

Benson, M. L., & Fox, G. L. (2004). *When violence hits home: How economics and neighborhood play a role* (NIJ Research in Brief Series 205004). Washington, DC: National Institute of Justice.

Berg, I. K. (1994). *Family based services: A solution-focused approach.* New York: Norton.

Bernal, G., & Shapiro, E. (2005). Cuban families. In M. McGoldrick, J. Giordano, & N. Garcia-Preto (Eds.), *Ethnicity and family therapy* (3rd ed., pp. 202–215). New York: Guilford Press.

Bien, N. Z., & Bry, B. H. (1980). An experimentally designed comparison of four intensities of school-based prevention programs for adolescents with adjustment problems. *Journal of Community Psychology, 8,* 110–116.

Biglan, A. (2015). *The nurture effect: How the science of human behavior can improve our lives and our world.* Oakland, CA: New Harbinger.

Billingsley, A. (1992). *Climbing Jacob's ladder: The enduring legacy of African-American families.* New York: Simon & Schuster.

Blase, K. A., Schroeder, J., & Van Dyke, M. (2014, April). *Tackling the wicked problems of implementing evidence-based programs.* Preconference workshop presented at the Blueprints Conference, Denver, CO.

Boots, S. W., & Geen, R. (1999). *Family care or foster care?: How state policies affect kinship caregivers* (New Federalism: Issues and Options for States, Series A, No. A-34). Washington, DC: Urban Institute.

Borduin, C. M. (2016, April). *MST update 2016, including published research findings 2014–present.* Paper presented at the Blueprints Conference, Denver, CO.

Borduin, C. M., Mann, B. J., Cone, L. T., Henggeler, S. W., Fucci, B. R., Blaske, D. M., & Williams, R. A. (1995). Multisystemic treatment of serious juvenile offenders: Long-term prevention of criminality and violence. *Journal of Consulting and Clinical Psychology, 63*(4), 569–578.

Bosworth, K. (2000). *Protective schools: Linking drug abuse prevention with student success.* Tucson: Arizona Board of Regents. Retrieved from *www.protective-school.org.*

Bowen, M. (1978). *Family therapy in clinical practice.* New York: Jason Aronson.

Boxer, P., Kubik, J., Ostermann, M., & Veysey, B. (2015). Gang involvement moderates the effectiveness of evidence-based intervention for justice-involved youth. *Children and Youth Services Review, 52,* 26–33.

Boyd-Franklin, N. (1989). *Black families in therapy: A multisystems approach.* New York: Guilford Press.

Boyd-Franklin, N. (2003). *Black families in therapy: Understanding the African American experience* (2nd ed.). New York: Guilford Press.

Boyd-Franklin, N. (2010). Incorporating spirituality and religion into the treatment of African American clients. *The Counseling Psychologist, 38*(7), 976–1000.

Boyd-Franklin, N., & Bry, B. H. (2000). *Reaching out in family therapy: Home-based, school, and community interventions.* New York: Guilford Press.

Boyd-Franklin, N., Cleek, E., Wofsy, M., & Mundy, B. (2013). *Therapy in the real world: Effective treatments for challenging problems.* New York: Guilford Press.

Boyd-Franklin, N., Franklin, A. J., & Toussaint, P. (2001). *Boys into men: Raising our African American sons.* New York: Plume.

Boyd-Franklin, N., & Lockwood, T. W. (1999). Spirituality and religion: Implications for psychotherapy with African American clients and families. In F. Walsh (Ed.), *Spiritual resources in family therapy* (pp. 90–103). New York: Guilford Press.

Boyd-Franklin, N., & Lockwood, T. W. (2009). Spirituality and religion: Implications for psychotherapy with African American families. In F. Walsh (Ed.), *Spirituality resources in family therapy* (2nd ed., pp. 141–155). New York: Guilford Press.

Boyd-Franklin, N., Steiner, G. L., & Boland, M. G. (Eds.). (1995). *Children, families, and HIV/AIDS: Psychosocial and therapeutic issues.* New York: Guilford Press.

Bradshaw, C. P., Waasdorp, T. E., Debnam, K. J., & Johnson, S. L. (2014). Measuring school climate in high schools: A focus on safety, engagement, and the environment. *Journal of School Health, 84*(9), 593–604.

Brezina, T., Agnew, R., Cullen, F. T., & Wright, J. P. (2004). The code of the street: A quantitative assessment of Elijah Anderson's subculture of violence thesis and its contribution to youth violence research. *Youth Violence and Juvenile Justice, 2*(4), 303–328.

Bridgeland, J. M., Dilulio, J. J., & Morison, K. B. (2006). The silent epidemic: Perspectives of high school dropouts (Report from Civic Enterprises). Retrieved from *https://eric.ed.gov/?id=ED513444.*

Bronfenbrenner, U. (1977). Toward an experimental ecology of human development. *American Psychologist, 45,* 513–530.

Bronfenbrenner, U. (1979). *The ecology of human development: Experiments by nature and design.* Cambridge, MA: Harvard University Press.

Bruce, M., & Bridgeland, J. (2014). *The mentoring effect: Young people's perspectives on the outcomes and availability of mentoring.* Washington, DC: Civic Enterprises and Hart Research Associates. Retrieved from *www.civicenterprises.net/Education.*

Brunk, M. (2016a, April). *Ensuring outcomes in the real world: Examples across family-based EBP's.* Paper presented at the Blueprints Conference, Denver, CO.

Brunk, M. (2016b, November 16). Multisystemic therapy is a top tier juvenile offender program [Web blog post]. Retrieved from *http://info.mstservices.com/blog/multisystemic-therapy-top-tier-juvenile-offender-program.*

Bry, B. H. (1982). Reducing the incidence of adolescent problems through preventive intervention: One- and five-year follow-up. *American Journal of Community Psychology, 10,* 265–276.

Bry, B. H. (1994). Preventing substance abuse by supporting families' efforts with community resources. *Child and Family Behavior Therapy, 16,* 21–26.

Bry, B. H. (2001a). *Achievement mentoring makes a difference: 1999–2001 Program Evaluation Results for Bry's Behavioral Monitoring and Reinforcement Achievement Mentoring Program.* Rochester, NY: Rochester City School District.

Bry, B. H. (2001b). *Revised manual for Bry's Behavioral Monitoring and Reinforcement/Achievement Mentoring Program.* East Stroudsburg, PA: Author.

Bry, B. H., & Attaway, N. (2000). *The Bry Behavioral Monitoring and Reinforcement Program evaluation summary report.* Rochester, NY: Rochester City School District.

Bry, B. H., Conboy, C., & Bisgay, K. (1986). Decreasing adolescent drug use and school failure: Long-term effects of targeted family problem-solving training. *Child and Family Behavior Therapy, 8*(1), 43–59.

Bry, B. H., & George, F. E. (1980). The preventive effects of early intervention on the attendance and grades of urban adolescents. *Professional Psychology, 11,* 252–261.

Bry, B. H., Greene, D. M., Schutte, C., & Fishman, C. A. (1991). *Targeted Family Intervention: Procedures manual.* East Stroudsburg, PA: Author.

Bry, B. H., & Krinsley, K. E. (1992). Booster sessions and long-term effects of behavioral family therapy on adolescent substance use and school performance. *Journal of Behavior Therapy and Experimental Psychiatry, 23,* 183–189.

Bry, B. H., McKeon, P., & Pandina, R. J. (1982). Extent of drug use as a function of number of risk factors. *Journal of Abnormal Psychology, 9*(4), 273–279.

Bry, B. H., & Witte, G. (1982, May). *Impact of a behaviorally-oriented, school-based, group intervention program upon alienation and self-esteem.* Paper presented at the annual meeting of the Eastern Evaluation Research Society, New York.

Bry, B. H., & Yadegar, M. (2013, November). *Increasing fidelity reporting in school-based, Achievement Mentoring Program dissemination: Time series analysis and participant feedback.* Paper presented at the Social Learning and Family Preconference of the Association of Behavioral and Cognitive Therapies Convention, Nashville, TN.

Buckner, J. C., Mezzacappa, E., & Beardslee, W. R. (2009). Self-regulation and its relations to adaptive functioning in low income youths. *American Journal of Orthopsychiatry, 79*(1), 19–30.

Burns, B. J., Phillips, S. D., Wagner, H. R., Barth, R. P., Kolko, D. J., Campbell, Y., & Landsverk, J. (2004). Mental health need and access to mental health services by youths involved with child welfare: A national survey. *Journal of the American Academy of Child and Adolescent Psychiatry, 43*(8), 960–970.

Burt, C. H., Simons, R. L., & Gibbons, F. X. (2012). Racial discrimination, ethnic-racial socialization, and crime: A micro-sociological model of risk and resilience. *American Sociological Review, 77,* 648–677.

Bushman, B. J., Newman, K., Calvert, S. L., Downey, G., Dredze, M., Gottfredson, M., . . . Webster, D. W. (2016). Youth violence: What we know and what we need to know. *American Psychologist, 71*(1), 17–39.

Carbonaro, W. J. (1998). A little help from my friend's parents: Intergenerational closure and educational outcomes. *Sociology of Education, 71,* 295–313.

Catalano, R. F., Oesterle, S., Fleming, C. B., & Hawkins, J. D. (2004). The importance of bonding to school for healthy development: Findings from the Social Developmental Research Group. *Journal of School Health, 74*(7), 252–261.

Center for Promise. (2015). *Don't quit on me: What young people who left school say about the power of relationships.* Washington, DC: America's Promise Alliance. Retrieved from *http://gradnation.org/report/dont-quit-me.*

Center for Supportive Schools. (2016). *Comprehensive achievement mentoring report: 2015–2016 end-of-year evaluation report.* Princeton, NJ: Center for Supportive Schools.

Centers for Disease Control and Prevention. (2009). *Violence prevention: Youth violence.* Retrieved April 17, 2009, from *www.cdc.gov/ncipc/dvp/YVP.*

Chassin, L., Hussong, A., & Beltran, I. (2009). Adolescent substance use. In R. M. Lerner & L. Steinberg (Eds.), *Handbook of adolescent psychology: Vol. 1. Individual bases of adolescent development* (pp. 723–764). Hoboken, NJ: Wiley.

Chipman, R., Wells, S., & Johnson, M. (2002). The meaning of quality in kinship foster care: Caregiver, child, and worker perspectives. *Families in Society: Journal of Contemporary Social Services, 83*(5), 508–520.

Christenson, S. L., Reschly, A. L., Appleton, J. J., Berman, S., Spangers, D., & Varro, P. (2008). Best practices in fostering student engagement. In A. Thomas & J. Grimes (Eds.), *Best practices in school psychology* (Vol. 1, pp. 1099–1120). Washington, DC: National Association of School Psychologists.

Chung-Do, J. J., Goebert, D. A., Hamagani, F., Chang, J. Y., & Hishinuma, E. S. (2015). Understanding the role of school connectedness and its association with violent attitudes and behaviors among an ethnically diverse sample of youth. *Journal of Interpersonal Violence, 32*(9), 1421–1446.

Cicchetti, D., Toth, S. L., & Maughan, A. (2000). An ecological-transactional model of child maltreatment. In A. Sameroff, M. Lewis, & S. M. Miller (Eds.), *Handbook of developmental psychopathology* (2nd ed., pp. 689–722). New York: Springer.

Clarke, L. O. (2009). Effects of a school-based adult mentoring intervention on low income, urban high school freshmen judged to be at risk for drop-out: A replication and extension (Order No. 3373362). Available from Dissertations & Theses @ Rutgers University. (305076792). Retrieved from *https://search-proquest-com. proxy.libraries.rutgers.edu/docview/305076792?accountid=13626.*

Cleary, T. J. (Ed.). (2015). *Self-regulated interventions with at-risk youth: Enhancing adaptability, performance, and well-being.* Washington, DC: American Psychological Association.

Cohen, J. A., Mannarino, A. P., & Deblinger, E. (2006). *Treating trauma and traumatic grief in children and adolescents.* New York: Guilford Press.

Comas-Díaz, L., & Griffith, E. E. H. (Eds.). (1988). *Clinical guidelines in cross cultural mental health.* New York: Wiley.

Connell, A. M., Klostermann, S., & Dishion, T. J. (2011). Family check up effects on adolescent arrest trajectories: Variation by developmental subtype. *Journal of Research on Adolescence, 22*(2), 36–38.

Cordero-Guzmán, H. R. (2005). Community-based organisations and migration in New York City. *Journal of Ethnic and Migration Studies, 31*(5), 889–909.

Cuddeback, G. S. (2004). Kinship family foster care: A methodological and substantive synthesis of research. *Children and Youth Services Review, 26*(7), 623–639.

Curry, G. D., Decker, S. H., & Egley, A. (2002). Gang involvement and delinquency in a middle school population. *Justice Quarterly, 19*(2), 275–292.

Daniels, A. C. (2016). *Bringing out the best in people: How to apply the astonishing power of positive reinforcement* (3rd ed.). New York: McGraw-Hill.

Dass-Brailsford, P. (2007). *A practical approach to trauma: Empowering interventions.* Thousand Oaks, CA: SAGE.

De Shazer, S., & Dolan, Y. (2007). *More than miracles: The art of solution-focused brief therapy.* New York: Haworth Press.

Deblinger, E., Mannarino, A. P., Cohen, J. A., Runyon, M. K., & Heflin, A. H. (2015). *Child sexual abuse: A primer for treating children, adolescents, and their nonoffending parents.* New York: Oxford University Press.

Deci, E. E., & Ryan, R. M. (1985). *Intrinsic motivation and self-determination in human behavior.* New York: Plenum Press.

Dishion, T. J., Ha, T., & Veronneau, M. H. (2012). An ecological analysis of the effects of deviant peer clustering on sexual promiscuity, problem behavior, and childbearing from early adolescence to adulthood: An enhancement of the life history framework. *Developmental Psychology, 48,* 703–717.

Dishion, T. J., Nelson, S. E., & Bullock, B. M. (2004). Premature adolescent autonomy: Parent disengagement and deviant peer process in the amplification of problem behavior. *Journal of Adolescence, 27*(5), 515–530.

Dishion, T. J., Nelson, S. E., & Kavanagh, K. (2003). The family check-up with high-risk young adolescents: Preventing early-onset substance use by parent monitoring. *Behavior Therapy, 34*(4), 553–571.

Dishion, T. J., & Patterson, G. R. (2016). The development and ecology of antisocial behavior: Linking etiology, prevention, and treatment. In D. Cicchetti (Ed.), *Developmental psychopathology: Vol. 3. Maladaption and psychopathology* (3rd ed., pp. 647–678). Hoboken, NJ: Wiley.

Dixon, A., Howie, P., & Starling, J. (2004). Psychopathology in female juvenile offenders. *Journal of Child Psychology and Psychiatry, 45*(6), 1150–1158.

Dodge, K. A., Dishion, T. J., & Lansford, J. E. (2006). *Deviant peer influences in programs for youth: Problems and solutions.* New York: Guilford Press.

Dodington, J., Mollen, C., Woodlock, J., Housman, A., Richmond, T. S., & Fein, J. A. (2012). Youth and adult perspectives on violence prevention strategies: A community-based participatory study. *Journal of Community Psychology, 40*(8), 1022–1031.

Dopp, A. R., Borduin, C. M., Wagner, D. V., & Sawyer, A. M. (2014). The economic impact of multisystemic therapy through midlife: A cost–benefit analysis with serious juvenile offenders and their siblings. *Journal of Consulting and Clinical Psychology, 82*(4), 694–705.

Dressel, P. L., & Barnhill, S. K. (1994). Reframing gerontological thought and practice: The case of grandmothers with daughters in prison. *The Gerontologist, 34*(5), 685–691.

Eccles, J. S. (2008). The value of an off-diagonal approach. *Journal of Social Issues, 64*(1), 227–232.

Eccles, J. S., Migdley, C., Wigfield, A., Buchanan, C. M., Reuman, D., Flanagan, C., & MacIver, D. (1993). Development during adolescence: The impact of stage-environment fit on young adolescents' experiences in school and in families. *American Psychologist, 48,* 90–101.

Eccles, J. S., O'Neill, S., & Wigfield, A. (2015). Ability self-perceptions and subjective task values in adolescents and children. In K. A. Moore & L. H. Lippman, *What do children need to flourish?: Conceptualing and measuring indicators of positive development* (pp. 237–249). New York: Springer.

Ehrle, J., & Geen, R. (2002). Kin and non-kin foster care—findings from a national survey. *Children and Youth Services Review, 24*(1–2), 15–35.

Ehrle, J., Geen, R., & Clark, R. (2001). *Children cared for by relatives: Who are they and how are they faring?* Washington, DC: New Federalism: National Survey of America's Families.

Eisenberg, N., Fabes, R. A., Carlo, G., & Karbon, M. (1992). Emotional responsivity to others: Behavioral correlates and socialization antecedents. In N. Eisenberg &

R. A. Fabes, (Eds.), *Emotion and its regulation in early development* (pp. 57–73). San Francisco, CA: Jossey-Bass.

Elliott, D., & Fagan, A. (2017). *The prevention of crime*. Malden, MA: Wiley.

Engstrom, M. (2008). Involving caregiving grandmothers in family interventions when mothers with substance use problems are incarcerated. *Family Process, 47*(3), 357–371.

Esbensen, F. A., Peterson, D., Taylor, T. J., & Freng, A. (2009). Similarities and differences in risk factors for violent offending and gang membership. *Australian and New Zealand Journal of Criminology, 42*(3), 310–335.

Fain, T., Greathouse, S. M., Turner, S. F., & Weinberg, H. D. (2014). Effectiveness of multisystemic therapy for minority youth: Outcomes over 8 years in Los Angeles County. *Journal of Juvenile Justice, 3*(2), 24–37.

Falender, C. A., Shafranske, E. P., & Falicov, C. J. (2014). *Multiculturalism and diversity in clinical supervision: A competency-based approach*. Washington, DC: American Psychological Association.

Falicov, C. J. (2005). Mexican families. In M. McGoldrick, J. Giordano, & N. Garcia-Preto (Eds.), *Ethnicity and family therapy* (pp. 229–241). New York: Guilford Press.

Falicov, C. J. (2014). *Latino families in therapy*. New York: Guilford Press.

Fall, A., & Roberts, G. (2012). High school dropouts: Interactions between social context, self-perceptions, school engagement, and student dropout. *Journal of Adolescence, 35*(4), 787–798.

Farrington, D. (2007). Origins of violent behavior over the lifespan. In D. J. Flannery, A. T. Vazsonyi, & I. D. Waldman (Eds.), *The Cambridge handbook of violent behavior and aggression* (pp. 19–48). New York: Cambridge University Press.

Fergus, E., Noguera, P., & Martin, M. (2014). *Schooling for resilience: Improving the life trajectory of Black and Latino boys*. Cambridge, MA: Harvard Education Press.

Fergus, S., & Zimmerman, M. A. (2005). Adolescent resilience: A framework for understanding healthy development in the face of risk. *Annual Reviews of Public Health, 26*, 399–419.

Ferguson, C. J., & Meehan, D. C. (2010). Saturday night's alright for fighting: Antisocial traits, fighting, and weapons carrying in a large sample of youth. *Psychiatric Quarterly, 81*(4), 293–302.

Figley, C. R., & Kiser, L. J. (2013). *Helping traumatized families*. New York: Routledge.

Finkelhor, D., & Dziuba-Leatherman, J. (1994). Victimization of children. *American Psychologist, 49*(3), 173–183.

Finn, J. D. (1989). Withdrawing from school. *Review of Educational Research, 75*, 117–142.

Finn, J. D., & Zimmer, K. S. (2012). Student engagement: What is it? Why does it matter? In S. L. Christenson, A. L. Reschly, & C. Wylie (Eds.), *Handbook of research on student engagement* (pp. 97–131). New York: Springer.

Fixsen, D. L., Naoom, S. F., Blase, K. A., Friedman, R. M., & Wallace, F. (2005). *Implementation research: A synthesis of the literature*. Tampa: University of South Florida, Louis de la Parte Florida Mental Health Institute, The National Implementation Research Network (FMHI Publication No. 231).

Flores, P. J. (2001). Addiction as an attachment disorder: Implications for group therapy (Special issue). *International Journal of Group Psychotherapy, 51*(1), 63–81.

Font, S. A. (2015). Is higher placement stability in kinship foster care by virtue or design? *Child Abuse and Neglect, 42*, 99–111.

Forehand, R., Breiner, J., McMahon, R. J., & Davies, G. (1981). Predictors of cross setting behavior change in the treatment of child problems. *Journal of Behavior Therapy and Experimental Psychiatry, 12*(4), 311–313.

Forman, S. G. (2015). *Implementation of mental health programs in schools: A change agent's guide*. Washington, DC: American Psychological Association.

Fox, J. A., & Swatt, M. L. (2008). The recent surge in homicides involving young Black males and guns: Time to reinvest in prevention and crime control. Retrieved on April 22, 2017, from *www.schoolinfosystem.org/pdf/2008/12/foxswatthomiciderpt122008.pdf*.

Franklin, A. J. (2004). *From brotherhood to manhood: How Black men rescue their relationships and dreams from the invisibility syndrome*. Hoboken, NJ: Wiley.

Franklin, A. J., Boyd-Franklin, N., & Kelly, S. (2006). Racism and invisibility: Race-related stress, emotional abuse and psychological trauma for people of color. *Journal of Emotional Abuse, 6*(2/3), 9–30.

Frazier, E. F. (1963). *The Negro church in America*. New York: Schocken.

Fruiht, V. M., & Wray-Lake, L. (2013). The role of mentor type and timing in predicting educational attainment. *Journal of Youth and Adolescence, 42*(9), 1459–1472.

Garcia-Preto, N. (2005). Latino families: An overview. In M. McGoldrick, J. Giordano, & N. Garcia-Preto (Eds.), *Ethnicity and family therapy* (3rd ed., pp. 153–165). New York: Guilford Press.

Gardere, J. (1999). *Smart parenting for African Americans: Helping your kids thrive in a difficult world*. Secaucus, NJ: Citadel Press.

Garmezy, N., Masten, A. S., & Tellegen, A. (1984). The study of stress and competence in children: A building block for developmental psychopathology. *Child Development, 55*(1), 97–111.

Geen, R., & Berrick, J. D. (2002). Kinship care: An evolving service delivery option. *Children and Youth Services Review, 24*(1–2), 1–14.

Gervan, S., Granic, I., Solomon, T., Blokland, K., & Ferguson, B. (2012). Paternal involvement in multisystemic therapy: Effects on adolescent outcomes and maternal depression. *Journal of Adolescence, 35*(3), 743–751.

Ghate, D. (2016). From programs to systems: Deploying implementation science and practice for sustained real world effectiveness in services for children and families. *Journal of Clinical Child and Adolescent Psychology, 45*(6), 812–826.

Gil, E. (1995). *Systemic treatment of families who abuse*. San Francisco: Jossey-Bass.

Gil, E. (1996). *Treating abused adolescents*. New York: Guilford Press.

Gilgoff, J. (2007). Boyz 2 men: Responsible empowerment of inner-city adolescent males. *Afterschool Matters, 6*, 35–43.

Gillen-O'Neel, C., & Fuligni, A. (2013). A longitudinal study of school belonging and academic motivation across high school. *Child Development, 84*(2), 678–692.

Gilman, A. B., Hill, K. G., Hawkins, J. D., Howell, J. C., & Kosterman, R. (2014). The developmental dynamics of joining a gang in adolescence: Patterns and predictors of gang membership. *Journal of Research on Adolescence, 24*(2), 204–219.

Gleeson, J. P. (2007). Kinship care research and literature: Lessons learned and directions for future research. *Kinship Reporter*, pp. 1–11.

Gleeson, J. P., Wesley, J. M., Ellis, R., Seryak, C., Talley, G. W., & Robinson, J. (2009). Becoming involved in raising a relative's child: Reasons, caregiver motivations, and pathways to informal kinship care. *Child and Family Social Work, 14*(3), 300–310.

Goddard, T. (2014). The indeterminacy of the risk factor prevention paradigm: A case study of community partnerships implementing youth and gang violence prevention policy. *Youth Justice, 14*(3), 1, 3–21.

Gomez, R., Cardoso, J. B., & Thompson, S. J. (2009). Kinship care with Hispanic children: Barriers and obstacles to policy and practice implementation. *Child Welfare Issues and Perspectives*, pp. 1–16.

Gorman-Smith, D., Henry, D. B., & Tolan, P. H. (2004). Exposure to community violence and violence perpetration: The protective effects of family functioning. *Journal of Clinical Child and Adolescent Psychology, 11*(3), 439–449.

Green, B. L., Miranda, J., Daroowalla, A., & Siddique, J. (2005). Trauma exposure, mental health functioning, and program needs of women in jail. *Crime and Delinquency, 51*(1), 133–151.

Green, E. (2014, July 27). Why do Americans stink at math? *The New York Times Magazine,* pp. 23–27, 40–41.

Greene, D. M., & Bry, B. H. (1991). A descriptive analysis of family discussions about everyday problems and decisions. *Analysis of Verbal Behavior, 9,* 29–39.

Gregory, A., Skiba, R. J., & Noguera, P. A. (2010). The achievement gap and the discipline gap: Two sides of the same coin? *Educational Researcher, 39*(1), 59–68.

Gregus, S. J., Craig, J. T., Rodriguez, J. H., Pastrana, F. A., & Cavell, T. A. (2015). Lunch buddy mentoring for children victimized by peers: Two pilot studies. *Journal of Applied School Psychology, 31*(2), 167–197.

Guerra, N. G., & Smith, E. P. (2006). *Preventing youth violence in a multicultural society.* Washington, DC: American Psychological Association.

Hadden, B. R., Toliver, W., Snowden, F., & Brown-Manning, R. (2016). An authentic discourse: Recentering race and racism as factors that contribute to police violence against unarmed Black or African American men. *Journal of Human Behavior in the Social Environment, 26*(3–4), 336–349.

Haley, J. (1976). *Problem solving therapy.* San Francisco: Jossey-Bass.

Hamre, B. K., & Pianta, R. C. (2006). Student-teacher relationships. In G. G. Bear & K. M. Minke (Eds.), *Children's needs III: Development, prevention, and intervention* (pp. 59–71). Washington, DC: National Association of School Psychologists.

Hardy, K. V. (1989). The theoretical myth of sameness: A critical issue in family therapy training and treatment. *Journal of Psychotherapy and the Family, 6*(1–2), 17–33.

Harris, J. (2014). Too poor to pay for peace of mind. Retrieved April 22, 2017, from *www.theroot.com/articles/culture/2014/11/mental_health_care_still_lacking_for_th%C2%A0ose_in_poverty.html.*

Hartman, A., & Laird, J. (1983). *Family-centered social work practice.* New York: Free Press.

Hawkins, J. D., Catalano, R., Kosterman, R., Abbott, R., & Hill, K. G. (1999). Preventing adolescent health-risk behaviors by strengthening protection during childhood. *Archives of Pediatrics and Adolescent Research, 153,* 226–234.

Hawkins, J. D., Catalano, R. F., & Miller, J. Y. (1992). Risk and protective factors for alcohol and other problems in adolescence and early childhood: Implications for substance abuse prevention. *Psychological Bulletin, 112,* 64–105.

Hawkins, J. D., Herrenkohl, T., Farrington, D. P., Brewer, D., Catalano, R. F., & Harachi, T. W. (2000). *Predictors of youth violence* (pp. 1–10). Washington, DC: U.S. Department of Justice, Office of Juvenile Justice and Delinquency Prevention.

Hebert, S., Bor, W., Swenson, C. C., & Boyle, C. (2014). Improving collaboration: A qualitative assessment of inter-agency collaboration between a pilot Multisystemic Therapy Child Abuse and Neglect (MST-CAN) program and a child protection team. *Australasian Psychiatry, 22*(4), 370–373.

Helms, J. E., & Cook, D. A. (1999). *Using race and culture in counseling and psychotherapy: Theory and process.* Needham Heights, MA: Allyn & Bacon.

Henggeler, S. W. (2016, April). *MST update 2016, including published research findings 2014–present.* Paper presented at the Blueprints Conference, Denver, CO.

Henggeler, S. W., & Borduin, C. M. (Eds.). (1990). *Family therapy and beyond: A multisystemic approach to treating behavior problems of children and adolescents.* Pacific Grove, CA: Brooks/Cole.

Henggeler, S. W., Cunningham, P. B., Rowland, M. D., Schoenwald, S. K., & Associates. (2012). *Contingency management for adolescent substance abuse: A practitioner's guide.* New York: Guilford Press.

Henggeler, S. W., Melton, G. B., & Smith, L. A. (1992). Family preservation using multisystemic therapy: An effective alternative to incarcerating serious juvenile offenders. *Journal of Consulting and Clinical Psychology, 60*(6), 953–961.

Henggeler, S. W., Rodick, J. D., Borduin, C. M., Hanson, C. L., Watson, S. M., & Urey, J. R. (1986). Multisystemic treatment of juvenile offenders: Effects on adolescent behavior and family interaction. *Developmental Psychology, 22*(1), 132–141.

Henggeler, S. W., & Schaeffer, C. M. (2016). Multisystemic therapy: Clinical overview, outcomes, and implementation research. *Family Process, 55*(3), 514–528.

Henggeler, S. W., Schoenwald, S. K., Borduin, C. M., Rowland, M. D., & Cunningham, P. B., (2009). *Multisystemic therapy for antisocial behavior in children and adolescents* (2nd ed.). New York: Guilford Press.

Henggeler, S. W., Schoenwald, S. K., Rowland, M. D., & Cunningham, P. B. (2002). *Multisystemic treatment of children and adolescents with serious emotional disturbance.* New York: Guilford Press.

Henggeler, S. W., & Sheidow, A. J. (2012). Empirically supported family-based treatments for conduct disorder and delinquency in adolescents. *Journal of Marital and Family Therapy, 38*(1), 30–58.

Hennessey, M., Ford, J. D., Mahoney, K., Ko, S. J., & Siegfried, C. B. (2004). *Trauma among girls in the juvenile justice system.* Los Angeles: National Child Traumatic Stress Network.

Henry, K. L., Knight, K. E., & Thornberry, T. P. (2012). School disengagement as a predictor of dropout, delinquency, and problem substance use during adolescence and early adulthood. *Journal of Youth and Adolescence, 41*(2), 156–166.

Herrenkohl, T. J., Maguin, E., Hill, K. G., Hawkins, J. D., Abbott, R. D., & Catalano, R. F. (2000). Developmental risk factors for youth violence. *Journal of Adolescent Health, 26*(3), 176–186.

Hines, P. M., & Boyd-Franklin, N. (2005). African American families. In M. McGoldrick, J. Giordano, & N. Garcia-Preto (Eds.), *Ethnicity and family therapy* (3rd ed., pp. 87–100). New York: Guilford Press.

Hoeve, M., Dubas, J. S., Eichelsheim, V. I., Van der Laan, P. H., Smeenk, W., & Gerris, J. R. (2009). The relationship between parenting and delinquency: A meta-analysis. *Journal of Abnormal Child Psychology, 37*(6), 749–775.

Holt, L. J., Bry, B. H., & Johnson, V. L. (2008). Enhancing school engagement in at-risk, urban minority adolescents through a school-based, adult mentoring intervention. *Child and Family Behavior Therapy, 30*(4), 297–318.

Howe, D. (2005). *Child abuse and neglect: Attachment, development, and intervention.* New York: Palgrave Macmillan.

Howell, J. C. (2003). *Preventing and reducing juvenile delinquency: A comprehensive framework.* Thousand Oaks, CA: SAGE.

Howell, J. C. (2012). *Gangs in America's communities.* Thousand Oaks, CA: SAGE.

Howell, J. C., Feld, B. C., Mears, D. P., Farrington, D. P., Loeber, R., & Petechuk, D. (2013). Young offenders and an effective response in the juvenile and adult justice systems: What happens, what should happen, and what we need to know (Study group on the transitions between juvenile delinquency and adult crime). Retrieved May 7, 2017, from *www.ncjrs.gov/pdffiles1/nij/grants/242935.pdf.*

Howell, J. C., & Griffiths, E. A. (2016). *Gangs in America's communities* (2nd ed.). Thousand Oaks, CA: SAGE.

Hurst, N. C., Sawatzky, D. D., & Pare, D. P. (1996). Families with multiple problems through a Bowenian lens. *Child Welfare, 75*(6), 693–708.

Imber-Black, E. (Ed.). (1993). *Secrets in families and family therapy.* New York: Norton.

Ivey, A. E., Ivey, M. B., Zalaquett, C. P., & Quirk, K. (2012). *Essentials of intentional interviewing: Counseling in a multicultural world.* Belmont, CA: Brooks/Cole.

Janosz, M., LeBlanc, M., Boulerice, B., & Tremblay, R. E. (2000). Predicting types of school dropouts: A typological approach with two longitudinal samples. *Journal of Educational Psychology, 92,* 171–190.

Jensen, B., & Sawyer, A. (2013). Regarding educación: A vision for school improvement. In B. Jensen & A. Sawyer (Eds.), *Regarding educación* (pp. 1–19). New York: Teachers College Press.

Johnson, W., McGue, M., & Iacono, W. G. (2006). Genetic and environmental influences on academic achievement trajectories during adolescence. *Developmental Psychology, 42,* 514–532.

Johnston, L. D., O'Malley, P. M., Bachman, J. G., & Schulenberg, J. (2011). *Monitoring the future national survey results on drug use, 1975–2010* (Vol. 1). Ann Arbor: Institute for Social Research, University of Michigan.

Jones, E. E., & Nisbett, R. E. (1971). The actor and the observer: Divergent perceptions of the causes of behavior. In E. E. Jones, D. E. Kanouse, H. H. Kelley, R. E. Nisbett, S. Valins, & B. Weiner (Eds.), *Attribution: Perceiving the causes of behavior.* Morristown, NJ: General Learning Press.

Jordan, W. J., Lara, J., & McPartland, J. M. (1994). *Exploring the complexity of early dropout causal structures.* Baltimore: Center for Research on Effective Schooling for Disadvantaged Students, Johns Hopkins University.

Junger-Tas, J., Ribeaud, D., & Cruyff, M. J. (2004). Juvenile delinquency and gender. *European Journal of Criminology, 1*(3), 333–375.

Jurbergs, N., Palcic, J. L., & Kelley, M. L. (2010). Daily Behavior Report Cards with and without home-based consequences: Improving classroom behavior in low income, African American children with ADHD. *Child and Family Behavior Therapy, 32*(3), 177–195.

Kagan, N. I., & Kagan, H. (1991). Interpersonal process recall. In P. W. Dowrick (Ed.), *Practical guide to using video in the behavioral sciences* (pp. 221–230). Oxford, UK: Wiley.

Kagan, R. (2012). *Rebuilding attachments with traumatized children: Healing from losses, violence, abuse, and neglect.* New York: Routledge.

Kagan, R. (2017). *Real life heroes: Toolkit for treating traumatic stress in children and families* (2nd ed.). New York: Routledge.

Kagan, R., & Schlossberg, S. (1989). *Families in perpetual crisis.* New York: Norton.

Kaur, P., Pote, H., Fox, S., & Paradisopoulos, D. A. (2015). Sustaining change following multisystemic therapy: Caregiver's perspectives. *Journal of Family Therapy, 39*(2), 264–283.

Kazdin, A. E., Kraemer, H. C., Kessler, R. C., Kupfer, D. J., & Offord, D. R. (1997). Contributions of risk-factor research to developmental psychopathology. *Clinical Psychology Review, 17*(4), 375–406.

Keller, T. E., Catalano, R. F., Haggerty, K. P., & Fleming, C. B. (2002). Parent figure transitions and delinquency and drug use among early adolescent children of substance abusers. *American Journal of Drug and Alcohol Abuse, 28,* 399–427.

Kelly, A., Butler, M., McDonnell, S., & Bry, B. (2013). The introduction of a formal mentoring programme in an Irish school setting—A process and outcome evaluation. In R. V. Nata (Series Ed.), *Progress in education* (Vol. 29, pp. 43–82). Hauppauge, NY: Nova Science.

Kelly, A., Butler, M., Twist, E., McDonnell, S., & Kennedy, L. (2011). Mentoring for Achievement: A pilot evaluation in an Irish school setting. *Procedia-Social and Behavioral Sciences, 29,* 1012–1031.

Korin, E. C., & Petry, S. S. (2005). Brazilian families. In M. McGoldrick, J. Giordano, & N. Garcia-Preto (Eds.), *Ethnicity and family therapy* (3rd ed., pp. 166–177). New York: Guilford Press.

Krinsley, K. E. (1991). *Behavioral family therapy for adolescent school problems: School performance effects and generalization to substance use* (Order No. 9125379).

Available from Dissertations & Theses @ Rutgers University. (303952046). Retrieved from *https://search-proquest-com.proxy.libraries.rutgers.edu/docvie w/303952046?accountid=13626.*

Krinsley, K. E., & Bry, B. H. (1991). Sequential analyses of adolescent, mother, and father behaviors in distressed and nondistressed families. *Child and Family Behavior Therapy, 13*(4), 45–62.

Kroll, B. (2007). A family affair?: Kinship care and parental substance misuse: Some dilemmas explored. *Child and Family Social Work, 12,* 84–93.

Kroll, B., & Taylor, A. (2003). *Parental substance misuse and child welfare.* London: Jessica Kingsley.

Kroneman, L., Loeber, R., & Hipwell, A. E. (2004). Is neighborhood context differently related to externalizing problems and delinquency for girls compared with boys? *Clinical Child and Family Psychology Review, 7*(2), 109–122.

Kropf, N. P., & Yoon, E. (2006). Grandparents raising grandchildren: Who are they? In B. Berkman & S. D'Ambruoso (Eds.), *Handbook of social work in health and aging* (pp. 355–362). New York: Oxford University Press.

Latzman, R. D., & Swisher, R. R. (2005). The interactive relationship among adolescent violence, street violence, and depression. *Journal of Community Psychology, 33*(3), 355–371.

Lebow, J. (Ed.). (2005). *Handbook of clinical family therapy.* Hoboken, NJ: Wiley.

Lee, E., & Mock, M. R. (2005). Asian families. In M. McGoldrick, J. Giordano, & N. Garcia-Preto, N. (Eds.), *Ethnicity and family therapy* (3rd ed., pp. 269–289). New York: Guilford Press.

Leos-Urbel, J., Bess, R., & Geen, R. (2000). *State policies for assessing and supporting kinship foster parents.* Washington, DC: Urban Institute.

Leos-Urbel, J., Bess, R., & Geen, R. (2002). The evolution of federal and state policies for assessing and supporting kinship caregivers. *Children and Youth Services Review, 24*(1–2), 37–52.

Li, Y., & Lerner, R. M. (2011). Trajectories of school engagement during adolescence: Implications for grades, depression, delinquency, and substance use. *Developmental Psychology, 47*(1), 233–347.

Liddle, H. A. (2005). *Troubled teens: Multidimensional family therapy.* New York: Guilford Press.

Liddle, H. A. (2016). Multidimensional family therapy. In T. Sexton & J. Lebow (Eds.), *Handbook of family therapy* (pp. 231–249). New York: Routledge.

Liddle, H. A., & Rowe, C. L. (2010). *Adolescent substance abuse: Research and clinical advances.* New York: Cambridge University Press.

Limber, S. P. (2004). Implementation of the Olweus Bullying Prevention Program: Lessons learned from the field. In D. Espelage & S. Swearer (Eds.), *Bullying in American schools: A social-ecological perspective on prevention and intervention* (pp. 351–363). Mahwah, NJ: Erlbaum.

Lochner, L., & Moretti, E. (2004). The effect of education on crime: Evidence from prison inmates, arrests, and self-reports. *American Economic Review, 94*(1), 155–189.

Loeber, R., & Farrington, D. P. (2012). Advancing knowledge about direct protective factors that may reduce youth violence. *American Journal of Preventive Medicine, 43*(2), S24–S27.

Logan, M., & Bry, B. H. (2013). *The Mentoring for Achievement Programme (MAP): Mentor's manual.* Dublin, Ireland: Archways.

Loseke, D. R., Gelles, R. J., & Cavanaugh, M. M. (Eds.). (2005). *Current controversies on family violence* (2nd ed.). Thousand Oaks, CA: SAGE.

Loseke, D. R., & Kurz, D. (2005). Men's violence toward women is the serious social problem. In D. R. Loseke, R. J. Gelles, & M. M. Cavanaugh (Eds.), *Current controversies on family violence* (2nd ed., pp. 79–96). Thousand Oaks, CA: SAGE.

Markman, H. J., Renick, M. J., Floyd, F. J., Stanley, S. M., & Clements, M. (1993). Preventing marital distress through communication and conflict management training: A 4- and 5-year follow-up. *Journal of Consulting and Clinical Psychology, 61*(1), 70–77.

Marks, H. M. (2000). Student engagement in instructional activity: Patterns in the elementary, middle, and high school years. *American Educational Research Journal, 37*, 153–184.

Massetti, G. M., Vivolo, A. M., Brookmeyer, K., DeGue, S., Holland, K. M., Holt, M. K., & Matjasko, J. L. (2011). Preventing youth violence perpetration among girls. *Journal of Women's Health, 20*(10), 1415–1428.

Masten, A. S., Garmezy, N., Tellegen, A., Pellegrini, D. S., Larkin, K., & Larsen, A. (1988). Competence and stress in school children: The moderating effects of individual and family qualities. *Journal of Child Psychology and Psychiatry, 29*(6), 745–764.

Mastroleo, N. R., Magill, M., Barnett, N. P., & Borsari, B. (2014). A pilot study of two supervision approaches for peer-led alcohol interventions with mandated college students. *Journal of Studies on Alcohol and Drugs, 75*(3), 458–466.

Mayer, G. R., Sulzer-Azaroff, B., & Wallace, M. (2013). *Behavior analysis for lasting change* (3rd ed.). Cornwall-on-Hudson, NY: Sloan Educational.

Mbiti, J. S. (1990). *African religions and philosophy* (2nd ed.). Portsmouth, NH: Heinemann Press.

McAdams-Mahmoud, V. (2005). African American Muslim families. In M. McGoldrick, J. Giordano, & N. Garcia-Preto (Eds.), *Ethnicity and family therapy* (3rd ed., pp. 138–152). New York: Guilford Press.

McGoldrick, M. (2011). *The genogram journey: Reconnecting with your family.* New York: Norton.

McGoldrick, M., Gerson, R., & Petry, S. S. (2008). *Genograms: Assessment and intervention.* New York: Norton.

McGoldrick, M., Giordano, J., & Garcia-Preto, N. (Eds.). (2005). *Ethnicity and family therapy* (3rd ed.). New York: Guilford Press.

McGoldrick, M., & Hardy, K. (2008). *Re-visioning family therapy: Race, culture and gender in clinical practice* (2nd ed.). New York: Guilford Press.

McMahon, S. D., Todd, N. R., Martinez, A., Coker, C., Sheu, C. F., Washburn, J., & Shah, S. (2013). Aggressive and pro-social behavior: Community violence, cognitive, and behavioral predictors among urban African American youth. *American Journal of Community Psychology, 51*, 407–421.

McNeely, C. (2005). Connection to school. In K. A. Moore & L. H. Lippman (Eds.), *What do children need to flourish?* (pp. 289–303). New York: Springer.

Mendel, C. A. (2016). *Training school counselors in Interpersonal Psychotherapy— Adolescent Skills Training (IPT-AST): An examination of barriers to and facilitators of implementation* (Order No. 10297488). Available from Dissertations & Theses @ Rutgers University. (1847936644). Retrieved from *https://search-proquest-com.proxy.libraries.rutgers.edu/docview/1847936644?accountid=13626.*

Meyer, P. J. (2003). "What would you do if you knew you couldn't fail?: Creating S.M.A.R.T. goals." In *Attitude is everything: If you want to succeed above and beyond.* Waco, TX: Meyer Resource Group.

Meyers, D. C., Durlak, J. A., & Wandersman, A. (2012). The quality implementation framework: A synthesis of critical steps in the implementation process. *American Journal of Community Psychology, 50*(3–4), 462–480.

Mihalic, S. F., & Elliott, D. S. (2015). Evidence-based programs registry: Blueprints for healthy youth development. *Evaluation and Program Planning, 48*, 124–131.

Miller, W. R., & Rollnick, S. (2009). Ten things motivational interviewing is not. *Behavioral and Cognitive Psychotherapy, 37*, 129–140.

Miller, W. R., & Rollnick, S. (2012). *Motivational interviewing: Helping people change* (3rd ed.). New York: Guilford Press.

Minuchin, P., Colapinto, J., & Minuchin, S. (2006). *Working with families of the poor* (2nd ed.). New York: Guilford Press.

Minuchin, S. (1974). *Families and family therapy*. Cambridge, MA: Harvard University Press.

Mitchell, H., & Lewter, N. (1986). *Soul theology: The heart of American black culture*. San Francisco: Harper & Row.

Monahan, K. C., Osterle, S., & Hawkins, J. D. (2010). Predictors and consequences of school connectedness. *The Prevention Researcher, 17*(3), 3–6.

Monahan, K. C., Rhew, I. C., Hawkins, J. D., & Brown, E. C. (2014). Adolescent pathways to co-occurring problem behavior: The effects of peer delinquency and peer substance use. *Journal of Research on Adolescence, 24*(4), 630–645.

Moore, S. E., Robinson, M. A., Adedoyin, A. C., Brooks, M., Harmon, D. K., & Boamah, D. (2016). Hands up—Don't shoot: Police shooting of young Black males: Implications for social work and human services. *Journal of Human Behavior in the Social Environment, 26*(3–4), 254–266.

Morgan, O. J., & Lizke, C. H. (2013). *Family interventions in substance abuse: Current best practices* (Vol. 26, No. 1–2). New York: Routledge.

MST Services. (2015). *MST delivers outcomes* (2015 MST Data Overview Report). Charleston, SC: Author.

Mumola, C. J. (2000). *Incarcerated parents and their children*. Washington, DC: Bureau of Justice Statistics Special Report. Retrieved May 7, 2017, from *https://eric.ed.gov/?id=ED448903*.

Murray, J., & Farrington, D. P. (2005). Parental imprisonment: Effects on boys' antisocial behavior and delinquency through the life course. *Journal of Child Psychology and Psychiatry, 46*, 1269–1278.

Murray, J., & Farrington, D. P. (2010). Risk factors for conduct disorder and delinquency: Key findings from longitudinal studies. *Canadian Journal of Psychiatry, 55*, 633–642.

Muthén, B. O., & Muthén, L. K. (2000). The development of heavy drinking and alcohol-related problems from ages 18 to 37 in a U.S. national sample. *Journal of Studies on Alcohol, 61*(2), 290–300.

Naar-King, S., & Suarez, M. (2011). *Motivational interviewing with adolescents and young adults*. New York: Guilford Press.

National AIA Resource Center. (2004). *Kinship care*. Berkeley, CA: Author.

National Center for Injury Prevention and Control. (2010). Ten leading causes of death, United States. Retrieved February 25, 2010, from *https://webappa.cdc.gov/sasweb/ncjpc/leadcaus 10.html*.

National Research Council. (2013). *Reforming juvenile justice: A developmental approach*. Washington. DC: National Academies Press.

Nevin, J. (2000). Behavioral momentum and the law of effect. *Behavioral and Brain Sciences, 23*, 73–130.

NewsOne. (2017). #SayHerName: 22 Black women who died during encounters with law enforcement. Retrieved August 8, 2017, from *https://newsone.com/3443796/sayhername-22-black-women-who-died-during-encounters-with-law-enforcement*.

Nichols, M. P. (2011). *The essentials of family therapy* (5th ed.). Boston: Allyn & Bacon.

Nobles, W. (2004). African philosophy: Foundation of Black psychology. In R. Jones (Ed.), *Black psychology* (4th ed.). Hampton, VA: Cobb & Henry Press.

Obando, D., Trujillo, A., & Trujillo, C. A. (2014). Substance use and antisocial behavior in adolescents: The role of family and peer-individual risk and protective factors. *Substance Use and Misuse, 49*(14), 1934–1944.

Ogden, T., Bjørnebekk, G., Kjøbli, J., Patras, J., Christiansen, T., Taraldsen, K., & Tollefsen, N. (2012). Measurement of implementation components ten years after a nationwide introduction of empirically supported programs–a pilot study. *Implementation Science, 7*(49), 1–11.

Ogden, T., & Halliday-Boykins, C. A. (2004). Multisystemic treatment of antisocial adolescents in Norway: Replication of clinical outcomes outside of the US. *Child and Adolescent Mental Health, 9*(2), 77–83.

Olweus, D. (1993). *Bullying at school: What we know and what we can do?* Malden, MA: Blackwell.

Pagani, L. S., Vitaro, F., Tremblay, R. E., Mc Duff, P., Japek, C., & Larose, S. (2008). When predictions fail: The case of unexpected pathways toward high school dropout. *Journal of Social Issues, 64*(1), 175–193.

Papadopoulou, M. (2016). The "space" of friendship: Young children's understandings and expressions of friendship in a reception class. *Early Child Development and Care, 186*(10), 1544–1558.

Paradisopoulos, D., Pote, H., Fox, S., & Kaur, P. (2015). Developing a model of sustained change following multisystemic therapy: Young people's perspectives. *Journal of Family Therapy, 37*(4), 471–491.

Parece, R. L. (1997). *Patterns of daily hassles and their appraisal in low-income single mothers: Effect of information on prevention workers* (Order No. 9815237). Available from Dissertations & Theses @ Rutgers University. (304415042). Retrieved from *https://search-proquest-com.proxy.libraries.rutgers.edu/docvie w/304415042?accountid=13626.*

Parker, M., & Bry, B. H. (1995, November). *Causal statements of clinic versus non-clinic families with adolescent problems.* Paper presented at the Social Learning and the Family Preconference, Association for the Advancement of Behavior Therapy, Washington, DC.

Parker, R. N., & Tuthill, L. (2006). Youth violence prevention among White youth. In N. G. Guerra & E. P. Smith (Eds.), *Preventing youth violence in a multicultural society* (pp. 199–218). Washington, DC: American Psychological Association.

Patterson, G. R., DeBaryshe, B. D., & Ramsey, E. (1989). A developmental perspective on antisocial behavior. *American Psychologist, 44*(2), 329–335.

Penney, S. R., Lee, Z., & Moretti, M. M. (2010). Gender differences in risk factors for violence: An examination of the predictive validity of the Structured Assessment of Violence Risk in Youth. *Aggressive Behavior, 36*(6), 390–404.

Peterson, C., Maier, S. F., & Seligman, M. E. (1993). *Learned helplessness: A theory for the age of personal control.* New York: Oxford University Press.

Pliszka, S. R., Sherman, J. O., Barrow, V., & Irick, S. (2000). Affective disorder in juvenile offenders: A preliminary study. *American Journal of Psychiatry, 157*(1), 130–132.

Pollack, G. H. (1970). Anniversary reactions: Trauma and mourning. *Psychoanalytic Quarterly, 39,* 347–371.

Portwood, S. G., Ayers, P. M., Kinnison, K. E., Waris, R. G., & Wise, D. L. (2005). Youth friends: Outcomes from a school-based mentoring program. *Journal of Primary Prevention, 26*(2), 129–188.

Poussaint, A., & Alexander, A. (2000). *Lay my burden down: Unraveling suicide and the mental health crisis among African Americans.* Boston: Beacon Press.

Pressley, M., & McCormick, C. B. (1995). *Advanced educational psychology for educators, researchers, and policymakers.* New York: HarperCollins.

Princeton Center for Leadership Training. (2012). *Achievement Mentoring: Mentor manual.* Princeton, NJ: Center for Supportive Schools.

Quin, D. (2017). Longitudinal and contextual associations between teacher–student relationships and student engagement. *Review of Educational Research, 87*(2), 345–387.

Ramnerö, J., & Törneke, N. (2008). *The ABCs of human behavior: Behavioral principles for the practicing clinician.* Oakland, CA: New Harbinger.

Real, K., & Poole, M. S. (2004). Innovation implementation: Conceptualization and measurement in organizational research. *Research in Organizational Change and Development, 15,* 63–134.

Reschly, A. L., & Christenson, S. L. (2012). Jingle, jangle, and conceptual haziness: Evolution and future directions of the engagement construct. In S. L. Christenson, A. L. Reschly, & C. Wylie (Eds.), *Handbook of research on student engagement* (pp. 3–19). New York: Springer.

Resnick, M. D., Ireland, M., & Borowsky, I. (2004). Youth violence perpetration: What protects? What predicts? Findings from the National Longitudinal Study of Adolescent Health. *Journal of Adolescent Health, 35*(424), e1–e10.

Reyes, O., Gillock, K. L., Kobus, K., & Sanchez, B. (2000). A longitudinal examination of the transition into senior high school for adolescents from urban, low-income status, and predominantly minority backgrounds. *American Journal of Community Psychology, 28*(4), 519–544.

Robin, A. L., & Foster, S. L. (2002). *Negotiating parent–adolescent conflict: A behavioral-family systems approach.* New York: Guilford Press.

Robinson, B. A., Winiarski, D. A., Brennan, P. A., Foster, S. L., Cunningham, P. B., & Whitmore, E. A. (2015). Social context, parental monitoring, and multisystemic therapy outcomes. *Psychotherapy, 52*(1), 103–110.

Roebroek, L., & Koning, I. M. (2016). The reciprocal relation between adolescents school engagement and alcohol consumption, and the role of parental support. *Prevention Science, 17,* 218–226.

Rogers, C. R. (1959). A theory of therapy, personality, and interpersonal relationships: As developed in the client-centered framework. In S. Koch (Ed.), *Psychology: The study of a science* (Vol. 3, pp. 184–256). New York: McGraw-Hill.

Rollnick, S., Kaplan, S. G., & Rutschman, R. (2016). *Motivational Interviewing in schools: Conversations to improve behavior and learning.* New York: Guilford Press.

Rosenkranz, T., de la Torre, M., Stevens, W. D., & Allensworth, E. M. (2014). *Free to fail or on-track to college: Why grades drop when students enter high school and what adults can do about it.* Chicago: University of Chicago Consortium on Chicago School Research.

Ruiz, D. S. (2004). Custodian African American grandmothers: Reasons for caregiving and assumption of the caregiver role. *African American Perspectives, 10,* 152–159.

Rumberger, R. W. (2004). Why students drop out of school. In G. Orfield (Ed.), *Dropout in America* (pp. 131–155). Cambridge, MA: Harvard Education Press.

Rumberger, R. W., & Rotermund, S. (2012). The relationship between engagement and high school dropout. In S. L. Christenson, A. L. Reschly, & C. Wylie (Eds.), *Handbook of research on student engagement* (pp. 491–513). New York: Springer.

Runyon, M. K., Deblinger, E., & Steer, R. A. (2014). PTSD symptom cluster profiles of youth who have experienced sexual or physical abuse. *Child Abuse and Neglect, 38*(1), 84–90.

Russell, D. M. (1979). *Predicting outcome in a school-based group treatment program for adolescents: Effects of controlling for non-treatment relationships and including interim measures.* Unpublished master's thesis, Rutgers, the State University of New Jersey, New Brunswick, NJ.

Rutter, M. (1985). Resilience in the face of adversity: Protective factors and resistance to psychiatric disorder. *British Journal of Psychiatry, 147*(6), 598–611.

Sawyer, A. M., & Borduin, C. M. (2011). Effects of multisystemic therapy through midlife: A 21.9-year follow-up to a randomized clinical trial with serious and violent juvenile offenders. *Journal of Consulting and Clinical Psychology, 79*(5), 643–652.

Schaeffer, C. M., & Borduin, C. M. (2005). Long-term follow-up to a randomized clinical trial of multisystemic therapy with serious and violent juvenile offenders. *Journal of Consulting and Clinical Psychology, 73*(3), 445–453.

Schaeffer, C. M., McCart, M. R., Henggeler, S. W., & Cunningham, P. B. (2011). Multisystemic therapy for conduct problems in youth. In R. C. Murrihy, T. A. Kidman, & T. H. Ollendick (Eds.), *Clinical handbook of assessing and treating conduct problems in youth* (pp. 273–292). New York: Springer.

Schneiderman, J. U., & Villagrana, M. (2010). Meeting children's mental and physical health needs in child welfare: The importance of caregivers. *Social Work in Health Care, 49*(2), 91–108.

Schoenwald, S. K. (2016). The Multisystemic Therapy® Quality Assurance/Quality Improvement System. In W. O'Donohue & A. Maragakis (Eds.), *Quality improvement in behavioral health* (pp. 169–192). Basel, Switzerland: Springer International.

Schoenwald, S. K., Henggeler, S. W., & Rowland, M. D. (2016). Multisystemic therapy. In T. Sexton & J. Lebow (Eds.), *Handbook of family therapy* (pp. 271–285). New York: Routledge.

Schoenwald, S. K., Sheidow, A. J., & Letourneau, E. J. (2004). Toward effective quality assurance in evidence-based practice: Links between expert consultation, therapist fidelity, and child outcomes. *Journal of Clinical Child and Adolescent Psychology, 33*(1), 94–104.

Schoenwald, S. K., Ward, D. M., Henggeler, S. W., Pickrel, S. G., & Patel, H. (1996). Multisystemic therapy treatment of substance abusing or dependent adolescent offenders: Costs of reducing incarceration, inpatient, and residential placement. *Journal of Child and Family Studies, 5*(4), 431–444.

Schwartz, D., & Gorman, A. H. (2003). Community violence exposure and children's academic functioning. *Journal of Educational Psychology, 95*(1), 163–173.

Sexton, T. L. (2011). *Functional family therapy in clinical practice: An evidence-based treatment model for working with troubled adolescents.* New York: Routledge.

Sexton, T. L., & Lebow, J. (2016). *Handbook of family therapy.* New York: Routledge.

Shlafer, R. J., McMorris, B. J., Sieving, R. E., & Gower, A. L. (2013). The impact of family and peer protective factors on girls' violence perpetration and victimization. *Journal of Adolescent Health, 52*(3), 365–371.

Siegel, L. J., & Welsh, B. C. (2014). *Juvenile delinquency: Theory, practice, and law* (12th ed.). Stamford, CT: Wadsworth, Cengage Learning.

Simmons, T., & Dye, J. L. (2003). Grandparents living with grandchildren: 2000. Census 2000 brief. Retrieved May 9, 2017, from *https://eric.ed.gov/?id=ED482412.*

Simon, P., & Ward, N. L. (2014). An evaluation of training for lay providers in the use of Motivational Interviewing to promote academic achievement among urban youth. *Advances in School Mental Health Promotion, 7,* 255–276.

Skiba, R. J., Michael, R. S., Nardo, A. C., & Peterson, R. L. (2002). The color of discipline: Sources of racial and gender disproportionality in school punishment. *Urban Review, 34*(4), 317–342.

Smith-Boydston, J. M., Holtzman, R. J., & Roberts, M. C. (2014). Transportability of multisystemic therapy to community settings: Can a program sustain outcomes without MST Services oversight? *Child and Youth Care Forum, 43*(5), 593–605.

Smithgall, C., Yang, D. H., & Weiner, D. (2013). Unmet mental health service needs in kinship care: The importance of assessing and supporting caregivers. *Journal of Family Social Work, 16*(5), 463–479.

Snyder, H. N., & Sickmund, M. (2006). *Juvenile offenders and victims: 2006 national report*. Washington, DC: Office of Juvenile Justice and Delinquency Prevention. Retrieved April 9, 2017, from *http://files.eric.ed.gov/fulltext/ED495786.pdf*.

Stepney, C. T. (2016). Hispanic ethnic identity and academic achievement for at-risk high school students: Examining the mediational role of self-efficacy and social support (Doctoral dissertation). Retrieved from *https://catalog-libraries-rutgers-edu.proxy.libraries.rutgers.edu/vufind/Record/5755847*.

Sternberg, J., & Bry, B. H. (1994). Solution generation and family conflict over time in problem-solving therapy with families of adolescents: The impact of therapist behavior. *Child and Family Behavior Therapy, 16*(4), 1–23.

Stoddard, S. A., Whiteside, L., Zimmerman, M. A., Cunningham, R. M., Chermack, S. T., & Walton, M. A. (2013). The relationship between cumulative risk and promotive factors and violent behavior among urban adolescents. *American Journal of Community Psychology, 51*, 57–65.

Suleiman Gonzalez, L. P. (2004). Five commentaries: Looking toward the future. *Future of Children, 14*(1), 184–189.

Sullivan, T. N., Helms, S. W., Kliewer, W., & Goodman, K. L. (2010). Associations between sadness and anger regulation coping, emotional expression, and physical and relational aggression among urban adolescents. *Social Development, 19*, 30–51.

Sundell, K., Hansson, K., Löfholm, C. A., Olsson, T., Gustle, L. H., & Kadesjö, C. (2008). The transportability of multisystemic therapy to Sweden: Short-term results from a randomized trial of conduct-disordered youths. *Journal of Family Psychology, 22*(4), 550–560.

Svensson, R. (2003). Gender differences in adolescent drug use: The impact of parental monitoring and peer deviance. *Youth and Society, 34*, 300–329.

Swenson, C. C., Henggeler, S. W., Taylor, I. S., & Addison, O. W. (2005). *Multisystemic therapy and neighborhood partnerships: Reducing adolescent violence and substance abuse*. New York: Guilford Press.

Symonds, J., Schoon, I., & Salmela-Aro, K. (2016). Developmental trajectories of emotional disengagement from schoolwork and their longitudinal associations in England. *British Educational Research Journal, 42*(6), 993–1022.

Szapocznik, J., Duff, J. H., Schwartz, S. J., Muir, J. A., & Brown, C. H. (2016). Brief strategic family therapy treatment for behavior problem youth. In T. Sexton & J. Lebow (Eds.), *Handbook of family therapy* (pp. 286–304). New York: Routledge.

Tatum, J., Moseley, S., Boyd-Franklin, N., & Herzog, E. (1995). A home based family systems approach to the treatment of African American teenage parents and their families. *ZERO TO THREE: Journal of the National Center for Clinical Infant Programs, 15*(4), 18–25.

Tavkar, P., & Hansen, D. J. (2011). Interventions for families victimized by child sexual abuse: Clinical issues and approaches for child advocacy center-based services. *Aggression and Violent Behavior, 16*(3), 188–199.

Taylor, A. L. (2010). *Testing a model of change in achievement mentoring for school behavior problems* (Order No. 3434857). Available from Dissertations & Theses @ Rutgers University. (847554084). Retrieved from *https://search-proquest-com.proxy.libraries.rutgers.edu/docview/847554084?accountid=13626*.

Testa, M. F., & Rolock, N. (2001). Professional foster care: A future worth pursuing. In K. Barbell & L. M. Wright (Eds.), *Family foster care in the next century* (pp. 107–124). New Brunswick, NJ: Transaction.

Thornberry, T. P. (1998). Membership in youth gangs and involvement in serious and violent offending. In R. Loeber & D. P. Farrington (Eds.), *Serious and violent juvenile offenders: Risk factors and successful interventions* (pp. 147–166). Thousand Oaks, CA: SAGE.

Thornberry, T. P., Huizinga, D., & Loeber, R. (2004). The causes and correlates studies:

Findings and policy implications. *Juvenile Justice-Causes and Correlates: Findings and Implications, 9*(1), 1–12.

Thornberry, T. P., & Krohn, M. D. (Eds.). (2003). *Taking stock of delinquency: An overview of findings from contemporary longitudinal studies.* New York: Springer Science + Business Media.

Thornberry, T. P., Krohn, M. D., Lizotte, A. J., Smith, C., & Tobin, K. (2003). *Gangs and delinquency in developmental perspective.* Cambridge, UK: Cambridge University Press.

Tolan, P. H., & Gorman-Smith, D. (2002). What violence prevention research can tell us about developmental psychopathology. *Development and Psychopathology, 14*(4), 713–729.

Tolan, P., Gorman-Smith, D., & Henry, D. (2006). Family violence. *Annual Review of Psychology, 57, 557–583.*

Trepper, T. S., & Barrett, M. J. (Eds.). (1986). *Treating incest: A multiple systems perspective.* New York: Haworth Press.

Tsai, M., Kohlenberg, R. J., Kanter, J. W., Kohlenberg, B., Follette, W. C., & Callaghan, G. M. (2009). *A guide to functional analytic psychotherapy: Awareness, courage, love and behaviorism.* New York: Springer.

Tuominen-Soini, H., & Salmela-Aro, K. (2014). Schoolwork engagement and burnout among Finnish high school students and young adults: Profiles, progressions, and educational outcomes. *Developmental Psychology, 50, 649–662.*

Turk, E. M., & Bry, B. H. (1992). Adolescents' and parents' explanatory styles and parents' causal explanations about their adolescents. *Cognitive Therapy and Research, 16,* 349–357.

Urga, P. A. (2003). *Understanding determinants of early adolescent academic achievement—A protective factor against substance abuse.* Unpublished Master's thesis, Rutgers, The State University of New Jersey, New Brunswick, NJ.

U.S. Department of Education, National Center for Educational Statistics. (2014). Status dropout rates. Retrieved from *http://nces.ed.gov/program/coe/indicator_coj.asp.*

Vance, J. D. (2016). *Hillbilly elegy: A memoir of a family and culture in crisis.* New York: HarperCollins.

Vazquez, C. I. (2005). Dominican families. In M. McGoldrick, J. Giordano, & N. Garcia-Preto (Eds.), *Ethnicity and family therapy* (3rd ed., pp. 216–228). New York: Guilford Press.

Veronneau, M., Dishion, T., Connell, A. M., & Kavanagh, K. (2016). A randomized controlled trial of the family check-up model in public secondary schools: Examining links between parent engagement and substance use progressions from early adolescence to adulthood. *Journal of Consulting and Clinical Psychology, 84*(6), 526–543.

Villagrana, M. (2010). Mental health services for children and youth in the child welfare system: A focus on caregivers as gatekeepers. *Children and Youth Services Review, 32*(5), 691–697.

Wagner, D. V., Borduin, C. M., Sawyer, A. M., & Dopp, A. R. (2014). Long-term prevention of criminality in siblings of serious and violent juvenile offenders: A 25-year follow-up to a randomized clinical trial of multisystemic therapy. *Journal of Consulting and Clinical Psychology, 82*(3), 492–499.

Wagner, E. F., & Waldron, H. B. (2001). *Innovations in adolescent substance abuse interventions.* Oxford UK: Elsevier Science.

Waldfogel, J., Garfinkel, I., & Kelly, B. (2007). Welfare and the costs of public assistance. In C. R. Belfield & H. M. Levin (Eds.), *Price we pay: Economic and social consequences of inadequate education* (pp. 160–176). Washington, DC: Brookings Institution Press.

Walker, M., & Glasgow, M. (2005). Parental substance misuse and the implications for children. In J. Taylor & B. Daniel (Eds.), *Child neglect: Practice issues for health and social care* (pp. 206–227). London: Jessica Kingsley.

Walsh, F. (2012). *Normal family processes* (4th ed.). New York: Guilford Press.

Walsh, F. (2016). *Strengthening family resilience* (3rd ed.). New York: Guilford Press.

Webster-Stratton, C. (2006). *The Incredible Years: A trouble-shooting guide for parents of children aged 2–8 years*. Seattle, WA: Incredible Years.

Webster-Stratton, C. (2016, April). *Incredible Years*. Keynote address presented at the Blueprints Conference, Denver, CO.

Webster-Stratton, C. H., Reid, M. J., & Marsenich, L. (2014). Improving therapist fidelity during implementation of evidence-based practices: Incredible Years program. *Psychiatric Services, 65*(6), 789–795.

What to know about MS 13 street gang. (2017). Retrieved from *http://time.com/4783163/ms-13-gang*.

Whitaker, D., Graham, C., Severtson, S., Furr-Holden, C., & Latimer, W. (2012). Neighborhood and family effects on learning motivation among urban African American middle school youth. *Journal of Child and Family Studies, 21*(1), 131–138.

Whitaker, T. R., & Snell, C. L. (2016). Parenting while powerless: Consequences of "the talk." *Journal of Human Behavior in the Social Environment, 26*(3–4), 303–309.

Widom, C. S. (2000). Motivation and mechanisms in the "cycle of violence." *Nebraska Symposium on Motivation, 46*, 1–38.

Williams, K. R., & Guerra, N. G. (2011). Perceptions of collective efficacy and bullying perpetration in schools. *Social Problems, 58*, 126–143.

Winokur, M., Rozen, D., Thompson, S., Green, S., & Valentine, D. (2005). *Kinship care in the United States: A systematic review of evidence-based research*. Ft. Collins: Social Work Research Center, Colorado State University. Retrieved May 12, 2017, from *https://pdfs.semanticscholar.org/ec6a/f186c738a1cdcff881fe5e-e5e13bf9f542cc.pdf*.

Wiseman, S. H., Chinman, M., Ebener, P. A., Hunter, S. B., Imm, P., & Wandersman, A. (2007). *Getting To Outcomes™: 10 steps for achieving results-based accountability*. Santa Monica, CA: Rand Corporation.

Woodcock, J., & Sheppard, M. (2002). Double trouble: Maternal depression and alcohol dependence as combined factors in child and family social work. *Children in Society, 16*, 232–245.

Yadegar, M., & Bry, B. H. (2014, November). *Ten years of program adherence across multiple settings, and associated developments in adherence assessment, program training, and ongoing consultation*. Poster presented at the Association of Behavioral and Cognitive Therapies Convention, Philadelphia, PA.

Ziminski, J. (2007). Systemic practice with kinship care families. *Journal of Social Work Practice, 21*(2), 239–250.

Author Index

361

Subject Index

Note. *f* following a page number indicates a figure.